LYNDHURST

MCGILL-QUEEN'S/ASSOCIATED MEDICAL SERVICES STUDIES IN THE
HISTORY OF MEDICINE, HEALTH, AND SOCIETY

SERIES EDITORS: S.O. FREEDMAN AND J.T.H. CONNOR

Volumes in this series have financial support from Associated Medical
Services, Inc. (AMS). Associated Medical Services Inc. was established in 1936
by Dr Jason Hannah as a pioneer prepaid not-for-profit health-care
organization in Ontario. With the advent of medicare, AMS became a
charitable organization supporting innovations in academic medicine and
health services, specifically the history of medicine and health care, as well as
innovations in health professional education and bioethics.

1 Home Medicine
The Newfoundland Experience
John K. Crellin

2 A Long Way from Home
The Tuberculosis Epidemic among
the Inuit
Pat Sandiford Grygier

3 Labrador Odyssey
The Journal and Photographs of
Eliot Curwen on the Second
Voyage of Wilfred Grenfell, 1893
Ronald Rompkey

4 Architecture in the Family Way
Doctors, Houses, and Women,
1870–1900
Annmarie Adams

5 Local Hospitals in Ancien Régime
France
Rationalization, Resistance,
Renewal, 1530–1789
Daniel Hickey

6 Foisted upon the Government?
State Responsibilities, Family
Obligations, and the Care of the
Dependant Aged in
Nineteenth-Century Ontario
Edgar-André Montigny

7 A Young Man's Benefit
The Independent Order of Odd
Fellows and Sickness Insurance in
the United States and Canada,
1860–1929
George Emery and J.C. Herbert
Emery

8 The Weariness, the Fever, and
the Fret
The Campaign against
Tuberculosis in Canada,
1900–1950
Katherine McCuaig

9 The War Diary of Clare Gass,
1915–1918
Edited by Susan Mann

10 Committed to the State Asylum
Insanity and Society in Nineteenth-
Century Quebec and Ontario
James E. Moran

11 Jessi Luther at the Grenfell Mission
Edited by Ronald Rompkey

12 Negotiating Disease
Power and Cancer Care,
1900–1950
Barbara Clow

13 For Patients of Moderate Means
A Social History of the Voluntary
Public General Hospital in Canada,
1890–1950
David Gagan and Rosemary Gagan

14 Into the House of Old
A History of Residential Care in
British Columbia
Megan J. Davies

15 St Mary's
The History of a London Teaching
Hospital
E.A. Heaman

16 Women, Health, and Nation
Canada and the United States since
1945
*Edited by Georgina Feldberg,
Molly Ladd-Taylor, Alison Li, and
Kathryn McPherson*

17 The Labrador Memoir of Dr Henry
Paddon, 1912–1938
Edited by Ronald Rompkey

18 J.B. Collip and the Development of
Medical Research in Canada
Extracts and Enterprise
Alison Li

19 The Ontario Cancer Institute
Successes and Reverses at
Sherbourne Street
E.A. McCulloch

20 Island Doctor
John Mackieson and Medicine in
Nineteenth-Century Prince Edward
Island
David A.E. Shephard

21 The Struggle to Serve
A History of the Moncton
Hospital, 1895 to 1953
W.G. Godfrey

22 An Element of Hope
Radium and the Response to
Cancer in Canada, 1900–1940
Charles Hayter

23 Labour in the Laboratory
Medical Laboratory Workers in the
Maritimes, 1900–1950
Peter L. Twohig

24 Rockefeller Foundation Funding
and Medical Education in Toronto,
Montreal, and Halifax
Marianne P. Fedunkiw

25 Push!
The Struggle for Midwifery in
Ontario
Ivy Lynn Bourgeault

26 Mental Health and Canadian
Society
Historical Perspectives
James Moran/ David Wright

27 SARS in Context
Memory, History, and Policy
*Edited by Jacalyn Duffin and
Arthur Sweetman*

28 Lyndhurst
Canada's First Rehabilitation
Centre for People with Spinal Cord
Injuries, 1945–1998
Geoffrey Reaume

Lyndhurst

Canada's First Rehabilitation Centre for People with Spinal Cord Injuries, 1945–1998

GEOFFREY REAUME

McGill-Queen's University Press
Montreal & Kingston • London • Ithaca

© McGill-Queen's University Press 2007

ISBN 978-0-7735-3212-0

Legal deposit second quarter 2007
Bibliothèque nationale du Québec

Printed in Canada on acid-free paper.

This book was commissioned by and has been published with the
help of a grant from the A.T. Jousse Appreciation Foundation,
Toronto.

McGill-Queen's University Press acknowledges the support of the
Canada Council for the Arts for our publishing program. We also
acknowledge the financial support of the Government of Canada
through the Book Publishing Industry Development Program
(BDIDP) for our publishing activities.

Library and Archives Canada Cataloguing in Publication

Reaume, Geoffrey, 1962–
   Lyndhurst: Canada's first rehabilitation centre for people with
spinal cord injuries, 1945–1998 / Geoffrey Reaume.

(McGill-Queen's/Associated Medical Services studies in the
history of medicine, health, and society; 28)
Includes bibliographical references and index.
ISBN 978-0-7735-3212-0

1. Lyndhurst Lodge (Toronto, Ont.) – History. 2. Spinal cord –
Wounds and injuries – Patients – Rehabilitation – Canada –
Disability – History. I. Title. II. Series.

RA645.S66R42 2007   362.19'74820860971   C2006-906194-7

Typeset by Jay Tee Graphics Ltd. in Sabon 10/13

Dedicated to Ken Langford and Mary Langford –
two participants in the history of Lyndhurst Lodge

Contents

Acknowledgments   xi
Introduction   3

1 Before Lyndhurst: Treatment of People with Spinal Cord Injuries up to 1945   9

2 From DVA to CPA, 1945–50   32

3 A Reputation for Rehabilitation: Lyndhurst Lodge, 1950–64   83

4 The Longest Decade, 1964–74   119

5 Lyndhurst on Sutherland: From Autonomy to Amalgamation, 1974–98   155

6 Conclusion: Lyndhurst's Legacy   191

Notes   199
Bibliography   243
Index   251

Acknowledgments

I would like to thank the original members of the A.T. Jousse Appreciation Foundation who hired me in spring 2001 to research and write this history book: Ken Langford, Dr William Geisler, Jill Nelson, and John Keeso. I would also like to thank fellow historians of medicine Michael Bliss, Pauline Mazumdar, and Geoffrey Hudson, for recommending me for this job. The above-mentioned members of the Jousse Foundation, along with Michael O'Brien, read drafts of my manuscript and provided comments for which I thank them. Two anonymous reviewers for McGill-Queen's University Press each provided a helpful critique of the manuscript, which was much appreciated. I also thank Philip Cercone and the editorial staff of McGill-Queen's University Press for being patient when the final revised manuscript was delayed longer than expected because of my new job at York University starting in 2004. Many thanks also to the copy editor, Lesley Andrassy.

Heartfelt thanks go to my colleagues and students at York University, School of Health Policy and Management, the Critical Disability Studies graduate program, and the Atkinson Faculty of Liberal and Professional Studies for allowing me to continue my work in disability history in such a supportive atmosphere. I also thank colleagues and students at Ryerson University, School of Disability Studies, for their support when I taught there part-time in 2002–03, while writing this book. I am grateful to the staff and students at the Institute for the History and Philosophy of Science and Technology, University of Toronto, for their support of my work as associate scholar of the institute since 2000.

I am most grateful to the many people who assisted me by providing access to archival material: Ken Hawkes and the staff of the Archives for Veteran's Affairs, Charlottetown, Prince Edward Island, provided an enormous amount of help by giving me complete access to a wealth of files on Lyndhurst Lodge, veterans, and paraplegia, which provided much of the documentary foundation for the early history contained in this book. Paul Banfield of the Queen's University Archives, Kingston, Ontario, was very helpful and I especially thank Jocelyn Allen for permitting unrestricted access to the records of her late father, Dr E.H. Botterell, which are held in these archives and contain a great deal of invaluable historical evidence about the early history of the treatment of paraplegia and the founding of Lyndhurst Lodge. Debbie Brentnell of the National Archives of Canada in Ottawa provided generous assistance, as did Yuri Shimpo and Mary Akenson, who were most helpful in providing timely access to files in the Archives of Ontario, Toronto. I also thank Magda Zakanyi, Bloorview MacMillan Centre Archives, Toronto, for her assistance. Lynne Lwow and the staff of the Canadian Paraplegic Association National Office in Ottawa, as well as Bill Adair and the staff of the Canadian Paraplegic Association Ontario Office in Toronto, were very welcoming and allowed me to research numerous documentary sources relating to Lyndhurst's history; their gracious support is much appreciated. I also thank Mark Rochon for permitting access to the Lyndhurst board of directors minutes, which are held by the Toronto Rehabilitation Institute.

As there is no one central archive for Lyndhurst history this research was given an incalculable degree of support by the following people, who have direct personal experiences of this history and who were very kind in providing access to documents in their possession that were essential to providing a more fully human portrait of this facility and the people associated with it. This includes material from the personal collections of Mary and Ken Langford, Dr William O. Geisler, James Burke, Bill Owen, Betty Brooks, Therese Proietti, Dorothy Naylor, Mary Tremblay, Dr Megan Wynne-Jones, and John Yaremko. The daughters of Dr A.T. Jousse, Eileen Jousse Woloshyn and Sheila Avery, were very generous in providing documents about their father. Loma Stone, who for twenty years was a nurse at Lyndhurst, was extraordinarily generous in providing a wealth of documentary evidence; she has done much to preserve the history of the period she was a part of. I thank them all for their help.

Above all else, I would like to thank the fifty-three people whom I interviewed for this book. Their memories of this history have provided the most important personal details that enliven the pages that follow and provide insights that I, as someone who is not physically disabled and who has never lived the history recounted here, could never provide through archival research alone. The greatest insights in this book are thanks to the generosity of the very large number of people who gave so freely of their time and of their memories of Lyndhurst Lodge Hospital. For their kindness, I would like to thank Ken Langford and the late Mary Langford; as well as the following former in-patients and out-patients of Lyndhurst: Tom Bailey, Katie Barton, Marjorie Bleasdell, Mabel Brown, James Burke (who experienced paraplegia as a pre-Lyndhurst patient), Kathy Drummond, Bev Hallam, the late Jack Higman, Myrll Jackson, Carmen Mobbs, Dorothy Naylor, Michael O'Brien, Bill Owen, Lucille Owen, Gordon Paterson, Therese Proietti, Kirby Rowe, Barbara Staton, Barbara Turnbull, and one person who has requested anonymity; the following former staff members of Lyndhurst and/or the Canadian Paraplegic Association: Betty Brooks, Bill Brown, Lloyd Charles, Lise Desrochers, Elizabeth Holman, Margaret MacDonald, Evelyn O. Paul, Ed Ratelle, Charlie Saso, Loma Stone, and Donna Walters; the following individuals who knew people that were closely associated with Lyndhurst or who themselves had dealings with this facility: Jocelyn Allen, Sheila Avery, Sadie Blain, Doreen Dunlop, Jane L. Glassco, Kathleen S. Griffin, Margaret Jousse, Eileen Jousse Woloshyn, and John Yaremko; the following doctors who either worked at Lyndhurst or who had contact with Lyndhurst patients and staff through their work at nearby health-care facilities: Henry Barnett, Nimmi Bharatwal, Wilfrid Bigelow, William O. Geisler, E. Peter MacDougall, Gavin Shanks, David Symington, Ron Tasker, Charles Tator, the late Delbert Wollin, and Megan Wynne-Jones. I would also like to thank two superb transcribers, Janet Bruch and Romi Mintchev, who did an immense amount of work transcribing interviews, all but five of which were recorded on tape. Last, but definitely not least, many thanks to my dear parents, Josephine Reaume and Nelson Reaume, for their comments on the manuscript at the earliest stages and for offering me much needed respite from my sweltering apartment when I was writing the first chapter way back in August 2002. Of course, any mistakes in this book are my responsibility alone.

I would like to dedicate this book to Ken Langford and the late Mary Langford – their dedication to working with people with disabilities in Lyndhurst Lodge and the Canadian Paraplegic Association, as well as to supporting one another over more than sixty-two years of marriage, much of which involved the history told in the following pages, is an admirable example for us all.

LYNDHURST

Introduction

This book is a history commissioned by the A.T. Jousse Appreciation Foundation, a group of former staff members and patients who named this charitable organization after the original medical director of Lyndhurst Lodge. Commissioned histories do not have a particularly good reputation among professional historians. They are often long on praise and short on critical assessment of whatever topic has been commissioned for publication. But this is not always the case in hospital histories. Some, like Elsbeth Heaman's study of St Mary's Hospital in London, England, are masterful studies that contribute significantly to our understanding of a particular health care institution and the people who were patients or staff there.[1] Others, such as Robert Neilsen's book on the Penetanguishene mental health centre in Ontario, provide a public relations-like presentation of the past that is of little use to a serious understanding of the people and place under consideration.[2] Still others fall somewhere in between, neither masterful survey nor puff piece propaganda but good solid books that provide both useful analysis and documentation on a particular facility, even though the authors are clearly setting out to write favourable accounts – Irene McDonald's history of St Michael's Hospital in Toronto is a good example of this kind of book.[3]

This present study includes views that are favourable to Lyndhurst Lodge and its operators as well as perspectives that are not flattering. I have tried to provide a range of views that would prevent it from being categorized as either an apologia or an attack, reflecting in large part the views of the people who lived and worked there and who were interviewed for this study. The purpose of this particular commissioned contribution is to provide an understanding of Lyndhurst Lodge

Hospital in the context of the development of services for people with spinal cord injuries over a half-century, largely through the insights of patients, staff, and physicians. Thus documentary archival history is supplemented with oral histories to provide more details on what it was like to live and work in this facility over the different periods being examined here, from the post-war growth in service provision to late twentieth-century cutbacks that led to another in a long series of transformations in Lyndhurst's organizational existence. This approach is also an attempt to bring to light some of the personal histories that deserve to be a major part of any study of this kind.

The history of people who are paraplegic and quadriplegic entails much more than their experiences in a particular rehabilitation facility. What their lives were like in the community and how physical and attitudinal barriers in the wider world affected them are also very much a part of this history. Thus, while this book is focused on the history of Lyndhurst Lodge in its various incarnations over a half-century, it also looks at the wider social context through the experiences of the people who lived in this facility, to enable readers to understand the systemic discrimination that has always existed for people with disabilities and how this has, or has not, been addressed.

Little about the history of people with paraplegia and quadriplegia has been written based on the experiences of people with these disabilities. John Russell Silver's book, *History of the Treatment of Spinal Injuries,* is the only published book-length study of this subject in English.[4] His study examines this topic from a clinical perspective in parts of Western Europe and North America, primarily from the late nineteenth century to the end of the twentieth century, with some earlier references. The personal experiences of people with spinal cord injuries are not a notable part of Silver's study. His book is in the tradition of a doctor-centred approach to medical history, reflecting the fact that the author himself is a physician who has worked in this field for five decades. Whatever its limitations as a study in the history of disability, Silver's book does provide a good deal of information about the overall development of the treatment of spinal cord injuries that is otherwise not available in one place. He therefore presents a more broadly based historical and geographical picture of spinal cord injuries over an extended period of time than do most other studies on this topic, including this one.

By far the most significant work on uncovering the perspectives of people with disabilities in the history of spinal cord injury is that of

Mary Tremblay, who has focused her research on Ontario. In her PhD dissertation and in a series of articles published since 1995, she has written about how advances in the treatment of spinal cord injuries in the 1930s and 1940s led to the establishment of Lyndhurst Lodge. She also provides a fascinating history of the early development of the folding wheelchair and the views of people with disabilities who used them.[5] This book owes much to Tremblay's work and follows her approach by providing a historical analysis of the medical developments in spinal cord injury treatment that took place during the period being studied here, while ensuring that the voices of people with disabilities who lived this history are included, along with those of the physicians, nurses, physiotherapists, and others who worked with them at Lyndhurst Lodge. This study also follows along the path trodden by other medical historians who have studied various hospitals and health-care facilities. Lyndhurst's emphasis on the rehabilitation of people with spinal cord injuries based on the intertwining of a medical model and a vocational approach clearly indicates that it fits within the general framework of a health-care institution and a facility for people with disabilities.

Hospital histories in Canada have included both academic studies and approaches meant for a non-academic audience, as some of the above references indicate. This book falls into the latter category of being commissioned for a general audience, while at the same time maintaining the essential basics of scholarly documentation. It is a familiar lament that medical history in Canada, as elsewhere, has been largely focused on doctors and administrators with little attention paid to the more common folk who were patients and staff in these facilities, though this is slowly changing.[6] In an attempt to help fill this void, this book includes discussion of the role of doctors, nursing and other staff, and patients in the history of Lyndhurst Lodge.

Lyndhurst is very much a crossover between two different approaches to interpreting the experiences of people undergoing medically directed treatment. It is part medical history, telling the story of clinical developments in the treatment of spinal cord injury, and part disability history, telling the story of how people with physical disabilities experienced Lyndhurst Lodge and its rehabilitation program. In contrast to medical history, disability history is a much more recently developed field in the sense that the perspectives of people with disabilities themselves are prioritized over those of people who are not disabled. Contributions in this field from Paul Longmore, Catherine Kudlick, and

Suzanne Burch, among others, provide a critical antidote to the more traditional scholarship in the history of medicine where people with disabilities are seldom heard from or understood as having views of their own, views that are often quite different from those of medical professionals overseeing their treatment.[7] Disability history scholarship is also important for helping to ensure that people with disabilities are not portrayed as the passive, silent recipients of medical treatment, something that the following pages aim to contribute to as well.

This book attempts to bridge both fields, with medical and disability history integrated as complementary to each other. Developments in treating people with spinal cord injuries are shown as leading to the long-term survival of more people who were paraplegic and quadriplegic than occurred before World War II. These developments, and the subsequent growth of a rehabilitation profession working at places like Lyndhurst, had a significant impact on the history of disability in Canada and elsewhere. The tension that exists between medical prerogatives to treat people with spinal cord injuries through rehabilitation programs, and the views of some people with these disabilities who feel they do not need to be "fixed" according to a medical model, but instead accepted as they are, will also come up in this book. It reflects some of the basic differences between approaches to how disability is to be understood, past and present. As with any other group of people anywhere, no one point of view can speak for all the people discussed here. Thus, some perspectives support the medical model approach as being essential to a person's understanding of their disability, as well as of their time at Lyndhurst and beyond. Tensions exist too between different ways of experiencing disability, just as tensions exist in various experiences of class, race, gender, sexual orientation, and so many other intrinsic dimensions of what it means to be human.

In recent decades, particularly since the 1990s, disability studies writers and researchers have provided greater understanding about how an environment is experienced as disabling, or inaccessible, thus forming the basis of inequality between people with and without disabilities. The work of Marcia Rioux, Michael Bach, John Hockenberry, Len Barton, Michael Oliver, Simi Linton, Marta Russell, Rod Michalko, and Tanya Titchkosky, among others, has provided significant insights into understanding the social dimensions of disability while also promoting disability rights as a basic part of the social contract between the state and society.[8] People with a host of disabilities are thus understood as having a host of abilities, something this study will demonstrate through the experiences of the people who lived at Lyndhurst Lodge. As well, this book looks at the historical developments related to social policies in regard to state support for people with physical disabilities through the advocacy work of the Canadian Paraplegic Association (CPA) from 1945. The involvement of World War II veterans first and then civilians who worked with veterans in creating and sustaining Lyndhurst Lodge and the CPA, highlights the important connections between war, disability, and provision of services, a link well known among historians of disability.[9] This history connects various strands together, from first-person accounts of disability experiences at Lyndhurst Lodge to the role of veterans and advocacy organizations in promoting greater access to social services at the local, provincial, and national levels for people who, in the not too distant past, had not been given much of a chance to live outside a confined environment – or not been given much of a chance to live at all after experiencing a spinal cord injury.

The care of people with spinal cord injuries in Canada and around the world went from the near universal fatalism that existed up to the 1930s to revolutionary changes in the following decades. These changes encompassed not only the medical treatment of paraplegia and quadriplegia but also the attitudes of and about people with disabilities. The role that Lyndhurst played in these changes is the focus of this study. Established in 1945 as the first centre in Canada to focus solely on the rehabilitation of people with spinal cord injuries, Lyndhurst became one of the most well-known facilities of its kind in the country.

Tracing this rehabilitation centre's history during its more than half-century of existence begins in chapter 1 with a pre-history about what life was like for people with spinal cord injuries prior to 1945. The role of veterans and interested physicians who advocated for the facility is especially important in leading to the opening of Lyndhurst Lodge during the final months of World War II. Chapter 2 discusses how the rehabilitation program was established, why activism by disabled veterans and allies was essential to keeping this facility from closing, and the overall importance of the shift from caring for military personnel to treating civilians at Lyndhurst. Chapter 3 covers the role of the veteran-founded Canadian Paraplegic Association in operating the lodge from 1950–64 and the continuing research programs and clinical developments during this period when Lyndhurst secured its wider reputation in the field. Chapter 4 focuses on the "longest decade" in Lyndhurst's history, 1964–74, when efforts to build a new facility were repeatedly delayed and the lodge continued to deteriorate while demand for its services continued unabated. Chapter 5 follows developments during the next quarter-century, from long-term studies into patient mortality, to wider activism among people with disabilities, to the ultimate amalgamation of Lyndhurst Lodge with two other Toronto facilities and the end of its independent existence.

This study includes many first-person accounts of people with disabilities who were patients at Lyndhurst, as well as the views of doctors, nurses, social workers, and physiotherapists – the personal perspectives of the people who were directly involved at all levels. By integrating clinical developments and studies of the overall patient population with first-person accounts of people who lived and worked at this facility, this book attempts to provide a widely based portrait of Lyndhurst's operation during its fifty-three-year existence as a stand-alone facility and how it affected the lives of the people with disabilities who lived there and made their own contributions to its history.

I

Before Lyndhurst:
Treatment of People with Spinal Cord
Injuries up to 1945

"Keep those spinal cord injuries in bed!"[1] That was the philosophy of treatment staff in the days before Lyndhurst Lodge was opened, according to Andy Clarke. A veteran of World War II, he recalled what is was like in April 1944 after he experienced a spinal cord injury while serving with the Royal Canadian Air Force in Britain. Less than a year later, he would be among the first group of patients to be admitted to Lyndhurst Lodge in Toronto on 15 January 1945. They entered a different world that would give a new lease on life to a group of disabled people, many of whom had previously been given up for dead. How Lyndhurst Lodge helped to make this change possible is the story of this book. To understand the background to this history, it is necessary to look at what it was like for people with spinal cord injuries prior to 1945 and why a few people were determined to change things for the better.

PEOPLE WITH SPINAL CORD INJURIES UP TO 1944

"An ailment not to be treated."[2] That sentiment existed for thousands of years when it came to considering the prospects for people with spinal cord injury. Whether the person was paraplegic (paralysis from the waist down including the legs) or quadriplegic (paralysis from the neck down including legs and arms), death was believed to be right around the corner. Over thousands of years complications claimed countless lives through the impairment of the nerves that traverse the spinal cord and transmit messages from the brain to other parts of the body. Thus the ability to move one's limbs and muscles, to control one's bladder and bowel, to maintain proper blood circulation and a healthy body temperature, and to have sexual function are all affected in a major, even fatal, way, starting from the location of the injury, or lesion, and continuing downwards throughout the rest of the body, which becomes paralysed.[3] A few statistics from the early twentieth century give an idea of the hopelessness that pervaded attitudes towards this group of disabled people.

In 1919 British physician J.W. Thomson Walker reported that 80 per cent of the paraplegic soldiers he had seen during the preceding two-and-a-half years had died from bladder infection.[4] Mortality rates for United States soldiers with spinal cord injuries from World War 1 were 80 per cent within two weeks of injury, while just 10 per cent lived beyond one year.[5] During the early twentieth century, medical schools taught their students that "patients with injured spinal cords seldom recovered from their paraplegia."[6] Ludwig Guttmann, a major figure in the British history of this topic, would later write that medical professionals in all countries during these years had a "profound defeatist attitude" about the long-term prospects for spinal cord injured people.[7] In spite of these odds, some people survived much longer than expected.

One person who beat the odds was a seventeen-year-old woman who was injured on 1 July 1900. She was the victim of a violent attack by a jealous male suitor, who shot her through the spine, killed the young man who had accompanied her to a lacrosse game, and then ended his own life. Though she was a complete paraplegic, with no movement in her lower body, and was given no chance of survival, this woman learned to take care of herself, with the help of a nurse. She lived another forty-eight years and found employment as a dressmaker, eventually dying in Toronto at the age of sixty-five. Unlike so many contemporaries with similar injuries, she never suffered from kidney infection, one of the prime causes of death among people with spinal cord injuries.[8]

Soldiers had no better prospects than civilians. Yet in spite of all the odds, some did survive. Four days before the end of World War 1 William P. became a paraplegic because of a bullet wound incurred while fighting in Belgium. Thirty years later he wrote a letter providing the only known first-person account of a Canadian veteran with a spinal cord injury from the 1914–18 war. He recalled being in hospitals in France, England, and Canada for two years after his injury. Eventually he married a "fine wife who takes the very best care of me in any way she can." They moved to a home on his brother's farm in the country near Sault Ste Marie, Ontario, where they lived "very comfortably" on a disability pension. Though there was no organized help for paraplegics during the pre–1945 period, William's letter provides a glimpse of how a person with spinal cord injuries survived at a time when so many others died.

My legs are just the same as when I left Christie St. [Hospital] in October 1920. I am paralyzed from the hip bones down, with no feeling in either leg, and no movement whatever. When lifted with hands and let go, I simply drop like a stone. I take enemas every other morning, as otherwise my bowels would move and I would not know they were moving, but by taking these enemas and being careful with my diet, I have very little trouble ... When I make water I have to strain a certain amount, but get along very well. I dress by rolling from side to side to get my clothes on, pants, underwear etc. and to get up out of bed I sit on side of bed and put one hand on arm of chair, other on bed, and lift myself in and out of bed that way.

I usually stay in bed till noon as I cannot stand to sit very long as my buttocks break out. I have had no bed sores since leaving Christie, but was very bad with them when I landed there, but they got them healed. I had two large ones, one on each side of the spine down quite low, but I couldn't feel them. I have to be very careful and watch closely at all times ... I have never had an x-ray of kidneys or bladder since I left Christie St. hospital in 1920 ... any place I can't go with my wheel-chair, such as up steps, I have to be carried. I drive my own car which is fixed up to operate all by hand.[9]

Many paraplegic veterans from both world wars were sent to Christie Street Hospital, where William P. was a patient. Canadian World War 1 paraplegic veterans were originally housed in Euclid Hall, a Toronto mansion converted by the government into a "home for incurables." They were eventually transferred to the roof ward at Christie Street Hospital, where at least one hundred wounded soldiers were domiciled.[10]

The first large-scale attempt to assist disabled veterans in Canada began during World War 1 when an artificial limb shop opened in Toronto in 1916. By the end of the war, Toronto had become the artificial limb-fitting centre for Canadian soldiers. The main location was eventually situated at the newly created Dominion Orthopaedic Hospital, Christie Street, known simply as Christie Street Hospital. It was set up specifically for veterans like those paraplegic servicemen who ended up on the roof ward. A workshop making orthopaedic devices was operated at this facility with veterans making up a majority of the staff.[11] However, delays in providing the necessary supportive services – artificial limbs and vocational training – led to anger and unemployment among disabled veterans in the post-war period.[12] These developments, while not directly affecting paraplegic soldiers, are nevertheless important to this story. They set a precedent of the first organized effort to assist physically disabled soldiers that policy-makers later referred to when developing plans during World War II.

For veterans of World War I who were paraplegic or quadriplegic, there were no policies geared towards helping them get on with their lives in Canada or anywhere else. They were expected to be dead within a short time. There are a few references from 1930–32 on the use of wheelchairs, splints, and drop-foot devices for veterans who were "totally disabled" or who had spinal cord injuries.[13] However, the near total absence, well into the 1930s, of any remotely serious discussion about assisting people with spinal cord injuries shows what could be expected by people who had this disability – beyond the most basic palliative care, there was no organized help at all for either soldiers or civilians.

During World War II, federal officials coordinating services for disabled veterans still held out little hope for veterans with spinal cord injuries. In May 1944 Ross Millar, medical assistant to the Deputy Minister of Pensions and National Health wrote: "There is a peculiar special casualty which for some reason or other we never thought of when we were setting up the [Rehabilitation] Committee ... men who have either had total severance of the spinal cord through direct gunshot or through severe injury."[14] Millar went on to note that some personal care attendants who knew a wounded veteran, such as a spouse or a male relative, might be trained to care for a person with spinal cord injuries at home. However, in general, he believed that the "great majority of them will be continuous Departmental hospital cases" so they should be institutionalized "under expert care in their own best interests."[15] Millar's views were based on the practices at that time and were not unusual. Considering the entrenched views about the negative prospects for paraplegics, getting federal planners to consider the needs of this group of veterans was no small achievement and was due in large part to the efforts of a wounded ex-soldier, John Counsell, and philanthropist L.M. Wood, as will be described shortly. It would take considerably less time to change these entrenched views for the better after 1945.

In the meantime, the future did not look very bright for most people with spinal cord injuries. One man's account reveals life for a paraplegic during the last years before a radical new approach took hold. James Burke was twenty-three when a car accident left him a paraplegic on 4 August 1940. He was in hospital for "seven years, four months and thirteen days," starting at St Michael's Hospital in downtown Toronto before being transferred to chronic-care facilities in the western part of the city – Queen Elizabeth's Hospital in Parkdale – where he remained for two years, and then Runnymede Hospital for several more years.

It took two years for Burke to be stabilized, as kidney problems and pressure sores were a frequent occurrence. Kept in bed, with little regular access to wheelchairs, most of which were the "old wicker type," Burke found Queen Elizabeth "a pretty static sort of situation ... not a good atmosphere. It was just end of the road stuff. Most people were quite elderly and not much time left to live and no activity whatever." Instead he provided his own activity – writing. He began to write short stories, which he read to eight other people with spinal cord injuries on his ward, who included both paraplegics and quadriplegics. His memories of this period were quite grim:

The atmosphere if you had a spinal injury in 1940 was dismal. I think you were written off pretty well because almost to a man you had infection and they couldn't do too much about it. I had sulfonamides, the first sulfa drugs in 1941. They were just coming in. They tried it on me and it worked. So that is why I am here and why I didn't succumb ...

You couldn't go out on the street, for instance, in one of these old wheelchairs if you managed to get one [at Queen Elizabeth Hospital]. I know there were some younger people there with spina bifida. They had their own little wheelchairs. They would head out onto the street and got caught. They were confined to bed for a couple of weeks ... They didn't care whether you soiled the bed. It didn't matter. "Don't worry about it." This is not exactly the way to increase your morale. I got into arguments that were that ridiculous about how many books you may have on your side table. They got heavy because they were really kind of brutal, they used to be intimidating. It was not a good place ... I had to declare myself a pauper. The City Government, Provincial Government and Federal Government each would pay a dollar a day for your maintenance in the hospital. So I started pretty low on the totem pole with a broken back.[16]

James Burke later went on to a successful writing career, including the publication of two novels, and also served for several years during the 1950s as editor of the Canadian Paraplegic Association magazine *Caliper*. He has lived with his wife, Laddie, in their suburban Toronto home for over fifty years. His story makes it clear that while important medical advances for treating paraplegia had been made by the time of his injury, the full impact was not felt for some years to come. While he credits sulfa drugs as being of crucial importance to his survival, he also shows that there was little understanding of other aspects of care. It would take the need for organized assistance to recently disabled veterans at the end of World War II to enable large numbers of civilians with spinal cord injuries to experience the benefits of the new ideas and treatments that were germinating by the early 1940s, but had not yet been felt among most people in chronic-care facilities.

E.H. BOTTERELL AND MEDICAL DEVELOPMENTS IN THE CARE OF SPINAL CORD INJURY, 1932–44

While most paraplegics or quadriplegics had a very poor prognosis at the time James Burke was disabled, medical developments that would improve survival prospects for thousands of people in years to come had already started. Developments in Canada during the 1930s were influenced by work done by neurosurgeon Donald Munro in Boston, which he published in 1937 and 1940. Munro had developed the "Munro Tidal Irrigator" to clean a person's bladder, a crucial development that allowed people with spinal cord injuries a greater chance of survival than before by reducing the rate of infection. He also promoted the view that pressure sores developed because of poor blood circulation in the affected area and could be prevented by regularly turning the person whenever they were in bed. Munro also said that these patients should receive an appropriate diet and physiotherapy program to assist their recovery.[17] These ideas would take some time to be used in wider practice, but already changes were starting to take place in Canada.

The first attempts in Toronto to try something different occurred at the Toronto General Hospital (TGH) in the fall of 1932. Dr Kenneth G. McKenzie, Canada's first neurosurgeon, used skull tongs for neck traction. A physician later wrote that this was "a great advance" as it ensured that the cervical fracture-dislocation was diminished, as was the stress on the spinal cord. This procedure also alleviated some of the pain experienced by the injured person.[18] Like Munro, during the mid-

1930s McKenzie advocated the importance of turning a paralysed bed patient within hours of hospital admission to prevent bed sores.[19] Dr E.H. (Harry) Botterell, the physician who lauded McKenzie's work, was to figure prominently in the history of paraplegia and in the early history of Lyndhurst Lodge. Born in Vancouver in 1906, he was raised and educated in Winnipeg, where he received his medical degree at the University of Manitoba before coming to Toronto. During 1932–33 Botterell was a tutor in physiology at the University of Toronto. The following academic year he held the post of resident surgeon at the TGH under W.E. Gallie, head of the surgery department, who had a great influence on Botterell.[20] After a year of study at the National Hospital in London, England, and another year at Yale University, Botterell came back to Toronto. It was during his time as a junior neurosurgeon at the TGH from 1936 to 1940 that he began to develop innovative treatments for spinal cord injuries and fractures.[21]

In 1936 Dr Gallie sparked Botterell's interest in this topic when he asked him to examine people who had spine fracture-dislocations and spinal cord injuries, these being either Gallie's own patients or those of a colleague elsewhere in the city.[22] While treating patient Frank C. in the spring of 1937 Botterell began to use the Munro Tidal Irrigator. It had just been brought back from Boston by Toronto doctor R.I. Harris.[23] Wilfrid Bigelow was a junior intern at the TGH who worked with Botterell during the late 1930s. He remembered patients with spinal cord injuries being considered a "write-off" when he was a medical student and saw some of them die from bladder infections, thus underlining the importance of this new treatment.[24]

After successfully using this technique on two patients, TGH colleague Dr Robin Pearse said, "My God, Botterell, these are the first clean bladders I have ever seen in paraplegic patients."[25] It was obvious that something new was taking place. Medical staff at the TGH began to take notice. Soon physicians across Canada would hear about these developments. Botterell compiled a list of sixteen "Broken Back Cases" from around Ontario who were injured between July 1936 and April 1939. He made a colour film of three of these individuals who became mobile after treatment for their injuries.[26] On 22 June 1939 Botterell and Gallie reported on this work to a meeting of the Canadian Medical Association in Montreal. Using both film and slides, Botterell read the paper at what proved to be a watershed moment in the history of paraplegia in Canada. Though the use of skull tongs by McKenzie and Munro's work in the United States were known by 1939, this was the first presentation, especially using films, to a national gathering of medical doctors about advances being made in a field that many of Botterell's colleagues did not understand and were skeptical about.[27] Underlining the largely uncharted territory he was getting into, Botterell's presentation and the unusual motion pictures he made provide a glimpse of the new treatment he was helping to pioneer, which Mary Tremblay would later identify as "the Canadian revolution in the management of spinal cord injury."[28] These people were among the first in Canada, indeed the world, to receive this new treatment, though as Botterell made clear at the time they did not all survive for long.

The experiences of four people, recounted below, illustrate both the hope and the difficulty encountered during those early years of finding the right treatment to improve the prospects for patients with spinal cord injuries. Botterell's film presentation of the three injured men was particularly important for the example he was trying to impress upon his colleagues from across the country.

Joe S. was a forty-five-year old man who was completely paralysed below the seventh cervical segment in a car accident in July 1936. Botterell did not see him until ten days after his accident, at which time he was placed in traction with skull tongs. He started to regain movement thirteen days after injury. Almost three years after the accident, Botterell reported that Joe's recovery was slow and gradual. The film presented to the CMA shows him going back to work at Tip Top Tailors, where he operated a press machine with both hands and feet, and later shows him walking up and down stairs outside. Some time after the June 1939 presentation, Joe S. died in a second car accident in which he was a passenger.[29]

Frank C., twenty-five, experienced complete paralysis of the legs immediately after a car accident in April 1937. The fracture was reduced by Dr Gallie with skull tongs. Within six months his legs began to gradually recover sensation and at 18 months the alignment of Frank's spine was showing improvement. Munro's tidal irrigator beat back the chills and fever that threatened his recovery and he was also able to voluntarily urinate. Before his discharge from the TGH in 1939, Frank C. was filmed walking with drop-foot braces and crutches.[30]

William M. was eighteen when his neck was broken by a tackle during a football game in November 1937. He became quadriplegic, with complete paralysis below the sixth cervical vertebra. Originally, a halter was used for traction for the first three days of treatment, but he found the pain intolerable. Botterell, who first saw William a day after his injury, then had him immobilized with fourteen pounds traction, using the skull-tong technique that Dr McKenzie had demonstrated in 1932. This relieved the teen's physical pain and allowed nursing care to take place. Eight days after his injury, the first signs of voluntary movement were noticed and thirteen days after he became a quadriplegic William was able urinate of his own accord. Botterell told his audience that "Slow, arduous progress has continued *throughout* the *19 months* since injury with tremendous effort by the patient and recovery from spastic paralysis."[31] The film shows him walking, riding his bike, and driving a car, as well as doing various exercises. Nearly half a century later, his former doctor reported that William M. had married, worked in the publishing industry and "lived for many years."[32]

In addition to the film of these three individuals, Botterell discussed the condition of these and other patients by using slides. He included a discussion of the experiences of one man whose outcome was not as favourable as some of the others, but whose treatment provided valuable lessons in understanding proper care for people with spinal cord injury. Hartley I. was a twenty-five-year-old truck driver who was injured in a highway accident in July 1938. Admitted to the TGH within a day after being injured, he was completely paralysed and had lost all sensation in his body. Pain was relieved when traction was used by means of skull tongs so that he could be turned every two hours to prevent bed sores. He was kept in traction for eight weeks and x-rays revealed good alignment of the cervical spine. To keep him from dying of respiratory failure, he was given intravenous treatment of saline and sucrose and then placed in an iron lung known as a Drinker respirator for four days until he was able to breathe again on his own. The tidal irrigator prevented infections for three months. Hartley died more than eight months after becoming quadriplegic from pulmonary collapse and bronchopneumonia.

Botterell told his audience, "The lesson taught us by this patient is that *no effort is too great to bring patients with acute spinal cord injuries through the state of spinal shock*. He showed us that it is possible to nurse extremely ill cases through the acute period of spinal shock. *The living importance of this principle is well demonstrated by three other patients*" – Joe. S., Frank C., and William M.[33] Forty years later, Botterell recalled the importance of all of these injured people in solidifying his interest in spinal cord treatment: "These four patients were really most exciting to a young man like me ... Oh, there were others, but these were the four."[34]

In June 1939 the message he was driving home to his fellow doctors was clear: treatments were possible for people with spinal cord injuries who had previously been considered hopeless. The main points that he stressed to his medical colleagues that day encapsulate the "revolution" in spinal cord injury treatment that would eventually transform the field:

- that reducing the fracture dislocation was crucial in the early stages of treatment;
- that "any remaining cord function" held out hope for recovery;
- that it was possible to prevent bladder infection and pressure sores;
- that their objective should be to get the person out of the hospital and back into the community, as had been done with the three men shown on film.[35]

This paper by Botterell and Gallie even attracted media attention. The *Toronto Daily Star* reported: "Applaud Surgeons For Spinal Success – Describe Recoveries Under Circumstances Which Once Meant Death."[36] The film made a particularly strong impression on the audience, as the newspaper reported that these people "would have been left to die a few years ago" and quoted Botterell's emphasis "never to give up in such spinal fracture cases."[37] While existing records of his speech focus on medical treatment by doctors, the newspaper story also mentions that he spoke about using physiotherapy and "all sorts of exercises" as part of the treatment.[38] Informing the nursing staff about these new forms of treatment was obviously crucial to their success, since nurses did most of the day-to-day work. In 1979 Botterell recalled: "I put McKenzie's skull tongs in him [patient William M.] to pull his neck out a little bit and then I looked after his bladder and I educated the nurses about the prevention of pressure sores and they really nursed him. That sounds easy, but believe me it is a lot."[39] Specialized nursing care was therefore an essential part of this program and was to become an integral part of the rehabilitation program at Lyndhurst Lodge. Since doctors had long believed that patients with spinal cord injuries died soon after their injury, it is not surprising that nurses would also have taken this view, like most other health-care professionals. Thus re-educating both doctors and nurses on these matters was a top priority for Botterell. Perhaps the most important lesson that Botterell drew from these experiences in 1936–39 was that people with spinal cord injuries did not have any one doctor assigned to their long-term care, as no physicians had previously specialized in treating people who were viewed as good as dead.[40] Continuous, organized care by a group of health care professionals trained in the needs of patients with spinal cord injuries was to replace the hodgepodge, uncoordinated treatment that had existed up until that time.

Botterell's Montreal presentation was his first major public talk on spinal cord injury. It also turned out to be the last major talk he gave before leaving the country for much of the next five years.[41] The outbreak of war in Europe was only weeks away and his services were needed elsewhere. But his work in this area was not put on hold by any means. He would spend most of 1940–44 in the Royal Canadian Army Medical Corps (RCAMC), stationed at the Canadian Neurological Hospital in Basingstoke, Hampshire, which he helped to establish.[42] During these years, the seeds were being sown for Lyndhurst Lodge. The idea of providing an organized plan to care for people with spinal cord injuries gradually took shape through the experiences and discussions Botterell had with colleagues and patients themselves in Britain. RCAMC Basingstoke Hospital was staffed by nurses and doctors from both Montreal and Toronto. They used this facility as headquarters for spinal cord injuries for both the Canadian armed forces and local civilian casualties. One of these casualties remembered the rather circuitous route he took to get to the Canadian neurosurgical hospital and the impression made on him by the chief neurosurgeon. Jack Higman was a twenty-one-year-old dispatch rider in the Canadian army stationed in southern England during the spring of 1944 when he was injured in a motorcycle accident that left him paraplegic.

Basingstoke ... it was just down the street from where I was stationed for heaven's sake ... I was picked up by an English truck and taken into a British hospital. He said: "What are you bringing him in here for?" He said: "He's not an Englishman." He said: "Take him to the Americans, that is where he belongs." He took me to another military hospital, an American one. He looked at me and saw the Canadian flag down on, you know, flash on there and he said: "And what are you bringing him here for? He's a Canadian. Take him to the Canadian hospital." So that is how I wound up there and seeing Dr Botterell. Botterell, the doctor, was smart, there was no doubt about it ... But we had a great, big doctor there that used to assist Dr Botterell on a lot of real tough operations, that sort of thing ... But he and Botterell used to fight like cats and dogs. Oh, oh jeez. It was something to listen to, you know. But I guess, all in all, they were two smart men and they both had two different roads to travel.[43]

Higman would later make his way back to Toronto and to Lyndhurst Lodge, where he would get to know other disabled veterans who were Botterell's patients at Basingstoke. In the course of his work in Britain, Botterell wrote that the Canadian hospital staff developed an "unshakeable conviction" about the need for "exemplary total care" for people with spine injuries.[44] They continued to develop their clinical knowledge and enhance treatments, such as by improving on Munro's tidal irrigator.[45] Botterell also met Dr Ludwig Guttmann and other physicians at the Stoke Mandeville Spinal Centre that opened in Aylesbury on 1 February 1944. After his first visit to this new facility in the fall of 1944, shortly before returning to Canada, Botterell wrote that Stoke Mandeville did not, at that time, have a clear idea of what people with spinal cord injuries should do after leaving the hospital. Guttman's significant work in wheelchair sports and rehabilitation would come in later years. A far greater influence on Botterell's thinking during the Basingstoke years was the eminent British neurosurgeon, Sir Geoffrey Jefferson, with whom he had "thought-provoking discussions" between 1940 and 1944 about the concept "that life outside hospital must be the primary objective for spinal cord injury patients."[46] In the midst of all this, Botterell met an injured veteran who would be instrumental in advancing the idea back in Canada that a special facility for paraplegics should be created based on these new principles of treatment.

JOHN COUNSELL, L.M. WOOD, AND THE EVEREST AND JENNINGS WHEELCHAIR, 1942–44

One of the central figures in this history is John Counsell, who became a driving force behind the establishment of Lyndhurst Lodge and who, along with six other veterans, went on to found the Canadian Paraplegic Association in 1945. Born in 1911 and raised in Hamilton, Ontario, Counsell was from a wealthy and well-connected family. His father was a lawyer and his mother was a friend of William Lyon Mackenzie King, Canada's Prime Minister for most of the 1920s and from 1935–48. Counsell's sister, Elizabeth, was married to Walter Gordon, a partner in the accounting firm Clarkson Gordon, who also worked in the Bank of Canada and Ministry of Finance during the war years and who would later serve as Canada's Minister of Finance from 1963–65. These connections, as well as others that would develop, were to prove invaluable to Counsell's work in the years to come and to the development of Lyndhurst Lodge. Counsell was educated at the exclusive Ridley

College in St Catharines, Ontario, as was Harry Botterell, five years his senior, who became another important connection as this story unfolds. Though he did not go to university, Counsell did study French in Europe and took a course in business insurance. From 1932–39 he worked as an insurance salesman in Montreal. He was married before the war, but the marriage did not last long after he returned from over-seas. In June 1940, the same month that France fell to Nazi Germany, he joined the Royal Hamilton Light Infantry and eventually rose to the rank of full lieutenant as commander of a platoon.[47]

While he was commander of this platoon the thirty-one-year-old Counsell was shot in the back during the Allied raid on the French coastal town of Dieppe on 19 August 1942. He was only able to return to the safety of Britain when another Hamilton soldier, John Gartshore, who was looking for a cousin, grabbed him off the beach and put his wounded comrade on one of the last landing craft taking men back across the English Channel.[48] Once back in Britain, he was transferred to the No. 1 Neurological Hospital, Royal Canadian Army Medical Corps, Basingstoke. In the months following his injury he developed a critical awareness of the prevailing situation for people with spinal cord injury and he learnt how to take care of himself. This newfound awareness would lead the Dieppe veteran to a pre-eminent place in the history of paraplegia in Canada generally and of Lyndhurst Lodge in particular. Decades later, Counsell's doctor at Basingstoke, Harry Botterell, wrote about the importance of their contact during this period:

[Lieutenant] Counsell remained in the hospital for a good many weeks. During this time, he became fully aware of the needs of the paraplegic patient for special hospital care and learned of the remarkable achievements of a few civilian patients in rehabilitating themselves, before World War II in Montreal and in Toronto. When, finally, Canadian Army policy required his return to Canada, he had acquired a remarkable understanding of the problems and needs of paraplegic patients. The Nursing Sisters, especially Jessie Jeffrey, were wonderfully supportive and encouraging throughout his hospitalization at the Neurological Hospital. Every effort was made by the neurosurgical staff to encourage [Lieutenant] Counsell to become a leader of a new and better program for the medical care and for rehabilitation of spinal cord injury veterans in Canada.[49]

After hospitalization in Basingstoke from August to early October 1942, Counsell returned to Canada and on October 14 he was admitted

to the Montreal Neurological Institute (MNI), where he stayed until late
March 1943. He was then transferred to the Toronto home of his sister
and brother-in-law, Elizabeth and Walter Gordon.[50] He lived there for
almost a year, until February 1944, when he returned to his hometown
of Hamilton and took up work in the insurance industry and as sales
agent for a local football club.[51] He was still living in Hamilton in late
1944 when he applied for a new job that brought him back to Toronto
and to a permanent association with the facility that he had a major
role in creating. But before he was able to take on the work for which
he became so well known, indeed before he returned to Hamilton in
early 1944, Counsell had to deal with a number of obstacles that were
directly related to his physical disability and to the absence of any rehabilitation program for paraplegics.

Though recognized as "a Dieppe hero" by his contemporaries and
decorated with the Military Cross by the Governor General while still
in Montreal, concerns were raised about Counsell's treatment by the
government ministry that was supposed to look after disabled veterans
in Canada.[52] Walter S. Woods, Associate Deputy Minister of the
Department of Pensions and National Health, noted that this wounded
soldier had not been provided with "information as to what his rights
were, what his pension would be" and that it took five months to process his discharge papers from the armed services.[53] The implication
was that this process needed to be speeded up to assist with the rehabilitation of disabled veterans, an emerging policy of increasing importance as more veterans returned home. Counsell was one of the early
disabled World War II veterans to return to Canada from overseas, and
was, according to Dr Botterell, the first Canadian to suffer a spinal
cord injury due to enemy action during the war.[54] Thus the problems he
encountered with government red tape back in Canada reflected the
evolving nature of rehabilitation policy during this period. The experiences of veterans like Counsell helped to iron things out in the long run
by showing officials which services needed to be improved, something
that he was eager to point out to them as time went on. Whether his
experience of bureaucratic negligence left any lasting impression on
John Counsell is impossible to say, though it is intriguing to speculate
on whether it gave him ideas about the need to create an effectively run
service for paraplegics with a minimum of delay.

In addition to the physical barriers that all people with spinal cord
injuries experienced, Counsell faced the attitudinal barriers in which
segregation was seen as the solution for a person with such a physical

disability. A few days after Counsell returned to Toronto in early 1943 Dr Charles McMane, Toronto District Administrator for the Department of Pensions and National Health, wrote, "I hope we are not establishing any precedent" by giving support to a paraplegic veteran living at home.[55] After listing the bed, wheelchair, related furnishings, and nursing care that was being provided for Counsell, McMane wrote: "Obviously, this man should be in an institution or, if not in an institution, he should be provided with a helplessness allowance and make his own arrangements for his care, because, if a number of patients similarly afflicted should demand the same sort of care, it would make a rather difficult situation."[56]

While a local government official was worrying about Counsell being a burden on the state, his niece Jane Glassco remembers quite a different side of him during this period: "He had a hospital bed set up in my mother's library. And he had nurses looking after him and a trapeze to pull himself up with ... All of his friends came to visit him and drink and smoke and play cards 'til three in the morning, which was a little hard on my mother ... But Lyndhurst began, I guess, around his bed thinking about other people in the same situation and deciding there had to be a place [for] rehabilitation plus life skills."[57]

Counsell was well known for his enjoyment of practical jokes. He was a good friend of Edward Dunlop, a fellow veteran of World War II who was blinded in that conflict and became head of the Department of Veterans Affairs (DVA) Casualty Rehabilitation Section in the postwar period. Some time after Counsell had moved to Toronto, both he and Dunlop had gone out for a night on the town. Counsell persuaded Dunlop to drive his car on a residential street. A policeman stopped them for driving without the car lights on. After being asked for his driver's licence, Dunlop responded, "Well I don't have a licence, I'm blind." Then after finding out that the car was Counsell's, the policeman demanded his license. The Dieppe veteran responded, motioning to the back seat, "Just a minute, it's in my wheelchair." They were arrested and towed to jail with both occupants laughing away. Both drivers were bailed out early the next day by Walter Gordon, Counsell's brother-in-law.[58] Although he enjoyed a good time with his friends, there is no doubt that John Counsell truly was in the driver's seat when it came to promoting the need for a new facility that came to be Lyndhurst Lodge.

His financial independence, constant nursing care, and awareness of the physical needs of paraplegics all allowed Counsell to effectively pursue a private rehabilitation program at a time when no such programs existed.[59] A crucial part of this rehabilitation process was becoming mobile and for that a wheelchair was needed; not just any wheelchair, but one particular type that he had found out about before returning to Ontario. While assistance from the Department of Pensions and National Health was rather slow in coming and even grudging from at least one official, the months Counsell spent in hospital before re-establishing himself back home were beneficial in ways that would later bear fruit for other paraplegics. In addition to Basingstoke hospital staff, who encouraged him to take on a leadership position among people with spinal cord injuries and who helped to educate him about self-care, Counsell was also greatly influenced by his doctor at the Montreal Neurological Institute, William Cone. This neurosurgeon had been stationed with the Canadian army hospital in Basingstoke in 1940–41 and was its first chief before he returned to Canada.[60] Dr Cone recommended to Counsell during his Montreal stay the new American-made Everest and Jennings wheelchair, which he considered "the best" as it was the first of the revolutionary folding wheelchairs, unlike the much more cumbersome older models.[61]

The first Canadian to purchase one of these new folding wheelchairs was Don Agnew. A paraplegic in Vancouver, Agnew had grown tired of strapping his wicker chair onto the back of his car. Since he was relatively close to the California-based company that made these lightweight chairs, Agnew was able to secure his own before they were widely available.[62] Making them more widely available was something Lyndhurst helped to achieve in years to come. In the meantime, it was necessary to establish why such a wheelchair was so important. Cone emphasized the importance of wheelchair use in re-establishing oneself after a spinal cord injury. He introduced Counsell to other paraplegics in Montreal who were proceeding down this new road to rehabilitation. One of these people, Jimmy Darou, was a former jockey who became a lifelong friend of Counsell's, as they both had a passion for horse racing.[63] Thus, increased mobility in a more practical wheelchair was linked with improved prospects for getting on with life out in the community.

Later in 1943 when he was living in Toronto, Counsell was able to get an E&J from California, with help from John McCarthy, a friend of his who was also the son of the Canadian ambassador to the United States.[64] His niece, Jane Glassco, remembers that this new wheelchair "made him mobile. We had a bunch of front stairs that he had to be hauled up and down into our house forever after." He then became one the first paraplegics to own a car that had hand controls. Now he could fold up his wheelchair in the back seat and drive away. "When he pulled up in front of the house he had a Bermuda bell [a special signal bell] that he pushed and everybody recognized his signal. My father would go out and help him up the stairs in his wheelchair ... He could get in and out of his car, and in and out of his wheelchair."[65]

With this new lease on life, Counsell was eager not only to drive around town but also to make more people aware of the possibilities that this new chair offered. Less than a year after returning to Toronto, he was modelling his new wheelchair – the first of its kind in Ontario – to a group of officials, including Dr McMane, who only eight months before had written that "this man should be in an institution." In doing so, the Dieppe veteran was helping to change minds about people with spinal cord injuries being "helpless."

Central to assisting with this work was L.M. (Lewis) Wood, a sixty-one-year-old wealthy businessman. A philanthropist, Wood was an early supporter, after World War I, of the Canadian National Institute for the Blind (CNIB), of which he was president from 1918–54. He was also involved in the National Society for the Deaf and Hard of Hearing and the Canadian Arthritis and Rheumatism Society, and during World War II he was chairman of the Toronto Rehabilitation Committee, which helped organize local services for disabled veterans.[66] His wealth and decades of involvement in these issues meant that he was quite influential with many well-placed people who took him seriously as a civic-minded businessman. Wood's attitude to this work was summed up in a remark he made to Dr Botterell in later years. Paraphrasing a famous remark by World War I French leader Georges Clemenceau about war and generals, Wood declared, "The spinal cord injury program is too important to be left to doctors."[67] But before this program could be initiated, Counsell and Wood would have to prepare some of the groundwork for what was to transpire at Lyndhurst Lodge beginning in 1945.

These two men first met through family connections. Wood was a card-playing friend of John Counsell's mother, from whom he learned about the younger man's disability. Besides an interest in disability, Wood and Counsell shared other common interests, including horse racing. As their friendship developed, they would go out to nearby Woodbine Race Track to bet on Counsell's horse, "Early Mischief." Years later, after Lyndhurst was established, another paraplegic veteran, Ken Langford, recalled going out to the track by taxi with Wood and spending the afternoon in the cab while a boy ran back and forth placing their bets.[68] Of such leisurely pursuits are rehabilitation centres built!

The Counsell and Wood campaign to provide improved services for people with spinal cord injuries began when they jointly informed government officials and medical personnel about the advances in wheelchair design. They linked this development with rehabilitation priorities for disabled veterans. In early December 1943 Wood contacted officials in the Department of Pensions and National Health in both Ottawa and Toronto, informing them about Counsell's new wheelchair which "impresses Mr Wood very much."[69] A meeting was arranged by Wood at Christie Street Hospital in Toronto on 13 December 1943 where Counsell modelled his new wheelchair. Six medical and military personnel attended this meeting, including Christie Street Hospital staff and Toronto area administrators and welfare officers who dealt with veterans' issues.[70] Meeting participants reported favourably on the folding wheelchair, which had removable arms and allowed for greater mobility outside a hospital. It was considered "a great improvement on the conventional type of indoor wheel chair, particularly for a case such as Mr Counsell."[71] Dr McMane thought it was the best wheelchair possible for someone living in the community, but believed that it was not so useful in an institution, which he felt required firmer, non-folding wheelchairs that would last longer.[72]

Two days after the wheelchair meeting, Wood arranged a meeting between Counsell and R. Wilson, Toronto district superintendent of the orthopedic division of the Department of Pensions and National Health. Using interest in the E&J wheelchair as a starting point, Counsell elaborated on the broader aspects of rehabilitation policy affecting people who use wheelchairs, arguing that it required "a new point-of-view" about rehabilitation in general.[73] At the same time, Counsell was offering his views on this subject to other officials, notably Captain J.A. Catto, Veterans' Welfare Officer in Toronto, and his colleagues. Out of this came the first official references about creating a facility (which eventually became Lyndhurst Lodge), an idea that was clearly linked to the new wheelchair: "Now the question has been brought up by Lieut. Counsell if it would not be possible for the government to provide a separate building, preferably within city limits, in charge of a competent neuro-surgical doctor, who is fully cognizant with the necessity of getting these men up and active ... We might say that it is only since obtaining the [Everest and Jennings] chair that Mr Counsell has been able to get around to any great extent. The way in which he handles himself, getting in and out of motor cars, and in and out of ordinary chairs, on to this wheel chair, is really amazing, and certainly I as a layman can see a great improvement in his physical well-being, since this chair has been obtained."[74]

These December 1943 meetings led to the idea of a specialized facility for people with paraplegia being taken seriously for the first time among federal rehabilitation officials. Plans were also made to design and manufacture a collapsible wheelchair, based on the Everest and Jennings wheelchair, in Toronto.[75] Counsell was frequently consulted about its design and use, so much so that one official eventually referred to it simply as "the Counsell chair."[76] However, problems with production and design led officials to scrap plans for a Canadian-made collapsible wheelchair. The first shipment of six Everest and Jennings wheelchairs arrived in Canada for distribution among disabled veterans in various parts of the country in January 1945, a little more than a year after Counsell and Wood first brought it to the attention of officials at Christie Street Hospital.[77] That these first few new wheelchairs arrived in the same month that Lyndhurst Lodge opened was a propitious quirk of timing.

THE ACQUISITION OF 153 LYNDHURST AVENUE, MAY 1944 – JANUARY 1945

Counsell and Wood had succeeded in getting federal authorities to take seriously the idea of setting up a building specifically for the rehabilitation of paraplegics. Now it was up to government officials to act. Within six months of the December 1943 meetings at Christie Street Hospital the wheels were set in motion. The first reference in official documents to the eventual site of Lyndhurst Lodge – 153 Lyndhurst Avenue – is in the form of an afterthought that occurred when an inspection was ordered of certain large homes as possible sites to house hospital patients. During the spring of 1944, with ongoing fighting in Italy and an expected invasion of France by the Allies, Canadian medical officials prepared to make room for more casualties. At the same time, all military districts across Canada were notified that "Joint Services Special Treatment Centres" were to be created in designated cities to serve army, navy, and air force personnel who required care for unspecified "special conditions."[78]

In this context, on 30 May 1944 the Deputy Minister of Pensions and National Health requested Toronto officials to inspect a house near

Casa Loma, a local landmark built in 1914 in the western, mid-town part of Toronto. It was important that the building should be in this area as it was supposed to be an adjunct of Christie Street Hospital, a few minutes away by vehicle. After discussing the Lennox Home, Deputy Minister Wodehouse wrote about "the home of a Mr Nathanson, deceased. I do not know the address, but it is in the vicinity of the hospital, and if you happen to know where it is, I am inclined to think it would be well to inspect it also and give me a report."[79] So began the next thirty years of the history of this building, built to house the fabulously rich, soon to be rich in history of an entirely different sort. Assistant District Administrator H.W. De Guerre and Chief Medical Officer A.C. Norwich examined both houses on a particularly memorable day during World War II – 6 June 1944 – D-Day on the Normandy beaches. In years to come, some of the men who were wounded in the Battle for Normandy would make their way to this house on a quiet Toronto street. De Guerre and Norwich reported back that the Lennox Home was rather dilapidated but the Nathanson home was in good shape with room for up to seventy-eight beds. Either place was judged as being only suitable if urgently needed for convalescent patients.[80]

On 26 June 1944, at a meeting in Ottawa, Health and Defence Department officials decided that the Nathanson home was the better of the two properties. Rather than using it for convalescent patients of a general type, who could already be accommodated, it was thought best to recommend its use for soldiers who had "paralgesia, or paralysis from the hips down."[81] The correct term eluded the writer, probably because a lack of knowledge about spinal cord injury was common at that time. Since twenty-six paraplegic patients were then at Christie Street Hospital and the Nathanson property was estimated to be able to house forty people (just over half of the original estimate), moving them to this new facility would allow more room for other types of patients at a regular hospital.[82] With this plan in mind, on 5 July 1944 the Wartime Committee on Hospitalization of the Department of National Defence approved a request made a day earlier by the Department of Pensions and National Health to obtain 153 Lyndhurst Avenue.[83] It was at that time occupied by Irene Nathanson, whose husband, Nathan Nathanson, had died the year before. With permission granted to buy the residence, officials spent the next four months negotiating with Mrs Nathanson's representatives to bring the price down from the original $75,000 to $45,000. This was agreed upon by all parties and approved by the federal government on 9 November 1944, the final sale to take effect on 1 January 1945.[84]

There were still some local hurdles to clear. Residents along Lyndhurst Avenue objected to changes in the by-law that restricted anything but residential housing in this area and were supported in this by some city officials. It was suggested that the paraplegic treatment centre should go to the Lennox house site that was already found to be unsuitable. To satisfy everyone, this building had to be assessed again as to its poor quality in comparison with the Lyndhurst property. Eventually, the neighbours said they did not object to having a veteran's hospital in their midst, as long as temporary structures were not erected on the property. Counsell, Wood, and several others appeared before the municipal Property Committee in late November to argue the case for the Lyndhurst site. Dr McMane even held out the prospect that paraplegic veterans might eventually all be sent to Sunnybrook Hospital, which was then under construction. Within a few weeks of this barrier arising, it just as quickly fell when the necessary by-law changes were passed and the neighbours were assured that every effort would be made to prevent a decline in their property values.[85]

What was so special about this thirty-year-old mansion that led the government to think that it would be suitable for disabled veterans? It was a three-floor, stuccoed brick building on three acres of wooded land on the side of a ravine in an upper-class neighbourhood, not far from St Clair Avenue and Bathurst Street – a major intersection – and only a few minutes from public transit. It was originally built as a home around 1914 for approximately $162,000 by Ralph Connable, chief executive of F.W. Woolworth Department stores in Canada. The short street that runs alongside the property is named after him. Perhaps 153 Lyndhurst's most famous house guest was Ernest Hemingway, who stayed there for several months in early 1920 as a tutor for Connable's son, during which time he also wrote for the *Toronto Daily Star*. Connable later sold the mansion for $100,000 to Nathanson, who was president of Famous Players Theatres.[86] Nathanson did extensive renovations on the site, so that by the time the Canadian government came calling in 1944 it was a grand place to live by most people's standards.

The dimensions of the house measured 170 feet by 295 feet and had 212 feet of frontage space, including a driveway and a tennis court. Inside it had, among other features, an eight-foot high ceiling in the basement where there was a fireproof vault; laundry, furnace, electrical, and storage rooms; a movie theatre that could seat about fifty people; and a bowling alley. The ground floor included reception and drawing rooms, music and ball rooms, dining rooms, two bedrooms, and a bathroom. The second floor had a large master bedroom, two smaller bedrooms, and a suite of three rooms along with bathrooms. On the third floor, which housed the servants' quarters, there was one large bedroom, four smaller rooms, and a bathroom. The two-storey brick garage on the property had five rooms and a bathroom on the upper floor for the chauffeur and his family. The three upper floors of the residence had hardwood floors, and various woodcarvings, fixtures, and paintings accented the decor in various parts of the house, especially in the first-floor rooms.[87]

While accommodation for paraplegic veterans was envisaged by those who were interested in purchasing this building, early documents made no reference to how people in wheelchairs were expected to get around the building, such as from the first to the second floor, which was then accessible only by a staircase. Undoubtedly, its proximity to Christie Street Hospital was considered essential. It would be an adjunct of medical services for veterans at the larger institution and it was important for administrative purposes that the two facilities be close to one another. But the main selling point was that the building had been very well maintained and had enough room to house a good number of people with spinal cord injuries, even though it was not made for this purpose.

Though the building was not designed with disabled people in mind – none was during the first half of the twentieth century – the first visitors after its purchase was approved included people with spinal cord injuries. In November 1944 Wood and some unnamed paraplegics, presumably including Counsell, visited Mrs Nathanson at 153 Lyndhurst Avenue. She poured tea and received them "most cordially" as she told them that though she was not moving out until the first of January, they were welcome to start moving in whenever they wanted.[88] Having taken a leading role in advocating for the creation of a separate paraplegic treatment facility, Counsell was hired by the federal government at the beginning of December as a Rehabilitation Officer, to act in an administrative and advisory role. At the same time, Counsell, along with Wood and three others, formed a committee whose job it was to oversee the organization of the unofficially named Lyndhurst Home for Paraplegics.[89] Even before this committee was established, plans were underway to make the building suitable for paraplegics. A request was made in November to pay for the installation of an elevator to service every floor, though it was recognized that patients would be moved in before this was completed.[90]

Hiring forty staff, including twelve each of nurses and orderlies as well as cooks and maids, was supposed to take place in the space of a few weeks. The first employee hired was Douglas Ford, starting on 18 December 1944, "who will be on duty continuously with Mrs. Nathanson's present staff who will make him familiar with all the utilities in the house."[91] It was soon recognized that it was not possible to hire all the staff while also getting the building prepared for its new purpose within such a short time. So it was decided that the building would be occupied gradually, with the initial accommodation to be no more than ten patients.[92] This plan was announced to the local press, who declared on 13 January 1945, two days before the first paraplegic veterans arrived, that the new facility was "Setting Pace For World To Help War Paralytics."[93] The newspaper story noted that the first administrative director of the yet to be named facility was John Counsell, "a living example of what can be done by a paralytic."[94] It was in no small measure through his efforts that this treatment centre had come into existence.

As the new facility was about to open, the world that it was leaving behind is perhaps best reflected in two documents written during negotiations to acquire the property the summer before. The first, written in July 1944, refers to using this "residential property for the care of bedridden paralytics ... [to] make them as comfortable as possible."[95] The second, written the following day, quotes Dr Bain, Director of Medical Services for the federal Health Department, who stated that the chief of the neurosurgery section wanted to "provide new forms of treatment for paralytics, and better results can be achieved by segregating this type of patient."[96] The first statement reflects the low expectations that were still held for people with a spinal cord injury, in which no serious effort at rehabilitation appears to have been considered. This was most likely a reflection of the memories of what happened to paraplegic veterans from World War I and to generations of civilians with spinal cord injuries. In contrast, the second statement offers the prospect that something new was afoot. The writer was not quite sure what this would entail, but compared to the statement made just a day earlier by another official involved in the same acquisition deal, more hope was being suggested for the future occupants of this property than was previously envisaged. Time would soon show in which direction history was moving.

2

From DVA to CPA, 1945–50

"The biggest change for the patients was no more lying in bed all day."[1] So wrote Theo Bullock, one of Lyndhurst's earliest patients in the spring of 1945. His memories encapsulate one of the basic principles that would come to govern the new facility – getting people with spinal cord injuries up and about rather than expecting them to be permanently immobile. This in turn was geared to preparing them for life back in the community. The first five years when this philosophy was put into practice were among the most important in Lyndhurst's history. By proving the validity of their approach, the operators of Lyndhurst Lodge ensured its continued existence for decades to come. As will become evident, the lessons learned during this early period would eventually benefit veterans and civilians alike across Canada.

THE OPENING OF LYNDHURST LODGE AND THE CHRISTIE STREET HOSPITAL CRISIS, JANUARY – MARCH 1945

On 15 January 1945 the first ten patients arrived at 153 Lyndhurst Avenue. Six of them were from Christie Street Hospital and four were from the Red Chevron, a nearby annex to Christie Street. Chief Medical Officer A.C. Norwich wrote a few weeks later that "despite the fact that conditions for their care at that institution are not ideal [the] patients ... expressed their willingness to be transferred and seem quite pleased with their new surroundings on arrival there."[2] Among this first group of wounded soldiers were two air force flight officers, Douglas Quirt and Andrew Clarke. Both of them had been paralysed in military plane accidents in England and they would both become founders of the Canadian Paraplegic Association a few months after arriving at Lyndhurst. Clarke recalled over thirty years later what the conditions were like during this period: "They had us stacked in there pretty closely. I happened to be housed on the second floor. There was no elevator. The orderly staff in those days carried us up and down the stairs."[3]

As work was underway to prepare the various rooms for occupation, Toronto Deputy Chief Fire Marshall Peter Herd visited a few days after the facility opened. After inspecting the entire building and recommending where improvements in fire safety could be made, he spoke to the patients about the part they needed to play in preventing a calamity from occurring. Noting that "more than anything else" fires in hospitals happened because of people falling asleep while smoking in bed, Herd "cautioned patients against such practice and promised to send us some special ashtrays."[4] Largely because of this visit, it was decided that no patients would be domiciled on the top floor. Herd pointed out that any paraplegic patients on the third floor would be in an especially dangerous predicament should a fire break out. It was decided that people with spinal cord injuries would occupy bedrooms on the first and second floors, which were to be fitted out with better emergency safeguards. As well, the cost of building an elevator and new fire escape to the third floor was significant, so limiting patient access to the first two storeys entailed less expense. The top floor was instead designated for staff use. Plans were made to build extensions on the first floor to make up for lost bed-space on the third floor. A smaller lift between the first and second floors, which would fit one wheelchair, was proposed in place of a larger elevator that would have had room for a hospital stretcher. By early February 1945 ramps had also been installed around the building to facilitate the coming and going of wheelchairs.[5] The former mansion was beginning to take on different dimensions.

While all of these plans were being made, John Counsell was actively involved in influencing the building design as well as continuing to advance his vision as to what purpose this place was supposed to serve. He also made it clear what he did not want it to become, a point that made a notable impression on one of the planners. Three weeks after the first patients moved in, Counsell discussed his ideas with A.E. MacGregor, superintendent of buildings in Toronto for the Department of Veterans Affairs. MacGregor wrote afterwards: "From my talk with Mr. Counsell, I was able to form a general idea of the purpose of this institution, and I must admit his viewpoint is quite new; not that I had any particular concept in mind, but rather that Mr. Counsell suggested the idea of purchasing Lyndhurst Lodge was so that it would be more of a training centre, rather than a permanent home for paraplegics. I understand that the patients that will be sent to Lyndhurst will be those that completed any surgical or particular medical treatment at Christie Street. These will then be sent to Lyndhurst where they will be instructed in the best methods of self-help and other such curative measures. This being the case, the institution will probably not be regarded as a permanent home."[6]

With the new facility rapidly taking shape, a decision to give it an official name was necessary. In February 1945 Major Edward Dunlop, head of the DVA Rehabilitation Division and a World War II veteran who had been blinded by a bomb blast, consulted Counsell about this matter. With the agreement of other departmental officials, it was decided that Lyndhurst Lodge would be the official title of 153 Lyndhurst Avenue.[7] This name reflected the name of the street on which the property was situated, the fact that it was in a former private residence that was quite unlike purpose-built health-care facilities, and the philosophy of Counsell. This place was intended to be a home-like, tranquil setting conducive to rehabilitation, not an institution where people stayed for years with little hope of returning to the community. A lodge suggested a stay in a pastoral setting, far from the sterile halls of large hospitals; impressions that were important to convey to future residents if their morale were to be restored. While Lyndhurst Lodge was far from being a rustic inn in the countryside, the name of the building came to play an important part in how people with spinal cord injuries perceived the building and their place in it in years to come.

Just as the name was being settled, so too was the choice of the first medical director of the newly christened Lyndhurst Lodge. Having influenced the creation of Lyndhurst Lodge through the efforts of John Counsell, Dr Harry Botterell would exercise great influence over who would run it. But before this was decided Botterell had to deal with a crisis at Christie Street Hospital, where he arrived for the first time to take up duties as head of the neurosurgical staff on 1 February 1945. In his unpublished memoir about this period, written forty years later, Botterell made clear his respect for the staff at Christie Street, notably Captain Joe Cluff, who was head of this unit at that time. However, he noted that veterans with spinal cord injuries who had previously received specialized care at Basingstoke were returned to "seriously overcrowded and understaffed wards" at the Christie Street Hospital. "The beds were so close together," Botterell wrote, "that physiotherapy was difficult if not impossible to carry out." Demoralized patients were rude to nurses, who in turn were "increasingly discouraged and seemingly indifferent to the welfare of the spinal cord injury group." The nurses had not been trained to care for them with anything other than the "fatalistic attitude" that was commonly held about this group of patients up until then. This crisis worsened when several new patients at Christie Street were treated with so much hostility by their peers who were already established there, that the new arrivals requested to be transferred back to the DVA hospital from whence they came. Botterell went to the ward where this took place and swore at the patients responsible for this behaviour, comments that elicited some attention in a "weekly scandal and gossip sheet."[8]

T.A. Bullock remembered the impression Botterell made when he showed up on his ward. Bullock was wounded in France in July 1944 by shrapnel from a German shell that left him with a spinal cord injury. He had been at Christie Street since August and recalled that with Botterell's arrival "The paraplegic wing was turned upside down!" The newly arrived doctor was very upset. Patients who had been treated by his staff at Basingstoke to ensure that they did not suffer from bed sores had been allowed to regress in Canada to the immobile state he had been trying to change. Staff at Christie Street Hospital who did not agree with Botterell's ideas about how to treat paraplegic patients were let go, which suited him fine – "To hell with them, get them out of here." He was similarly blunt in his talk to the veterans, as Bullock recalled:

When he strode into the room to introduce himself to us he told us we wouldn't believe what he had to say right now, but that within three months, we would be out of beds and into wheelchairs and able to look after ourselves. In fact, he said, most of us would be on our way home. He went on to say that he did not have time for men who would not help him and themselves to make this come true, and those that did not work at this would be lost by the wayside. Then he left the room. Naturally this caused quite a few comments, but most of the boys felt things could not get any worse and were willing to go along with the doctor. The house was thoroughly cleaned and Botterell brought in his own crew. He was a no nonsense man and charged right on ahead. The [Everest and] Jennings wheelchair started to appear, and some of the boys got out of bed for the first time ... The treatment of paraplegics was turned upside down and

I was one of the guinea pigs who set the way for their treatment for years to come.[9]

Botterell wrote out a detailed report for the DVA on the "intolerable situation" at Christie Street, setting out his ideas on how to improve matters, including specialized care for patients with spinal cord injuries. Shortly thereafter, he was told to appear in Ottawa before the committee in charge of Joint Services Special Treatment Centres. What transpired from this was a greater appreciation of the needs of veterans with spinal cord injuries among a wider group of influential people in Ottawa, a recognition that would directly benefit the staff and patients at both Christie Street and its annex, Lyndhurst Lodge, in the weeks and months to come. After the committee meeting was over, Botterell met Dr W.P. Warner, who had just been appointed as the first DVA director general of treatment services, an extremely important figure in the history of disabled World War II veterans. They agreed on the importance of setting up a rehabilitation program for people with spinal cord injuries, including plans to integrate them back into the community and to eliminate the neglect that Botterell had found at Christie Street Hospital.[10]

Crucial to achieving this goal was the hiring of specialized nursing staff and the employment of expert medical consultants at Christie Street, along the lines that Botterell had envisaged before the war. Dr Carl Aberhart was hired on a part-time basis to oversee the urological care of patients, thus ensuring that care of bladders was consistently maintained. Dr Clifford Ash was also employed on a part-time basis as a neuro-radiologist to be in charge of x-ray work. Isabel Wilson was hired full-time in early 1945 as head of nursing staff in charge of patients with spinal cord injuries at Christie Street. In this position, she made recommendations on how to improve conditions for this group, which led to "first class patient care," according to Botterell. Many of the patients who came under her care went on to Lyndhurst, where her influence was felt, though she did not work there. To better organize care of these patients, space was found at Christie Street Hospital for a spinal cord injury unit on the ground floor.[11]

As would become routine in years to come with other hospitals, patients would first receive care at a general hospital to stabilize their condition and to receive acute care in the weeks after their injury. From there they would be sent for rehabilitation to Lyndhurst when and if their condition had improved enough. If complications arose requiring intensive medical intervention after a patient arrived at Lyndhurst, they would be transferred back to the hospital, where staff at the paraplegic unit would care for them (Christie Street and later Toronto General or Sunnybrook Hospital). Ideas, which been germinating in the mind of Botterell and others with whom he had consulted since the late 1930s, were now about to be put into practice. To a greater degree and on a broader scale than had ever happened before in Canada, developments began to move away from neglect towards a more positive, active approach. At this critical juncture in February–March 1945 A.T. Jousse arrived on the scene. He was to come to personify Lyndhurst Lodge for the next thirty years. Like his colleague and friend Botterell, Jousse would make significant contributions to the care of paraplegics and quadriplegics in the decades to come.

DR A.T. JOUSSE AND THE EARLY MONTHS OF THE LYNDHURST LODGE EXPERIMENT

Albin Theophile Jousse was born on 21 July 1910 in Vankleek Hill, Ontario, a small town near the Quebec border, halfway between Ottawa and Montreal. His father was born in Quebec and his mother was born in Ontario. From them, he inherited an Anglo-French background, though he could not speak French. Jousse was raised in Vankleek Hill, where he attended primary school and high school. After graduation in 1928, he moved to Toronto, where he studied for two years at the College of Optometry. Upon completion of his optometry studies in 1930, he returned to Vankleek Hill where he was unemployed for a year during the depths of the Great Depression. In July 1931 Jousse found employment in Lindsay, Ontario, where he worked for the next three years as an optometrist in McCarthy's Jewelry Store. In 1934 he enrolled at McMaster University in Hamilton, from which he graduated in 1937 with a bachelor's degree in science. From 1937 to 1942 Jousse attended the University of Toronto, where he earned his medical degree. During eight years of university studies, 1934–42, he found summer work as an optometrist in his hometown, as well as in Hamilton, Brantford, St Catharines, and Niagara Falls, Ontario. After obtaining his MD, Jousse was an intern at the Toronto General Hospital in 1942–43 and found employment in the fields of neurosurgery and neuropsychiatry. He worked half-time at two different jobs from the autumn of 1943 until February 1945: as an "instructor in clinical examination to final year medical students" in the Department of

Surgery, University of Toronto, under the supervision of Dr Kenneth McKenzie; and as a supervisor of nursing and orderly staff in "psychiatric and medical care of patients including shock therapy" at Ontario Hospital, Toronto, the city's largest mental institution. He left these jobs, he wrote, "to assume a more responsible position."[12] It was a responsibility he would maintain for the rest of his professional life.

As a youth, he developed a limp that stayed with him all of his life. In 1947 Jousse attributed this disability to "lameness resulting from syringomyelia," a progressive disease of the spinal cord that causes muscle wasting, spasticity, and loss of sensation.[13] As years went by, his limp became more noticeable and he began to use canes and then crutches in the latter part of his life. His disability affected him in other ways. Though Jousse tried to join the armed services during World War II, he was turned down as "not physically acceptable."[14] His daughter, Eileen Woloshyn, said that her father "had always … been quite chagrined that he wasn't able to do anything in the war. So he considered this [working at Lyndhurst] his war effort."[15] Jousse himself had said to Botterell when the position of medical director was offered to him, "My war effort had not been much and I am glad to accept the job."[16] He had been about to leave Toronto to work as an internist in Sudbury when this job prospect opened up. The ongoing crisis on the overcrowded wards at Christie Street Hospital and the urgent need to find someone to take on the specialized care of patients with spinal cord injuries formed the backdrop to this offer.

Botterell consulted with Dr McKenzie, who recommended Jousse to him, based on his work at the TGH during the preceding years. Jousse's work in neurology, psychiatry, and internal medicine indicated to both McKenzie and Botterell that he was the best candidate available, given the complex and largely uncharted waters the new medical director was heading into.[17] Since there was, as yet, no entrenched field dealing with the care of spinal cord injuries, it seemed wise to choose someone who had skills in a number of areas, predicting, in a way, the interdisciplinary approach that would later develop. Chief Medical Officer A.C. Norwich felt that there was "no one in the [Armed] Forces more suitable" for the Lyndhurst job, though Jousse had been cautioned that he could be replaced by a physician returning from the war, should any candidates come forward.[18] At the end of February 1945 Jousse was appointed by the Department of Veterans Affairs as temporary medical officer, with a salary of $375.00 a month, to "treat all paraplegics under the care of the [DVA]."[19] This entailed responsibility for veterans with spinal cord injuries at Christie Street Hospital as well as overall supervision of Lyndhurst Lodge. The close coordination between these two facilities, the main hospital and its annex, was essential to the development of the rehabilitation program.

Jousse recalled several decades later that Lyndhurst staff and medical consultants came primarily from Christie Street (and later Sunnybrook) Hospital with Dr Botterell being the key support behind the scenes: "He was the man who conceived [Lyndhurst], planned it in detail and really set the pattern for fulfillment of our goals of rehabilitation."[20] This guidance was essential for Jousse. In 1979 he of spoke of how much he had to learn on the job and also offered a picture of these early days at Lyndhurst:

I must say that the patients and myself had about equal knowledge of para-plegia at that time and they probably knew more about it really, except ana-tomically from a textbook point of view. I had no idea about rehabilitation ... I thought it was a great idea of course, but how was it going to be done?... I did the only thing I knew that I should do and this is I went around in the first few weeks and I examined each one, talked to them a great deal and encouraged them to get up or be gotten up, to get into a program of exercises, because we did have some physiotherapists there who really knew more than I did at the time and nurses who were really good. The head nurse was a charming old woman from the [First] World War. I don't mean old in years but settled in her ways, old in experience and quite convinced that to try and get the poor boys up from bed was unkind. We had a struggle with her too.[21]

This first head nurse, Miss Mabel Lawrence, had been the day-to-day supervisor of the lodge between the arrival of the first patients in mid-January and Jousse's official start on 1 March 1945. She lived on the premises until her living quarters were needed for three patients in the summer of 1945.[22] While sources for patient and staff activity in January–February 1945 are scant, greater documentation of daily life at the new facility is provided by regular monthly reports written by the medical officer in charge from March to October 1945. In his first report written at the end of March 1945, Jousse reported that there were seven nurses, one nurse's aide, and five orderlies on duty to look after twenty-one patients. Eleven of these patients, Jousse wrote, would never regain movement in the lower part of their bodies, while ten wounded soldiers did have the ability to move their legs, five of them being able to stand. Jousse reported that most of the patients lived on the main floor because of the absence of an elevator, a difficult situation since only one bathroom was available on this level, while four bathrooms were accessible on the second floor.[23]

In spite of these difficulties, he wrote that the morale of this group of patients was "surprisingly good." At the same time, however, the incidence of depression amongst some patients was also mentioned. But with two exceptions, Jousse felt most of them could be "fired with the desire to be re-established." To help relieve the monotony, movies were shown two evenings a week, which was a popular diversion. On three other nights each week, young women came in to socialize, such as by playing cards, though they were not as popular with the servicemen as were the movies. Several patients were also transported to see a hockey game at Maple Leaf Gardens, a form of entertainment that would become something of an institution at Lyndhurst in the decades to come. Another aspect of life at the lodge that was established during these first few weeks and would be felt for years to come was getting patients to bed at 9 p.m. Entertainment had to be concluded by this time, though people who had gone off the property had to be back by 10 p.m. unless permission to stay out longer had been granted. Weekend passes could also be granted for people who had families or friends who were planning to take them home for a few days. If any patient found it disturbing, keeping lights on in the bedroom or listening to the radio was not permitted late at night.

Of the staff, six nurses worked the day shift, as did two orderlies, one nurse worked the night shift with help from a nurse's aide and two orderlies who worked until 11 p.m., and an orderly worked from 11 p.m. to 7:30 a.m. The primary goal of nursing staff during these first few weeks was the prevention of pressure sores. Patients had to be turned every two hours, all day and night long, with rubbing alcohol applied to the back every night. Both male and female staff worked together to do this job, though Jousse noted that the night nurse was especially busy with this task. Anticipating the important psychological dimension of rehabilitation work that would develop in the years to come, Jousse wrote of the essential role nurses performed in "maintaining the morale of patients and of instilling optimism in those who have a gloomy outlook." Noting that there was "great individual variation" in the abilities of the present employees to carry out this part of their job, with three nurses being particularly adept, he recommended that those nurses who showed promise in this regard be kept as permanent staff at Lyndhurst and not transferred elsewhere. In this way, a professional rehabilitation nursing staff would be created at Lyndhurst, something that Jousse planned from the very first days of his new job. Since folding wheelchairs were the most urgent need "from the patients' point of view" in March 1945, it can be surmised that patients spent most of their time in bed during this period. Physiotherapy was instituted, but there were some problems in getting it established. One male physiotherapist was employed in early 1945, but Jousse wanted him replaced as he "is unable to command cooperation from patients ... He appears to be afraid of incurring their ill-will, as though his purpose at the Lodge is to gain their favor [rather] than to make them well." In the second half of March, patients did become more active in group physiotherapy activities in the recreation room, though not because of the staff member assigned to this job. Instead it was due to "the active lead taken by one of the patients, who is a trained [physiotherapy instructor], a capable leader and an excellent example."[24] By May the original male physiotherapist had been replaced by Jean Sharpe and a full-time male assistant. Their work was praised as "there is no friction between patients and operators" as there had been.[25]

That first spring at Lyndhurst, Theo Bullock remembered that it was understood by patients that "as long as you were breathing you had to get up and dress." Meals, using the washroom, exercise in the gym, all required formerly bed-bound veterans to be up and about regularly. They were also encouraged to get out in the neighbourhood in wheelchairs, an unusual sight at that time. "This was quite the change from Christie and what the doctors were trying to do was working. Everyone was much happier and healthier. During this period John Counsell would come up in the driveway in his car, pull his wheelchair out from behind him, get himself into it, then buss [sic] around Lyndhurst. John was a great one for the horse races, and after he would put on his show he would say, 'I'm off to the races, see you tomorrow' and away he'd go. What a sight for the boys who would be spending the rest of their lives in a wheelchair."

Bullock also recalled the anguish that patients faced day in and out. Infected bladders led to chills which caused sufferers to "shake like mad," while penicillin, sulpha drugs, and extra blankets were used to combat this potentially life-threatening condition – "the threat of death was not far away." Indeed, while at Lyndhurst Bullock bled profusely from where his suprapubic tube was inserted and required emergency surgery at Christie Street. The tube was replaced by a catheter.

Though he was able to walk with two canes by this time, loss of blood left Bullock in a weakened condition when he was returned to Lyndhurst a few days after surgery. Worst of all, his bladder was badly infected. "I knew at this point that I was not going to make it, which was very hard to take after getting this far. I got really down in the dumps." After further attempts to improve his condition failed, Botterell, who was regularly assisting Jousse on rounds at Lyndhurst during these first months, offered a possible solution. He told Bullock they were trying out a new drug, streptomycin, that had never been tested on people before. Botterell told his patient that this drug might kill him and wanted to know whether or not he wanted to have it injected. Bullock responded: "What have I got to lose?" He was then transferred back to Christie Street Hospital. Every eight hours for ten days, Bullock and several other patients had this drug shot into their arms and buttocks. Its effect was like "a good kick in the butt." At the end of the treatment, Bullock had his catheter removed to see what the results would be. "I climbed into my wheelchair, took my jug and away I went. I stood and started to go in the jug. I kept going and going and began to think the jug would not be able to handle it, but it stopped at eleven ounces. Everything was as clear as a bell, I couldn't believe the difference the ten days made. Then it hit me that I was going to make it, and I do not mind in the least saying that I sat back in my wheelchair and cried like a baby. My God I had made it! When I was able to pull myself together I went to the nurses' station, set down my jug and everyone came running over and took a look. They all knew what this meant to a paraplegic. Back in the room I told Ted [Higginbottom] what had happened and we all had a good cry because Ted knew he would be next."

A few days later, shortly before his twenty-third birthday on 6 June 1945, Bullock was discharged, ten months after being wounded in France. As for the physician who offered him this treatment: "Dr Botterell was a no-nonsense man, I suppose one might say he was a bit rough, but he knew what he was doing, and every paraplegic owes their life to him."[26]

Several days after these momentous events in the life of this veteran, a crucial meeting was held about Lyndhurst's future. On 8 June 1945 a status report meeting was held at Lyndhurst Lodge while Jousse was away on a study trip. Botterell was in attendance along with Wood, Counsell, and DVA officials W.P. Warner of the Rehabilitation Branch and Brigadier Murray Dillon, who was there to consult on building design. While medical requirements still had to be determined, a high priority was placed on making more space available, so a sixteen-bed extension to the facility was agreed upon. There were twenty-five patients resident at Lyndhurst in June 1945 and the people in charge wanted to accommodate forty to forty-five as soon as possible. When staff and visitors were added, there were as many as sixty-five people in the building for the noon meal.[27] In other words, the place was crammed full. In spite of difficulties with physical arrangements at the new treatment centre, Wood said the attendees at this meeting were "thrilled" with the progress made so far. Dr Warner wrote: "It was the general feeling at the meeting in Toronto that the Lyndhurst Lodge experiment should be continued and that no one was in a position at present to clearly outline what was the best set up for the rehabilitation of this group."[28] Trying to determine what was "the best set up" for patient care at Lyndhurst was being looked into at the very moment that Warner wrote these words by the man who would have otherwise been present at this meeting. On his return, plans for the rehabilitation program in Toronto had come into much clearer focus.[29]

ESTABLISHING A REHABILITATION PROGRAM AT LYNDHURST LODGE

Jousse and Botterell were in New York City on 30 April and 1 May 1945 to study treatment techniques at the Institute for the Crippled and Disabled. This privately funded out-patient facility opened in 1917 for the rehabilitation of physically disabled veterans. Eventually civilians made up most of its clientele. Paraplegics only began to be included in 1943, but within two years a good deal had been accomplished to spread its reputation north of the border. So impressed were the two Toronto doctors with its program, that Jousse returned to learn more from the New York Institute for two weeks in June with physiotherapists Jean Sharpe from Lyndhurst and Ruth Nettlefield from Christie Street. From this trip they returned with a better understanding of how to organize treatment services for people with spinal cord injuries. Central to this was ensuring that staff were trained to work with patients at different stages of rehabilitation. The main points that they gleaned from the June trip to New York was the need to organize a rehabilitation program in three inter-related areas: self-care, mobility (or "locomotion"), and vocational re-training. These ideas would soon make their way back to Toronto.

Considering its importance in the history of Lyndhurst Lodge, it is worth describing what Jousse observed on this trip. Paraplegics began their rehabilitation as bed-patients with lifting exercises to develop their upper body strength – pectoral girdle, arm, and hand muscles. This was essential for a person with a spinal cord injury to do their own transfers, that is, going from bed to wheelchair and back again as well as to and from wheelchair and toilet. Practising transfers became a standard part of the rehabilitation program. Learning to dress and undress was also emphasized from the earliest stage. Mat classes taught the patient balance and exercises developed forward and backward motion.

Walking techniques were also used in New York, beginning with trying to walk between parallel bars. Crutches were tried when a person was leaning against a wall and later when they could move away from the wall, while a physiotherapist stood by each step of the way. If the person was able to walk, they would then learn various sitting and standing routines, as well as going up and down stairs, curbs, and the like. However, Jousse was very cautious about employing crutch-walking techniques. He pointed out that it was "extremely strenuous" for people with spinal cord injuries and could literally make them sick or be inappropriate for a number of physiological reasons. After touring a ward for in-patient paraplegics at New York's Bellevue Hospital, he suggested that long-term bed-patients suffered weakening of muscles "due to a prolonged rest in bed rather than [due] to the severity of the injury." This point in particular would become one of the most basic goals of rehabilitation at Lyndhurst – to get people out of bed and physically active so their muscles would not deteriorate. When noting the work done by speech therapists at the institute, Jousse observed how this re-training included teaching a person to write again, a practice that was later used at Lyndhurst for people whose hands had become disabled. A film of the paraplegic rehabilitation program had been shown to the Canadian visitors. In July it was viewed by patients and staff back in Toronto at both Christie Street Hospital and Lyndhurst Lodge.[30]

Jousse and Botterell began to implement the concepts used at the New York institute immediately after their first visit. As a result patients had shown a "marked change" in their involvement in physiotherapy. Whereas in the first few months of Lyndhurst's existence, patients were not systematically assessed as to their needs or capabilities this now began to be done. Lyndhurst patients began to be categorized into two distinct groups for rehabilitation purposes: those with complete lesions who would never walk again; and those who had partial use of their lower limbs. Treadmills, wall bars, and punching bags were installed to facilitate physiotherapy in May, 1945. A rope was also fixed to the ceiling of the gym for climbing exercises. The primary obstacle confronting rehabilitation efforts had at first been the persistence of serious bladder problems, according to Jousse. However, by the spring of 1945 the use of tidal irrigators improved this situation. No doubt because of these developments, more patients were reported out of bed for longer periods of time, with increased physical training. Occupational therapy during these early months was stymied, with the person employed in this job reporting lack of interest among the patients. However, two unnamed patients did find some work while still at Lyndhurst, one repairing watches and another fixing golf clubs. Classes in hand dexterity were also offered by the OT department with assistance from physiotherapists. By late summer, OT work at Lyndhurst was ended as it was not seen to be of much use.[31] The emphasis in re-training was instead placed on physiotherapy.

In 1946–47 Jousse and his colleagues published several articles describing how they approached the treatment of people with spinal cord injuries. These treatments started to be put into practice during the summer of 1945 through the new paraplegic services organized in Toronto. Out of this developed the team approach to overall medical care of paraplegics and quadriplegics initiated at Christie Street Hospital by Botterell in early 1945 and further refined in the following months. Of crucial importance was consistent genito-urinary care to prevent the bladder infections that had caused so many deaths. This was the specialty of urologists, notably Dr Carl Aberhart with assistance from Dr Joe Cluff. Neurosurgeons under the direction of Botterell operated on nerve roots and the spinal cord to relieve intolerable pain and to stop flexor leg spasms, as these conditions made it impossible for an injured person to get into a wheelchair. Plastic surgeons were called upon to close severe pressure sores that would otherwise have prevented a patient from getting out of bed and commencing physical retraining. Orthopaedic surgeons dealt with fractures in which stabilizing the spine was essential to allow a person to participate in rehabilitation. Nursing care was paramount to monitoring the progress at each stage of patient care and ward staff had to be specially trained in these areas. All of this acute medical care took place at Christie Street Hospital, along with some preliminary physical retraining. The overall retraining program that developed from this stage on straddled both Christie

Street and Lyndhurst. Though these later stages were not strictly separate from one another, they focused on the following five areas: exercises while in bed; transferring to and from a wheelchair; gym classes and getting ready for brace-walking; walking between parallel bars; using crutches to walk with braces.[32]

The physiotherapist began to work with the patient right after their arrival in hospital, by massaging and carefully manipulating paralysed parts of the body to prevent them from becoming deformed, decalcified, and fractured. Such consequences could lead to death. While a patient was still in bed, tension exercises were initiated to improve upper body strength in the chest, arms, and hands. Dressing and self-care, such as washing, were the next stage. With the help of bars attached above their beds, patients were accustomed to turning every two hours, 24 hours a day, to prevent pressure sores; some woke up on their own, others had alarm clocks or staff to assist them. Teaching patients to sit up on their own was also important as they first became dizzy because of the months of lying on their back while becoming stabilized. When patients could sit up they would be able to practise transfers between bed and a wheelchair and between wheelchair and a toilet.

When patients could independently complete their wheelchair transfers they were considered suitable for transfer from Christie Street to Lyndhurst Lodge, as long as space was available. Physiotherapists, orderlies, and nursing staff were crucial throughout this day-to-day physical retraining and teaching of self-care at both facilities. At Lyndhurst, wheelchair exercises included flexing arm and hand muscles with weight pulleys attached to the wall and hitting a punching bag. Mat class exercises included having patients transfer from their wheelchairs to the mat and back again by themselves. Once on the mat, the patients exercised their trunks and arms, and did buttock walking to improve their physical balance and build up their muscles in that part of the body. These classes lasted six to eight weeks. Wearing of braces while trying to walk between parallel bars was also attempted, as was crutch walking. Some patients also exercised by playing golf, archery, and croquet.[33]

Some of these approaches were found to be less effective than others. During these first months of Lyndhurst's operation a great deal of emphasis was placed on brace-walking, as a way of improving the chances of getting veterans with spinal cord injuries back into the community. Botterell reported in June that no patients had been able to walk so far because of substandard braces. During the spring of 1945 the orthopaedic department that served Lyndhurst at Christie Street Hospital had been working on improved leg-braces for which two patients had volunteered to be test models, one of whom was John Counsell.[34] By the following year, it was reported that out of ninety-six paraplegic veterans who had been at Lyndhurst, thirty-nine were undergoing brace-walking training, though six of this number were said to find it of "no practical value" and twenty-one others were able to walk without braces at all.[35] While later years would see a departure from this focus on use of braces for paraplegics, during the experimental days when rehabilitation was starting to take off in Toronto, it was a major area of research. It reflected the influence of efforts in the United States, as was seen during the trips to New York City. Botterell later wrote that leg-braces were seldom of long-term benefit for most patients, though there were some exceptions, as discussed later in this book. Botterell wrote, "We, the medical staff and Donald Munro, had mistaken the usefulness and importance of brace-walking."[36] The caution that Jousse had originally recorded about using this approach, after his second trip to the Institute for the Crippled and Disabled, was eventually confirmed.

The Lyndhurst retraining program varied depending on the ability of the person to participate and the extent of the spinal cord injury. Jousse and physiotherapist Ruth Nettlefield wrote in 1946 about the three different groups of patients they worked with. People who had flaccid leg paralysis and significant sensory loss but maintained control of muscles in their abdomens, and who could even move their thighs, formed the first group. Another group had spastic paralysis in their legs and portions of their trunks, though their shoulders and arms were unaffected by the injury. The last group had spastic paralysis in their legs and upper body, as well as paralysis of the arms and hands, a condition that came to be called quadriplegia. All people in these various conditions experience bowel and bladder paralysis. Jousse and Nettlefield noted that the "psychological shock" of finding oneself in this condition was common amongst all patients. But they were surprised that most of these disabled people were not even more despondent, considering the unexpected and traumatic change that had overtaken their life. They concluded by stating that "the physiotherapist's responsibility to these patients is to prevent deformity, to re-educate and to maintain morale."[37] These basic principles formed the core of the physiotherapy program for patients with spinal cord injuries in Toronto.

The essential part of the rehabilitation program at Lyndhurst was reintegration into society, something that began even before the new system was worked out. At the end of May 1945 the first patient in Lyndhurst history was discharged back into the community. A part-time job was found for this man after Jousse had taken him to Selective Service in Toronto to help him find work. This is revealing in itself: the work that rehabilitation officers and social workers would later undertake – finding jobs in the community for Lyndhurst alumnae – was initially done by the head of the lodge. Jousse wrote at the time that this "precedent ... should be of considerable value in the future." By August Ken Purchase was employed as Casualty Rehabilitation Officer (CRO), a crucial job. In consultation with the medical officer in charge, the CRO was responsible for helping patients to find employment or vocational retraining in the community. Purchase, and those who succeeded him, such as Jim Bartlett, who was hired four years later, were to be a vital link for reintegrating people with spinal cord injuries into jobs and homes.[38]

Other aspects of the rehabilitation program were also being developed at this time. While the dignity that work could bring was important to a person's morale and well-being, so too was the ability to maintain some dignity over control of basic physiological functions. With the assistance of orderlies, laxatives were administered to most patients on the toilet rather than in bed, except in a few instances. This was preferred by patients for obvious reasons of hygiene and personal privacy. As well, Jousse reported on the use of a condom and a drainage bag for urination, which was meant to help keep a person dry, though it did not always work properly.[39] In time, this attention to basic daily needs allowed more people to return to the community able to look after themselves.

In July 1945 an out-patient department had been set up to treat five people with spinal cord injuries, two from Christie Street, the first of many hundreds of out-patients who would make their way to Lyndhurst for regular treatment in the years to come. Six months after Lyndhurst's opening, patients' daily routine had changed from largely bed-bound activities to one in which only "3 or 4 of the 25 patients" remained in bed past 9 a.m. and six to ten of them were up early enough for daily breakfast. As patients' bladder care had improved with tidal irrigators, more of them were able to take baths on their own and more were able to care for themselves. We get a glimpse of the food available to patients during this time in Jousse's report that "some of the patients do not care for salads and cold meat in the evenings, preferring a hot dinner twice a day." It was later explained that because many of these men had worked at heavy labour prior to their injury and were used to hearty meals criticism of green meals was to be expected. Beginning in the summer of 1945 the use of the therapeutic pool at Divadale convalescent hospital began for patients who were able to control their bladders and bowels. Hydrotherapy was used for patients who had partial paraplegia; the warm water offered "temporary relief from spasm."[40] Hydrotherapist Charles (Chuck) Reeve was to become the resident expert in this treatment, first at Divadale and after 1950 in the new pool at Lyndhurst.

Since mobility was an essential part of rehabilitation and re-establishing independence outside of the hospital, access to wheelchairs was crucial. Initially, a steady supply of the folding wheelchairs that John Counsell had done so much to promote was slow in coming. Efforts to make an acceptable Canadian-made collapsible continued throughout 1945 with Lyndhurst patients being asked to try them out to see how good they were. Everest and Jennings chairs won out as more comfortable, lighter, and sturdier, though people discharged to rural areas found it hard to manoeuvre on gravel. A bigger wheel was required for this surface. Up to the summer of 1945 wheelchairs were in short supply in Toronto. However, by the end of the year, when there were twenty-five in-patients at Lyndhurst, twenty-nine wheelchairs were available and twenty of these were the coveted Everest and Jennings chairs. A little over a year later, the E & J was reported by Jousse to be the "wheel chair of choice for well over 90% of all paraplegic patients."[41] Its place at Lyndhurst, and in the lives of people with spinal cord injuries, was secure for years to come.

Ken Langford, who was responsible for Lyndhurst wheelchair purchases in the latter part of the 1940s, offered insight into why wheelchair supplies were initially rather difficult to predict. He found that Everest and Jennings supplied only about 10 per cent of the wheelchairs ordered. So when wheelchairs were needed, ten times as many were ordered. Eventually, the supplier "caught up" with his math, though unexpectedly so. Lyndhurst needed eight wheelchairs. So, as he had done before, Langford ordered ten times the number, expecting to get a fraction of those requested. Instead, eighty wheelchairs showed up! Fortunately, Conn Smythe, owner of the Maple Leaf Gardens and a major supporter of Lyndhurst, found space for the excess wheelchairs at the local hockey arena, where they remained in reserve for future owners.[42] Re-working the driving mechanisms of cars, so that hand-controls would enable a person with a spinal cord injury to drive an automobile, was also an important advance closely allied to the spread of collapsible wheelchairs. Learning to drive with hand-controls, as well as to transfer back and forth between wheelchair and car, with the wheelchair folded up for the ride, also came to be an important part of retraining in the years ahead.[43]

In the meantime, Lyndhurst's patient population was in constant flux as veterans were transferred between the two DVA paraplegic units in Toronto in the spring and early summer of 1945. It was a busy place. However, its operators were not yet able to provide the full range of services that they were planning. Indeed, those services that were supposed to be available could come up short. Jousse had trouble getting radiologists to interpret x-rays during the summer vacation period at Christie Street Hospital, leaving it up to him to frequently go to non-DVA hospitals in the city for analysis. Even getting patients to have a fifteen minute x-ray often took up the better part of the day because of transportation problems with Christie Street. He estimated that at times it to took up to three weeks from the time an x-ray appointment was requested until it was actually completed.[44] However, the program was moving forward. As some of the participants recalled more than a half-century later, rehab could be both work and relaxation.

Jack Higman had been one of Botterell's patients at Basingstoke in 1944 after his army injury left him paraplegic. The following year, he was among the first group of patients at Lyndhurst, a group of men he fondly recalled as "a bunch of characters ... Playing tricks on each other and things like that ... We had a lot of fun together." Higman remembered too that there was a lot of work for them to do. "I know that they used to exercise the hides off of us everyday trying to build us up. And they figured that that was the most important thing. That was to build yourself up so that you could make a life for yourself, so far so good ... They had these exercises and I know that they had that rope in the middle of the ballroom. When you had gone through all these courses and that, the day that you can crawl up that rope and tap the roof, you are a graduate and that sort of thing. Well, I think that it was thirty feet high ... And we got some people to show that it could be done."

He also recalled a one-day fishing trip to Algonquin Park by pontoon plane, arranged by the Ontario Department of Lands and Forests for paraplegic veterans from Toronto. "We had a very nice day ... All of the planes took off and brought us back to Toronto again. It sort of makes me laugh about those old days to hop on an airplane to fly up North just to have a picnic ... There wasn't a lot of drinking or anything like that. We just had a good time and a darn good dinner ... In fact we just ate outside right with our plates on our laps ... We enjoyed it very much."[45]

Ken Langford recalled that patients and staff were all new and were not too sure what to expect. A lieutenant in the Calgary Highlanders, he had been wounded in Holland by shrapnel in the right chest and spinal cord that left him paraplegic in February 1945. He was originally given scotch instead of penicillin when he was wounded, since "I guess that they wanted to save the penicillin for people who had a better chance of surviving." Over two months later, he was admitted to Christie Street Hospital on 26 April 1945. From there he was transferred to Lyndhurst on 12 November 1945.[46] He recalled his initial association with the facility he would come to know very well.

Lyndhurst had no facilities for acute care. It was strictly rehabilitation so that graduating from Christie Street to Lyndhurst was a big step ... Dr. Jousse's attitude generally was that the patients should try to do anything they wanted to do and to try everything that they could. That was probably the best way to rehabilitate them and get them ready to go home. But at that time living accommodation for wheelchairs was fairly hard to find so patients tended to be there for quite a long while. And they used Lyndhurst as their home until such time as they could find some place to live ... The program that Dr. Jousse had developed fell into place and it was somewhat unusual. Patients were quite free to go out of hospital and do anything they wanted to. It was by no means an institution, which was unusual at that time for hospitals. And it was very effective because it gave patients a chance to see what they could do and certainly speeded up their recovery.

In one example of the unorthodox rehabilitation program just getting underway, when Ken Langford was experiencing a difficult period Jousse encouraged Mary Langford to take her husband away from Lyndhurst for a summer at a rented cottage. "So we did, we were a couple of hundred miles away from the nearest doctor that knew anything about it. We spent the summer there and I never looked back, which was an interesting example of his methods of treatment."[47]

As the rehabilitation program as Lyndhurst took shape, the building was being transformed to suit its new purpose, though not without significant, albeit temporary, hitches. By May 1945 a lift between the first and second floors had been installed to enable a single wheelchair user to move between the two floors. However, it did not at first pass a safety test by the city building inspector. On top of this, the fire chief had reversed the earlier inspector's finding that gave the go-ahead for occupation of the second floor by patients. He insisted more emergency escapes were needed. Chief Medical Officer Norwich refused the fire chief's request to evacuate patients from the second floor of Lyndhurst which he said was "impossible" because of the overcrowded state of all Toronto DVA facilities. Though these problems were worked out with the installation of more safety features in the months to come, an idea of the desperate attempt to resolve these difficulties can be found in the suggestion to attach ropes from some upper floor windows to provide a means of emergency escape until enough fire escapes were built.[48]

Other problems also needed to be dealt with before the lodge could take on a larger group of patients. While it was possible to hold rehabilitation exercises outside in the warm weather, with the return of the cooler temperatures the building would become more crowded as people stayed inside. Jousse expressed concern that the welfare of Lyndhurst patients was not being fully considered: "This matter of lack of space can seriously hinder our project which is that of re-training patients and restoring them to health, not merely offering them a place to live." By the fall of 1945 construction of a new sixteen-bed addition was underway, and though this did not alleviate the cramped conditions for retraining rooms, it did help to provide badly needed space for more in-patients beginning in early 1946. Rehabilitation services at Lyndhurst were given a significant boost in September 1945 when six physiotherapy students from the University of Toronto began to help. Some of the nursing staff were also being hired as permanent employees as the professionalization of nursing care at Lyndhurst began to be consolidated. Of particular long-term importance was the hiring at this time of George White as a "physical educationalist" to replace Douglas Whittle, who had left of his own accord a few months after he started work. White was himself a veteran of World War II during which he lost a leg in combat. Jousse wrote of the newly hired instructor, "This man works conscientiously and is well-liked by the patients. He shows some initiative in devising games and exercises. He is willing to learn and is acquiring some knowledge of remedial work about which he knew nothing at the start."[49] In the years to come, George White became something of an institution at Lyndhurst among those who knew him as will be seen in the next chapter. Thus in late 1945 the rehabilitation program was established on a firm footing both in concept and in the hiring of people who would come to form the nucleus of a professional staff trained to care for individuals with spinal cord injury. However, the physical space requirements would remain a constant problem in the decades to come and would never be completely satisfactorily resolved at 153 Lyndhurst Avenue.

By the fall of 1945 the rehabilitation program at Lyndhurst was in full gear. John Counsell reported that most of the veteran paraplegics were "embarked on one course or another preparing them for the time when they will be going home."[50] This included complete paraplegics starting classes at a radio school two blocks south of the CPA office in downtown Toronto, which Wood had introduced them to the previous July. Casualty Rehabilitation Officer Ken Purchase travelled to Ted Higginbottom's hometown of St Thomas, Ontario, where his pre-war job at a local department store was set up for his return. "Things are really beginning to move at Lyndhurst" Counsell wrote in November.[51] Edward Dunlop, DVA supervisor in the Casualty Rehabilitation Section, wrote back to Counsell acknowledging the "beginnings of actual success" at Lyndhurst and stating: "I believe that you have been the 'catalyst' in that your example has been a major factor in determining the attitude of both this Department and of the paraplegics themselves."[52] An article in *The Globe and Mail* offered an impression of the facility at this time. The report noted that the atmosphere was "friendly, cheerful ... which is considerably more like that of a fraternity house than that of a hospital. It's something like a Y.M.C.A. gymnasium too, particularly when the boys get to work on their parallel bars, punching bag, wall weights and mat exercises."[53] This hive of activity was not limited to physical retraining. For while all of this was going on, a group of Lyndhurst patients was also busy establishing a new disability organization that would significantly affect the history of paraplegia far beyond the halls of this facility.

THE FORMATION OF THE CANADIAN PARAPLEGIC ASSOCIATION AND THE DEVELOPMENT OF FEDERAL POLICY ON PARAPLEGIA

During these early months patients with spinal cord injuries were more than observers of the plans being made for this new facility. On 16 January 1945, the day after Lyndhurst Lodge accepted its initial group of patients, the first meeting of the Paraplegic Committee met at Christie Street Hospital. Of the eight people in attendance, two were veterans with paraplegia: John Counsell, chairman of the meeting, and Andy Clarke, who was among the ten veterans who had arrived at Lyndhurst Avenue the day before. The rest of the attendees were DVA medical officials, except for L.M. Wood, the philanthropist businessman who by this time had become good friends with Counsell. At this meeting Wood suggested, and other participants agreed, "that the Paraplegics should form an association similar to that of the Amputation Association, and incorporate with the Dominion Government." It was recommended that membership in this group should be limited to people with paraplegia, except for honorary members who could help to advance its work. It was also agreed at this meeting to set up a Patients' Council at Lyndhurst Lodge that would offer advice on "the care and comfort of patients."[54] Two months later, in his first report, Jousse noted that this patient-initiated body had indeed been organized, with an executive that held weekly meetings where "complaints, criticisms and suggestions are [afterwards] brought to the Medical Officer." Jousse wrote that he felt this initiative in "Self-Government" was a good idea, allowing patients to "assume responsibility for disciplining errant members of the group."[55]

The most important long-lasting effect of this meeting sprang from Wood's suggestion: the creation of an organization run by and for paraplegics. Though Wood was not himself disabled, his experiences over the preceding quarter of a century in disability organizations helped to shape the foundations of what was to come. On 10 May 1945 the Canadian Paraplegic Association (CPA) was incorporated by the Canadian government. On 23 May 1945 the first meeting of its directors was held at Lyndhurst Lodge. All of the original seven charter members of the CPA were veterans of World War II and were connected with Lyndhurst Lodge as current or former patients: John Counsell, elected president, who was one of the founders of Lyndhurst and at times also an in-patient for treatment there; Lieutenant Colonel Arthur Hay, who had been wounded during the Battle of Normandy; Flight Officers Joseph Wrangham, Douglas Quirt, and Andrew Clarke (Quirt and Clarke were among the original ten patients brought to Lyndhurst in January 1945); Sergeant Major Edward Higginbottom; and Signalman Jack Higman, who was destined to be the longest-surviving member of this group at the time of his death in 2002.[56] Higman recalled the day the CPA was formed and the start of his involvement in it: "I know then that they formed the Canadian Paraplegic Association and I was late getting away that day. They sort of caught me going by the door and got me to sign up because you needed seven members to have this charter. I didn't know that. But anyway that is how I got on the Paraplegic Board. I guess that I was just the last boy out and I got caught (laughs). I enjoyed it. My association with the men and that was very good. They are a lot of pretty wonderful fellows."[57]

Of the founding members, Arthur Hay became vice-president and Andy Clarke was secretary. John Counsell had been a DVA employee working out of Lyndhurst since the previous December as an assistant rehabilitation officer, in which position he helped to influence its operation. At their June meeting members of the association felt that he could do his job more effectively as full-time head of the CPA, not in a government job, acting as a liaison between both groups. The DVA was asked, and eventually agreed, to pay any expenses incurred in the future when Counsell traversed the country to promote the care of paraplegic soldiers.[58] This change was crucial, for it brought Counsell into a national position, with contacts across the country in the years to come. The CPA soon became an important part of the overall national disability program that was then being devised, with Counsell and Lyndhurst playing a leading role. As Jousse put it in May 1945, when referring to the Dieppe veteran: "The most important fact in the development of [a] successful plan of re-establishment is, and will continue to be, the leadership available from the casualties themselves." He stressed the importance of a close working relationship between the CPA and DVA and was prescient when he predicted the association's future role, only four days after it was incorporated: "I am confident they will eventually open the door of opportunity to many civilian casualties in this field, and will become a tremendous factor in the rehabilitation of the physically handicapped."[59] Counsell's high profile in the CPA, and the fact that it was started and staffed by paraplegics who went through the treatment centre, would help to spread Lyndhurst's reputation far and wide. Thus Lyndhurst Lodge and the CPA came to be inseparable, to the point that the organization founded within its walls in the spring of 1945 would become its owner within five years.

In the meantime, the association had to get established. Its purpose in 1945 was to fraternally support Canadian paraplegics through vocational, educational, and professional training; to ensure proper medical services were available and medical research was carried out for all people with spinal cord injuries; and to establish offices and branches to assist with all aspects of this work.[60] Though the CPA was founded by veterans in a veteran's special treatment centre, those who started it intended to welcome both civilian and soldier paraplegics into its ranks. It included people who were not disabled among its members from the outset; honorary members whose contacts made things happen. The first able-bodied members were several new directors who were appointed that spring: L.M. Wood, whose suggestion back in January paved the way for the CPA's founding four months later; E.W. Bickle, president of the Toronto Board of Trade; and Walter Gordon of Clarkson Gordon accountants, who would become the auditors of the association and eventually of Lyndhurst itself. Appropriately, Gordon was made honorary treasurer. Perhaps the most rambunctious new director was Conn Smythe, a major in the Royal Canadian Artillery who had served in both World Wars and walked with some difficulty as a result of a disabling bullet wound. Smythe was most famous as the owner and builder of Maple Leaf Gardens where Toronto's National Hockey League team played in the downtown core. Because of his own experiences and interest in supporting disabled veterans, Smythe was instrumental in providing the seed money to get the CPA financially afloat with just over $4500 from Maple Leaf Gardens in May 1945. By August the CPA opened a small store-front operation out of Maple Leaf Gardens at 46 Carlton Street. This was its first National Office. It was provided at low rent and was wheelchair accessible, as the entrance was level with the sidewalk.[61] Smythe also arranged for Lyndhurst patients to see free hockey games at Maple Leaf Gardens, a practice that began in March 1945. Within two years this expanded to include paraplegics being flown in from across Canada for a weekend visit at the Royal York Hotel to see teams play at the fabled building, all expenses paid by the Maple Leafs' owners.[62]

The rehabilitation program, which encouraged disabled people to venture out into the community, enabled a Lyndhurst in-patient to become involved in the CPA by volunteering at the office on Carlton Avenue. Eventually this in-patient, Ken Langford, a graduate lawyer, was employed by the CPA from 1946–77, as general secretary and managing director. As will be seen in subsequent chapters, he was significantly involved in the operation of the facility where he had been a patient.

In the same month that the CPA set up shop in downtown Toronto, a crucial meeting about people with spinal cord injuries was held at the

Department of Veterans Affairs in Ottawa. Among the fifteen participants were three people deeply involved in the setting up and operation
of Lyndhurst: Dr Botterell, Dr Jousse, and John Counsell. The participants at this August 15 meeting, chaired by Dr Warner, head of the DVA
Rehabilitation Branch, agreed that there would be four centres across
Canada to treat paraplegic veterans: Shaughnessy Hospital in Vancouver,
which would serve patients from British Columbia and Alberta; Deer
Lodge in Winnipeg, which would be responsible for Saskatchewan,
Manitoba, and northwestern Ontario; Lyndhurst Lodge in Toronto,
which would serve the rest of Ontario; and Ste Anne de Bellevue outside
Montreal, which would cover Quebec, New Brunswick, Nova Scotia,
and Prince Edward Island (though by the late 1940s Maritime patients
would also come to Toronto). At that time there were 162 paraplegic
veterans across Canada, with Toronto recording the largest concentra-
tion, sixty-four: thirty-seven at Christie Street with eleven empty beds;
and twenty-seven at Lyndhurst Lodge, where there were no empty beds.
As the first such facility in Canada specifically set up for paraplegics,
Lyndhurst's influence was already obvious during its first summer: "It
was the opinion of the meeting that each paraplegia centre should have
one doctor appointed to look after the overall care of the paraplegic
from his admittance to ultimate rehabilitation and discharge, to co-
ordinate the work of the surgical specialists, the occupational specialists
and the Casualty Rehabilitation Officers, such doctor to follow along
the system employed by Dr. Jousse at Toronto ... [Regarding Winnipeg]:
The Doctor appointed would go to Toronto for two or three weeks to
study the set-up and then organize a similar one in Winnipeg."[63]

The CPA's work was also furthered by the recommendation that
Counsell and Wood should travel to Vancouver and Winnipeg to set up
branches there. Thus DVA staff would go to Lyndhurst to get ideas
about how to set up paraplegic centres elsewhere in Canada, while people who helped to found Lyndhurst would travel around the country to
"spread the word" about the work that was being done at this new
facility and to offer advice as to how the CPA could help. A mutually
supportive relationship was developing between the DVA and the CPA
as post-war rehabilitation efforts intensified. The August 15 meeting
made it clear that no definite national guidelines were being established
as to how paraplegic veterans should be employed or what kind of
vocational training should be implemented. This was largely because of
widespread problems with lack of space and staff in all DVA hospitals.
However, the urgent need to do something was apparent to all. Enough

was known to move forward with what was the first federal policy in Canada on the organization of treatment for people with spinal cord injuries. Lyndhurst's example would be at the centre of this through its pioneering role in Canada and, in the years to come, through the advocacy of the CPA. It would also become more widely known through the pages of *The Caliper*, the CPA's national quarterly magazine, which made its debut in 1946.[64] The plans, which were at that time focused on disabled veterans, would soon begin to apply to the civilian population and to the operation of Lyndhurst itself.

FROM VETERANS TO CIVILIANS

The paraplegic acute care unit at Christie Street Hospital and the rehabilitation program at Lyndhurst Lodge succeeded in proving their effectiveness to such an extent that their future purpose came into question. They were so successful in treating veterans that they very nearly worked themselves out of existence. Whereas in the post-World War I period 80 per cent of soldiers with spinal cord injuries died within two years, after World War II the story was quite different. Casualties were not only surviving beyond all previous experience but they were returning home in significant numbers. In December 1945 Botterell reported that the last paraplegic World War II casualty had been admitted to Christie Street Hospital the previous summer. By the following spring the number of paraplegic veterans who remained as active patients in Toronto had declined from a high of 103 to 59. Of the remaining patients, twelve were expected to go home within two months. This meant that 71 out of 103 paraplegic patients would no longer require active care by mid-1946. Of this number seven had died, four from complications related to their spinal cord injuries, three from other causes. The sixty-four patients who survived and were no longer under active care represented 62 per cent of the total. At Lyndhurst Lodge, of the sixty patients who had gone through its doors in the first year and a half of operation, thirty-nine "are either doing some useful work, or are at school," meaning 65 per cent were on the road to rehabilitation.[65] All of this presented a good news, bad news scenario. The good news was that a majority of paraplegics were both surviving and getting on with life back in the community. The bad news was that with the decreasing number of paraplegic veterans, the paraplegic services of Christie Street and Lyndhurst were in danger of being broken up before they could benefit the biggest group of people with spinal cord injuries: civilians. In December 1945 Dr Botterell, with the support of his superiors at Christie Street Hospital, expressed concern that this program would "disintegrate" within eighteen months without the admission of new patients who were not veterans. The CPA also supported extending medical services to civilians.[66]

During the following weeks, negotiations were undertaken with the Workmen's Compensation Board (WCB), the Ontario agency that looked after people injured on the job, DVA officials, and patients at Lyndhurst itself to see whether some agreement could be reached. The DVA director of medical services, Dr T.D. Bain, expressed support for this idea. He suggested that they experiment with "one or two" patient admissions and noted that the WCB had five or six people per year who would be suitable for this treatment. They were presently hospitalized at the Toronto General Hospital. Bain wrote that veterans who were still at Lyndhurst at this time, twenty-five in-patients and thirteen out-patients, were also consulted: "I discussed this proposal in a recent visit in Toronto with Mr. Counsell in an endeavour to obtain the reaction of the service patients. Mr. Counsell expressed the opinion that with the exception of two patients who were prone to complain about most things, such an extension of the facilities would be welcomed by the remainder of the paraplegic group."[67] By late January they agreed to accept two WCB patients, but as no beds were available, this matter was left in abeyance until later in the year.[68] In the meantime, word started to get around that the future of Lyndhurst Lodge was uncertain. G. Woodrow Bradford, a civilian member of the CPA, wrote to the Minister of Veterans Affairs in March 1946:

I would like to express to you my heartfelt thanks for the splendid work your Department is doing at Lyndhurst Lodge in Toronto not only for veterans directly but also for countless unfortunate civilians with spinal injuries which have caused paralysis. I for one have been greatly encouraged by the publicity of the results of Dr. Joesse [sic] and his staff and since last fall have been able to help myself to get into a wheelchair by following some of the methods of Lyndhurst. I have been stricken by Transverse myelitis since May 1942 and apparently the medical profession had nothing to offer except staying in bed on your back. I am now 31 years of age. I finally got in touch with Dr. Jousse who greatly encouraged me and told me there was no reason why I couldn't do what the boys at Lyndhurst were doing. I have been very fortunate to be in a position to have the best of attention but I often wonder what the poor less fortunate victims of paralysis caused by spinal troubles do. To make a long story short, I would like to add my humble support to asking for continuance of Lyndhurst Lodge and opening its splendid facilities to the civilian population who require this treatment.[69]

Botterell reiterated in May that WCB patients and other civilians should be admitted "in an increasing degree" to DVA paraplegic facilities in Toronto "regardless of their individual capacity to pay."[70] A few weeks later, a doctor in Sudbury, R.V. Chapple, began writing to DVA officials about a sixteen-year-old boy, Frank C., who became paralysed in November 1945. Another doctor in Sudbury had originally written to the Ontario government for support. However, the non-committal response from the province, according to Chapple, was something "I wish to discard as the first obstacle in the boy's future."[71] Instead, he wrote to Botterell, who offered his help; Botterell recalled that he had examined Frank during ward rounds while on a visit to Sudbury in mid-May.[72] Chapple explained that the boy's parents had exhausted their finances but the local Rotary Club had raised enough funds to underwrite his medical care. Included in his letter-writing campaign was his local Member of Parliament, J.L. Gauthier, to whom he mentioned the uncertainty surrounding the Toronto treatment centre: "The organization which has been working at Lyndhurst ... is apparently about to be disbanded. This is a most unfortunate circumstance as there are a large number of civilians who could be treated by the same organization."[73]

The pressure that was building is reflected in the comments of Dr Norwich, who wrote to the DVA deputy minister in mid-June: "Treatment of this nature to civilians, if accepted by the department, of course constitutes a complete inovation [sic] in departmental policy. Doubtless there are numerous civilian cases throughout the country who would benefit by the form of treatment applied by this Department, and should it become generally known that we are accepting civilians there would probably be a great many applications."[74] Three days after Norwich wrote this letter, Jousse wrote to Botterell informing him that since May seven paraplegic patients had been discharged from Lyndhurst, allowing more room for patients who had been in the preliminary acute care stage at Christie Street Hospital. Noting that three WCB patients who were then hospitalized in the TGH would "benefit greatly" if they were transferred to this paraplegic unit, Jousse concluded: "In the course of the next six weeks more paraplegic patients must be admitted to this service at Christie St. Hospital, else it may cease to exist and it will only be a matter of time before the same situation arises at Lyndhurst Lodge."[75]

Botterell wrote to his superiors about Jousse's letter. He noted that his earlier warnings about the "disintegration" of paraplegic services was on the verge of being proven correct and asked that six beds each, instead of the earlier agreed-upon two, be set aside for civilian and WCB patients. Within days DVA officials were recommending that this proposal go ahead, as long as care for the veterans continued unimpeded. However, it was not until 22 August 1946 that official approval was granted for the admission of non-veterans. This decision was directed not just to Toronto but to all four paraplegic treatment centres in Canada. This allowed for the admission of a sufficient number of civilians to keep all of them operating. Admission was to be based on a guaranteed payment of $6 per day to the DVA.[76] On 2 October 1946 sixteen-year-old Frank C. of Sudbury was admitted to Lyndhurst Lodge as the first civilian patient with a spinal cord injury. He remained there for five months' rehabilitation until his discharge on 4 March 1947. L.M. Wood called the DVA in Ottawa to let them know about this development: "They were all delighted to be able to give this service on a re-payment basis."[77] The campaign to get civilians into Christie Street and Lyndhurst Lodge had paid off, thanks to pressure exerted from both doctors and lay-people. They ended up influencing the survival of Lyndhurst Lodge and, most importantly, the survival of people across Canada with spinal cord injuries. Their experiences during these first years of the Toronto paraplegic unit provide a ward's eye view of how these policies translated into reality for patients and staff.

As civilians began to be accepted into Lyndhurst in the fall of 1946, both males and females arrived for treatment as in-patients and out-patients. The different experiences that men and women patients had in Lyndhurst during these early years notably reflects the overwhelming influence of male military culture in the facility's foundation, both in terms of the original clientele for whom it was created and in the therapeutic ethos, which was anything but subtle. First-person accounts and archival evidence indicate the intensity of macho physical performance, where a perception of impressing one's peers with being physically and emotionally "tough" was part and parcel of what was expected of all people undergoing the therapeutic regimen at Lyndhurst. The military experiences of the founders and veteran patients during the formative months when Lyndhurst "proved" its worth to the wider world also connected to the sense of needing to "prove" one's ability to "tough it out" in therapy by "bucking up" and getting on with what was expected by those who were in charge – doctors, nursing staff, physiotherapists – and by many fellow patients. To do otherwise could spell dismissal from the rehabilitation program, which in the context of the times could mean social oblivion with no further options for most people to turn to for support in wider society. The male-centred physical toughness of treatment was ingrained in both mind and body among staff and transmitted to patients during everyday life at Lyndhurst, particularly in regard to therapy but also in informal social networks that affected women in their experiences just as it affected men.

The second floor was specifically designated for the use of female patients with spinal cord injuries. Five of the twenty-four civilian patients admitted to Lyndhurst Lodge up to the end of April 1947 were women, three of whom were out-patients. The first women patients were admitted to the out-patient department in November 1946 and the first in-patients followed in January.[78] Ruth Clark of Chatham, Ontario, arrived at Lyndhurst shortly after this first group of women patients. She had been paraplegic since 1929, when an infection caused her disability. During this period her sister Lola had cared for her at home. Clark had first read about Lyndhurst Lodge in a newspaper at the beginning of 1946. "Amazed," she wrote to Dr Jousse requesting admission, but had to wait until permission was granted in June 1947; she was at first turned down because of being a civilian and because of a policy of no women patients. The local newspaper reported that at Lyndhurst she participated in mat and wheelchair classes and "what men call 'bull sessions'" where she found out that she did not have to remain "helpless." "The psychological effect upon a civilian after seeing what has been accomplished for the veteran, and what he has accomplished for himself, can hardly be overrated. The experience, in Miss Clark's own words 'was revitalizing'." She returned to Chatham where she started to do things "she had forgotten how to do." Within the next few months, she had taken up selling magazines and had moved "from her own room where she spent nearly 18 years" into a new home from which Clark ran her own business.[79]

People who had contracted polio also went through the rehabilitation program at Lyndhurst starting in the late 1940s. Jousse said this group was focused on people with "serious polio disabilities who most need assistance."[80] Marjorie Bleasdell was a twenty-nine-year-old married mother of three children when she became disabled with polio on 11 November 1948. This eventually led to her going to Lyndhurst after time in other local hospitals and at home. One memory of her arrival at the lodge in 1949 always stayed with her: "We all had our own little radio. The first radio music that I ever heard was: 'A Slow Boat to China' ... That was the music. But I thought: 'I'm a slow boat here' ... I'll never forget that when they sing that song. It reminds me of going into Lyndhurst." She shared a room with eight women on the second floor. When they went down for exercises to stretch "cramped up" limbs Marjorie remembered hearing howls of "It hurts" by some of the other women. "I thought: 'Damn, I am not going to make a noise.' Oh it was my own fault because they just stretched this leg so far it broke the hamstrings." Anxious to do things on her own, one time she went into a brick wall while going down a ramp in a wheelchair; fortunately someone was there to catch her. When she insisted on walking between parallel bars, Jousse told her to go ahead. She fell down, as the medical director anticipated. He "caught me before I even hit the ground." It was his way of letting patients find out what they could and could not do.

Marjorie Bleasdell particularly liked working with hydrotherapist Charles (Chuck) Reeve, "a perfect gentleman." Floating in the pool gave the feeling that, "Oh, I can use this leg. Great!" Even though she was paralysed from the neck down and could not move her legs once out of the pool, it gave her the confidence to keep trying. Marjorie also recalled some of the relationships between patients. Several women patients were in stryker frames, body-length metal sheets used to stabilize the spine by keeping a patient immobile. One woman she remembered talking to "would be crying. Her husband was supposed to come and see her but he never came." In another instance, when visiting with male patients, awkwardness mixed with laughter could lighten the difficult times people endured.

I met some of the boys ... And they said: "Come on down Marj, we are going to play cards tonight." So I thought: "OK, I'll go down" ... Then of course, a little while later I had to go to the bathroom. And I thought: "God, if I go to the bathroom, they won't let me go back to the boys." Because mine and the girl's room was way down further ... One of the boys said: "OK, Marj use our bathroom." Well, in those days, they didn't have the nice bars to get up and down ... They only had a big rope from the ceiling, with a bar across ... and you hold onto that and you swing yourself onto the toilet ... So, of course, one of the boys went in with me, but they were thinking that it would be too high for me. So this chap just lowered [the rope] for me. I was going to get on so it was fine.

Half an hour later, somebody said: "Where's Marj?" "God, she's in the bath-room!" They pushed the wheelchair too far away and they couldn't hear me calling ... These were fun days way back ... I didn't realize that I was in a hospital. It wasn't a hospital ... It gave you a nice homey feeling, a nice comfortable feeling.

After approximately six months in Lyndhurst Marjorie Bleasdell returned to her family. Her husband, Harry, was a source of constant support throughout this period and afterwards. She left Lyndhurst on crutches, and had braces made, but when she changed to cane-walking, Mrs Bleasdell decided to try something different: using umbrellas with a steel shaft for her cane. Eventually she collected thirty-six umbrellas, which the local department store happily supplied, even calling whenever a new shipment came in. She even had umbrellas made to match her dresses with material from the bottom of her clothes.[81]

Dorothy Naylor, a married twenty-five-year-old mother of two children, was a roommate of Marjorie Bleasdell in 1949. The two women became friends and both had supportive husbands and families. Mrs Naylor recalled how her husband, Walter, visited each day after work during her four month stay at the lodge, even though they had no car and he worked and lived at the opposite end of the city. Before going to Lyndhurst, she was at Toronto General Hospital, where she was a patient of Dr Botterell. He operated on her in May 1949 for a slipped disk that caused her to be partially paralysed. When her husband asked the doctor why his wife was being sent to Lyndhurst, which neither of them had heard of before, she says that Botterell responded: "'If I send her home now I might as well send her to commit suicide. She has got to get strength back in them legs before she goes any place. So she is going to go to Lyndhurst and don't think that she is just going to lay around and get sun burnt ... Oh no. Where she is going she is going to work and she has got to get herself back on her feet.' That is what I did and that's why I went there and I am glad I did really."

Like others, Dorothy Naylor said she found Lyndhurst quite unlike a hospital, such as the TGH, which she had just left. The physical environment was "so beautiful" overlooking a ravine with plenty of birds chirping away. Most importantly, she was encouraged to learn to take care of herself and not to depend on the staff to do things like washing and going to the toilet. One day after she arrived, she remembers Jousse said to her, "'I'll give you three weeks to get out of that chair,' and I did." The person who helped her the most in this regard was staff member Bert Hanson. Hanson's comments about Dorothy taking so long to touch her toes, as well as his refusal to take her out of the wheelchair for mat class, leaving her to do it herself, "made me so mad" that she felt like throwing things at him. But she never did. Instead, she said he "took a lot of trouble with me" by motivating her to walk along a ramp with a bar. "It was that [that] I really think helped me, really and truly." After discharge, she returned as an out-patient three times each week for some time. It was not easy. She walked on crutches along the sidewalk, travelling "on that rickety old street car, down to St. Clair," and did two hours of mat class. The staff at Lyndhurst insisted on independence even as an out-patient – when Naylor returned the first time with her mother-in-law, the matron told them: "Well this is the first time and the last time. She is to come by herself."

Some weeks after she began her out-patient therapy, Jousse took away her crutches and replaced them with canes. "I will never forget coming home as long as I live. I just wondered how I would get home." Around 1950, about one year after entering Lyndhurst, Dorothy Naylor no longer needed canes to walk. What did these experiences mean to her? "I always said that there was [four] men in my life to give me back my life ... That was Dr Botterell, Bert Hanson, Dr Jousse and my husband because without him I don't know what I would have done."[82]

While some patients, such as Ken Langford, Marjorie Bleasdell, and Dorothy Naylor were already married when they came to the lodge, others met their future spouses while receiving treatment at Lyndhurst. Katherine Cassels was disabled with polio when she was ten. As a girl, she went for therapy at the polio treatment centre in Warm Springs, Georgia, at the beginning of the 1930s. There she met its founder, Franklin Roosevelt, then Governor of New York, who "swam in the pool with us and joined in many other activities. A most wonderful man was he." From 1946 into the early 1950s Miss Cassels worked as medical secretary for Jousse and later did clerical work at the CPA office. She had to take leave at times to go to New York for operations on her leg. During this period she also went through rehabilitation at Lyndhurst Lodge. It was while she was at the lodge that an aspect of life that happened everywhere outside blossomed inside the walls of the paraplegic centre: romance. "It was at rehab at Lyndhurst that I met my husband, Grenville. My husband was in a wheelchair, too. And it was just meant to be ... We surprised everyone. The staff were aghast that they hadn't seen this coming, that they hadn't spotted our romance before. We were very cagey about going out. I would pick him up in my car at the back door where his room was ... [He] had dermatomyositis ... But he was a very proud man and a very wonderful man ... It took several years before we were married ... We were married for almost forty-four years, a most happy time [until Grenville Barton's death in 1995] ... When we became engaged [people] felt that the marriage probably would not last because we had such different backgrounds. It made no difference at all."[83]

The romance that started between Katie Cassels and Grenville Barton at Lyndhurst Lodge in 1947–48 led to their marriage in 1951, at which time soon-to-be Katherine Barton said: "I feel very strongly about two people with a disability being married ... It's almost a blessing in disguise. I know that sounds terribly self-assured, but I believe they can make a go of it. They understand each other's problems and they are determined to make it work and therefore they do make a pretty good job out of it."[84] Other couples met at Lyndhurst Lodge and made their way to the altar – something the media made much of. A report about the wedding of Alphonsus Diemer and Nora Byrnes exclaimed, "Wedding Sets Town Agog, Bride and Groom Paraplegics."[85] Ken Langford recalled that people at Lyndhurst did not find these marital unions as sensational as the press did: "Well, we were brought up on the philosophy that the disability really wasn't that important. If there was something that you wanted to do go ahead and do it. So we didn't really think too much of it ... The graduates of Lyndhurst were trying new things every day."[86]

Current and former Lyndhurst patients also helped to pave the way for post-secondary education for disabled persons at a time when few thought such things were possible. With the help of vocational counsellors like Ken Purchase and Jim Bartlett at Lyndhurst Lodge, connections were made in the community that provided dividends for people preparing for post-rehabilitation life. In June 1949 four Lyndhurst alumnae became alumnae of the University of Toronto: A.D. McEwan, Andy Clarke, Bill O'Connor, and Doug Quirt. Theo Bullock was a fellow patient at Lyndhurst when Clarke and Quirt went off to study: "There were no ramps in those days of course, so people at the College would pick up them and the chairs and carry them up the stairs. I can well remember Andy writing his exams suffering from an infected bladder. During the night the doctors would pump him full of penicillin and sulpha drugs and in the morning away he went for another day at school."[87]

Overseeing all of these changes, of course, was Dr Jousse. Evelyn Paul was the only Lyndhurst staff member from the 1940s who was able to be interviewed for this book. A physiotherapist, she worked at Lyndhurst briefly as a student in 1946 and again from 1949–53.

Everyone adored Dr. Jousse generally. Across the board the patients admired him and respected him. I think that they felt a sort comradeship with him because he did have a disability and I think that was a real plus for his position in Lyndhurst. He was very, very supportive to the nurses and the physios and he was very supportive to anyone who worked there. He was very good with the patients and he spoke to them and he was very helpful with them. He stayed a little bit aloof from them, like he didn't come down and become a brother to them. He maintained an atmosphere of being the doctor and yet he was very good with patients especially the ones who had been in the services. They would actually flaunt the rules a bit and maybe got drunk and Dr. Jousse would speak to them quite firmly but he always laughed about it because he knew that they were just doing what they would have done ordinarily. I think that was his whole method of treatment; making them develop their lives as they would have developed them. So he was tolerant about drinking and raising cain.[88]

The esteem in which Jousse was held by the first group of patients who went through Lyndhurst Lodge is perhaps best expressed by their presentation of a new car to him on 31 October 1947. To prevent him knowing about what was coming, the medical director was informed that a Halloween party was going to take place that day, lest he become suspicious about the unusually large number of current and former Lyndhurst residents gathered at the building. Ninety paraplegic veterans of World War II had contributed to a collection to buy him a new Chevrolet. Jousse was "paraded" to the car where fifty of the ninety veterans were waiting in front of the building; they had come from all over southwestern Ontario for the event. He thanked them and said: "You are a wonderful bunch." One of the presenters, Tony Bagnato, told a reporter, "He has been a pal to all of us as well as a good doctor. There have been hundreds of occasions when he went out of his way to help us ... We are all very thankful for his help."[89]

By this time the native of Vankleek Hill, Ontario, was firmly established as an expert on paraplegia both at Lyndhurst Lodge and across

Canada. While Botterell had been essential to getting the facility up and running and guiding it through its first chaotic months, Jousse soon had matters in hand as trial and error showed the way to improving treatment for people with spinal cord injuries. Botterell continued as the expert neurological consultant. However, during 1946 he gradually withdrew from his earlier intense involvement with Lyndhurst Lodge, "I presume because he felt that I was handling it reasonably well," according to Jousse.[90] The two physicians remained close personally and professionally for the rest of their lives. Jousse's second wife, Margaret, recalled "Al felt like a brother to Dr. Botterell."[91] As the decade drew to a close, the facility that both doctors had done so much to shape was about to be influenced by new developments over who funded and owned it.

FROM DVA to CPA

In the spring of 1947 the Ontario provincial government agreed to provide the CPA with $25,000 to help finance the care of civilian paraplegics in Toronto DVA facilities. The CPA medical board would vet all civilian applications before a patient could be admitted.[92] This financial support became all the more urgent when the DVA increased the daily rate for non-veteran paraplegics to $9 per day, effective 1 July 1948.[93] As a result of this increase, for the 1948–49 fiscal year Ontario increased its funding for civilian paraplegic patient care with an annual grant of $40,000 and the City of Toronto provided another $9,000. That year the remaining treatment expenses of almost $7,400 were recovered through patients and municipalities outside Toronto.[94] Thus by the late 1940s regular funding from the province and local governments had been secured to enable people who were not veterans or WCB patients to be treated at Lyndhurst. This in turn was crucial to allowing the lodge to remain open.

Numbers reveal how the patient population of Lyndhurst Lodge had changed within a few years of its opening, while also indicating that though most veterans had gone home quite a few still came back for acute care when the need arose. Christie Street Hospital and Lyndhurst Lodge had treated a combined total of 103 armed service personnel with spinal cord injuries, of whom only nine were still in hospital by the spring of 1948. Five of these veterans were slated to be discharged that same year. By mid-1948 twenty ex-servicemen and one ex-servicewoman from World War II who had sustained spinal cord injuries after returning to civilian life, as well as eleven former World War I soldiers, three of whom were injured during wartime service, had also undergone treatment in Toronto. During the preceding year, fifty veterans had been re-admitted after discharge to deal with acute medical problems, such as pressure sores or bladder problems. In October 1947, one year after the first civilian had been admitted to Lyndhurst, twenty-five civilians were going through the paraplegic treatment program in Toronto. This figure had jumped to forty-six civilians by the end of May 1948. Thus, the CPA Medical Advisory Committee reported: "The need for the continuance of the organization for the benefit of those wounded while on service, for those ex-service personnel who became paraplegic by accident or disease following discharge, and for civilians who can obtain this type of service through no other source, requires no further emphasis."[95] Three years after opening Lyndhurst Lodge had proven itself as being needed on a permanent basis. Its survival was no longer in question. But with veterans no longer making up its in-patient population in large numbers, its days as a federal departmental facility were coming to an end.

By 1949 preliminary acute care for spinal cord injuries had shifted from Christie Street Hospital, which had closed with the opening of the new Sunnybrook Hospital in the city's eastern suburbs. Toronto General Hospital continued to serve WCB patients with spinal cord injuries; they were hospitalized there before being sent to Lyndhurst. Sixty-three WCB patients had been treated in Toronto by the end of the 1940s.[96] As the old Christie Street Hospital closed its doors to make way for a new veterans' hospital, so too the DVA decided to end its control of Lyndhurst Lodge, now that it was primarily used for civilian patients. Of 388 patients with spinal cord injuries treated in Toronto between early 1945 and the spring of 1949, 120, or nearly 31 per cent, were veterans.[97] When more than two-thirds of all patients in this specialized service were non-veterans, it is easy to understand why this change in ownership came about. Accordingly, negotiations began in March 1949 after the DVA informed a meeting at Lyndhurst Lodge that the federal government wanted to end its operation of this facility. Over the following months negotiations continued until it was announced in November that the building would be transferred to the ownership of the CPA effective 1 April 1950.[98]

The property at 153 Lyndhurst was sold to the CPA by the Canadian government for the nominal sum of $1, including all medical equipment purchased and installed by the DVA. The agreement also stipulated that should a national emergency arise during which the department required the building again, it was to be returned to its former owner.[99] This change, however, did not mean an end to Lyndhurst's liaison with the DVA. Through the CPA, collegial cooperation between the DVA and Lyndhurst Lodge continued when treatment of veterans with spinal cord injuries was required, particularly in regard to services at Sunnybrook Hospital. After ownership changed hands, it was agreed that veteran in-patients at Lyndhurst Lodge would continue to have their treatment paid for by the DVA at the agreed-upon per diem rate.[100] During its final year of operation under the DVA, the paraplegic Special Treatment Centre was full to capacity, as 134 people were in-patients and out-patients in 1949–50.[101] One of these patients was G. Woodrow Bradford, who had written a letter to the Veterans' Affairs Minister in March 1946 pleading for the continued operation of Lyndhurst Lodge. Four years later at the CPA annual meeting held a few weeks after the transfer in ownership had taken place, Bradford publicly "expressed appreciation both personally and on behalf of other civilian patients" for the rehabilitation program that had been provided at the former DVA facility.[102] As a facility operated by a disability service agency, Lyndhurst Lodge would continue on the path clearly laid down under the DVA of innovative treatment for people with spinal cord injuries. Employees of the DVA now became employees of the CPA. The organization that had formed within its walls had become the owner of its birthplace, and in the years ahead would continue to improve upon these first years of rehabilitation.

The story of those who inhabited the halls of Lyndhurst during its first years of operation would resonate in the lives of future occupants in the years to come. Most of the first group of patients were living out in the community, getting on with their lives, by 1950. But it is important to remember that not all of Lyndhurst's alumnae survived to see this changing of the guard. Lieutenant Colonel Arthur John Hay was one of the original seven founders of the CPA in May 1945, eventually becoming chairman and vice-president. He had been wounded during the Battle of Normandy the summer before, when a German shell blew off one of his legs and left him a paraplegic. Hay remained hospitalized until 1947 and was an in-patient at both Christie Street Hospital and Lyndhurst Lodge before returning to live with his wife, Edith, in Hamilton, where they had resided before the war. There, he worked as a car salesman until ill health forced him back into hospital several months before he died at Sunnybrook. He was forty-one years old.[103]

The rehabilitation program that Lyndhurst was pioneering enabled Arthur Hay to work on behalf of other disabled people and to live with his family for a few brief years before he succumbed to complications from his war wounds in June 1949. That the organization he helped to found would take ownership of the facility where he was once a patient, less than a year after his death, was a fitting tribute to the legacy of Lieutenant Colonel Arthur Hay and his comrades, who demonstrated just how much people with spinal cord injuries could achieve.

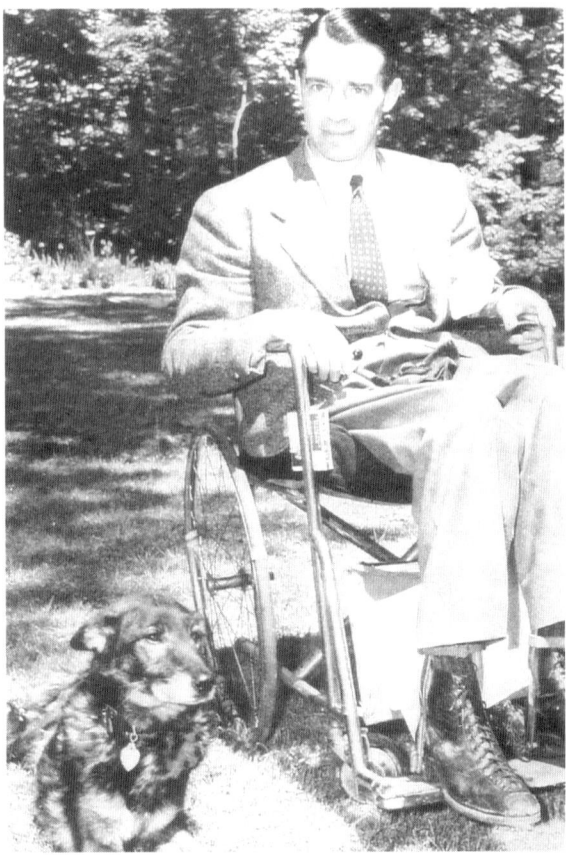

John Counsell in an Everest and Jennings wheelchair
on the grounds of Lyndhurst Lodge, 1947. The dog
Mike, a Lyndhurst pet, had a spinal cord injury that
left him partially paralysed. Originally published in
The Globe and Mail, 21 June 1947. Photo courtesy of
Ken Langford.

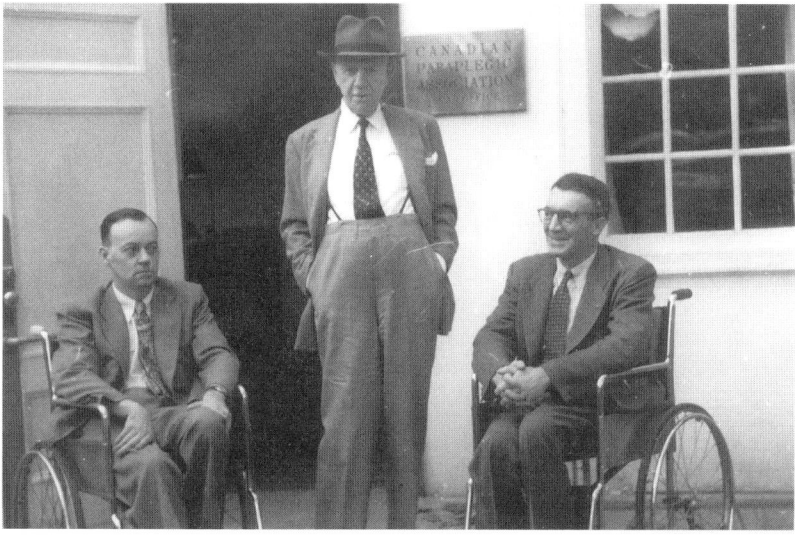

From left to right: Ken Langford, L.M. Wood, and John Counsell in front of the head office of the Canadian Paraplegic Association on the grounds of Lyndhurst Lodge, circa 1950. Photo courtesy of Ken Langford.

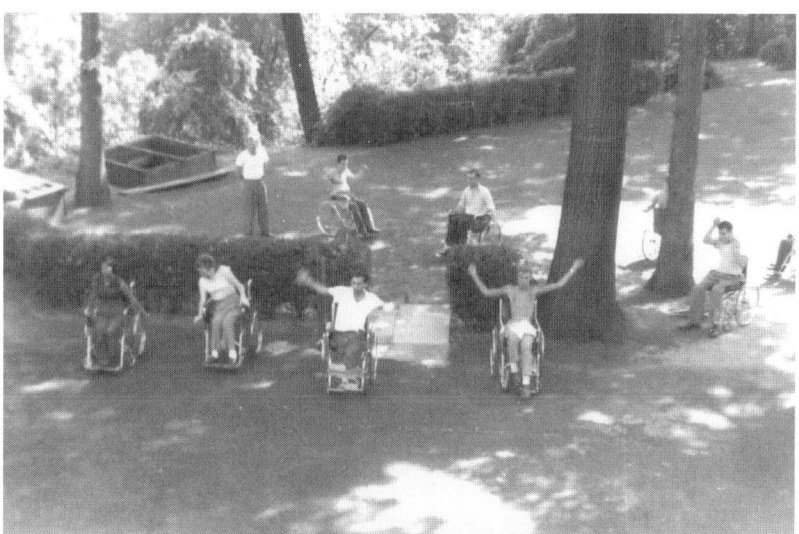

George White and an outdoor physiotherapy chair class at Lyndhurst Lodge, circa 1960.
Photo courtesy of Ken Langford.

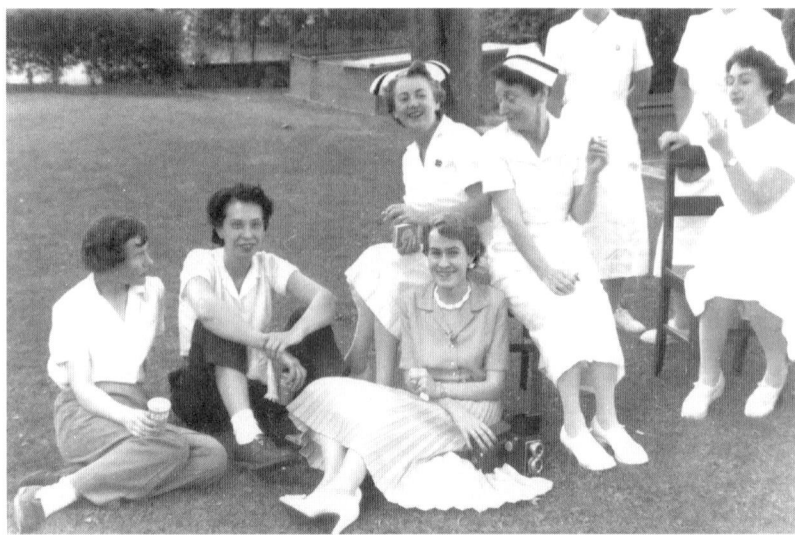

Barbara Duffin, head physiotherapist (second from left), with physiotherapy and nursing staff and Vi Arnold (seated in the centre), Dr Jousse's secretary, circa 1960. Photo courtesy of Ken Langford.

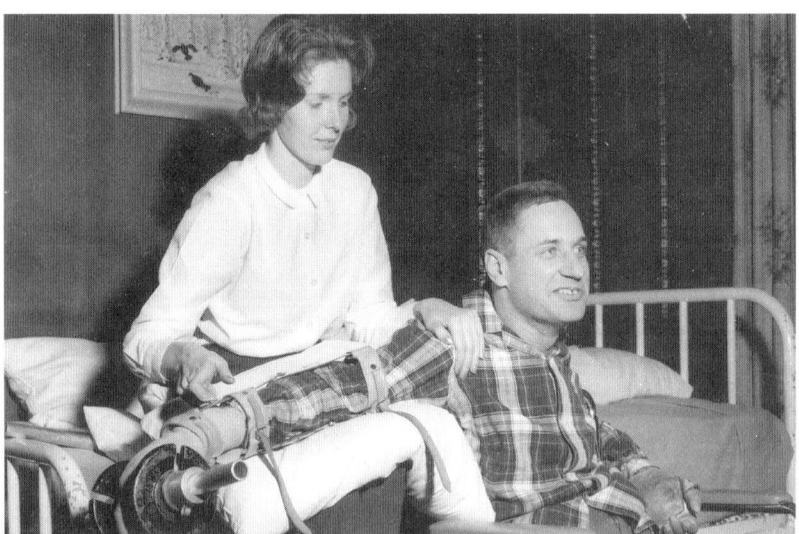

Gerald McHaffie being assisted with exercises by physiotherapist Betty Brooks in early 1964. He was injured on the job in a car accident while working for a Canadian company in England. First published in the *Workmen's Compensation Board News Bulletin*, March 1964. Photo courtesy of Loma Stone.

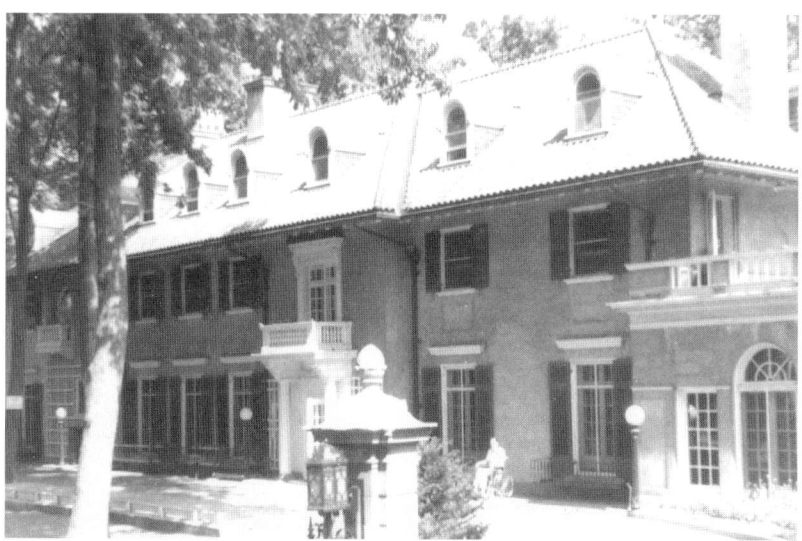

Lyndhurst Lodge, circa 1960. Photo courtesy of Ken Langford.

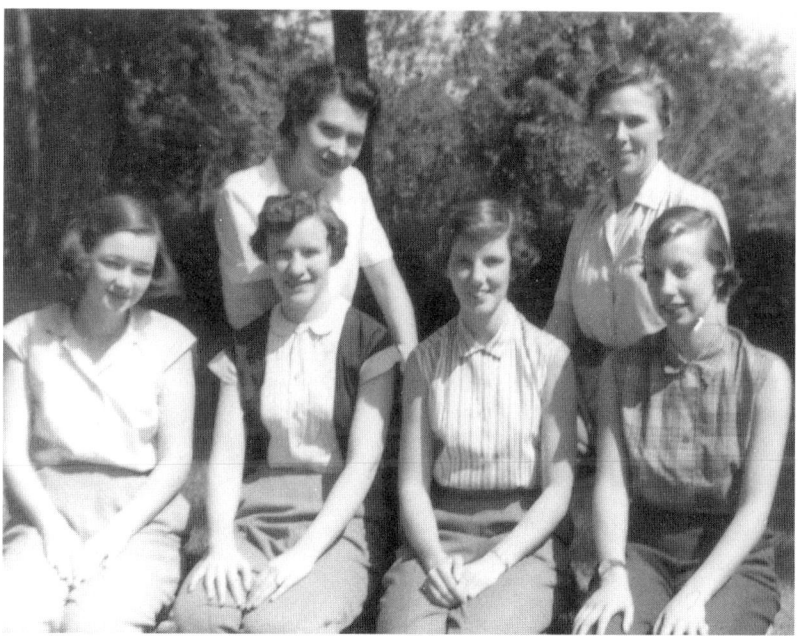

Barbara Duffin, head physiotherapist (second row on the left), with physiotherapy staff, Lyndhurst Lodge, circa 1960. Photo courtesy of Ken Langford.

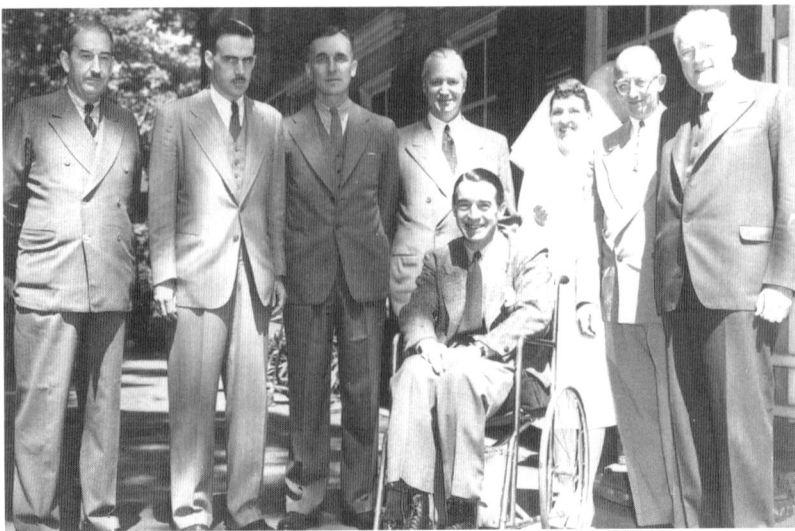

Group photo in front of Lyndhurst Lodge, 1947. From the left: Dr Joseph A. MacFarlane, dean of medicine, University of Toronto; Dr A.T. Jousse, medical director, Lyndhurst Lodge; Dr E.H. Botterell, neurosurgeon, Toronto General Hospital and co-founder Lyndhurst Lodge; George Drew, premier of Ontario; John Counsell, president of the Canadian Paraplegic Association, co-founder Lyndhurst Lodge; Marie Pilon, head nurse, Lyndhurst Lodge; Dr Carl Aberhart, urologist; Dr William Gallie, professor of surgery, University of Toronto. Photo courtesy of Ken Langford; originally appeared in the *Globe and Mail.*

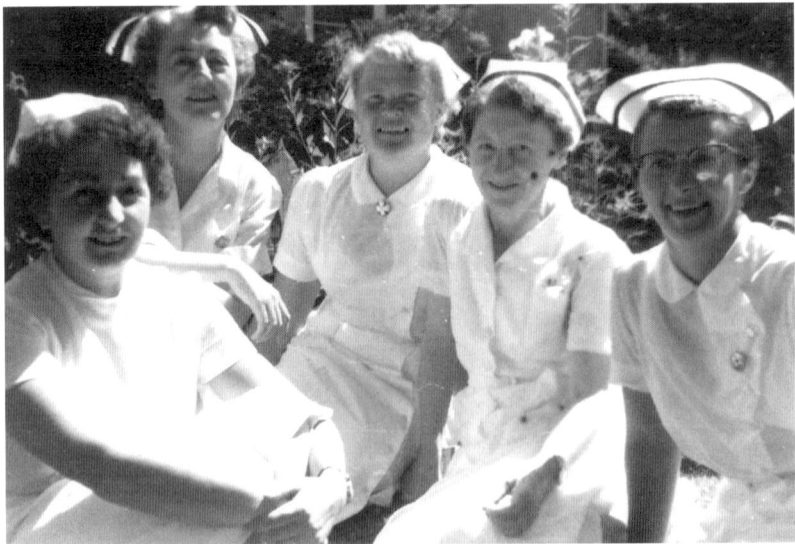

Nursing staff, Lyndhurst Lodge, circa 1960. Photo courtesy of Ken Langford.

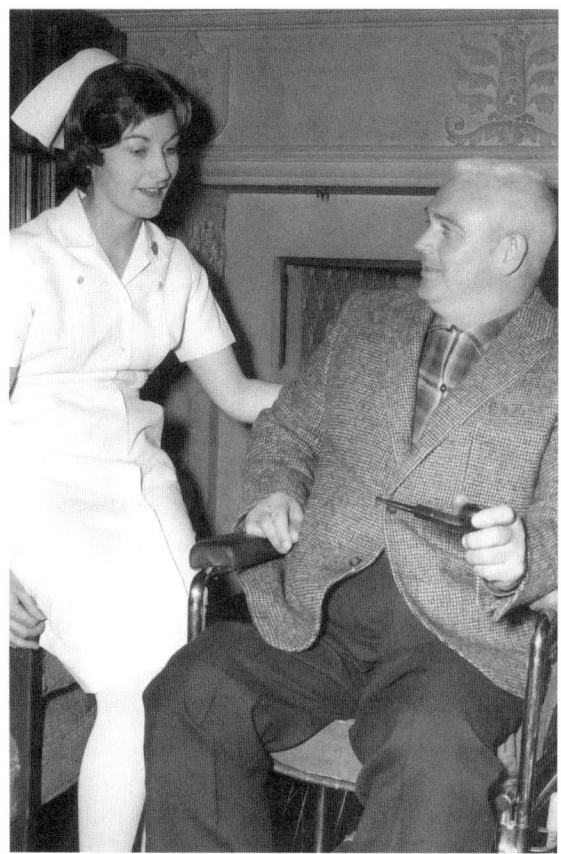

Nurse Elizabeth Truscott with Ted Cole, a truck driver
who was injured in 1953. This photo is from early
1964 when he made a return visit to Lyndhurst. First
published in the *Workmen's Compensation Board
News Bulletin*, March 1964. Photo courtesy of Loma
Stone.

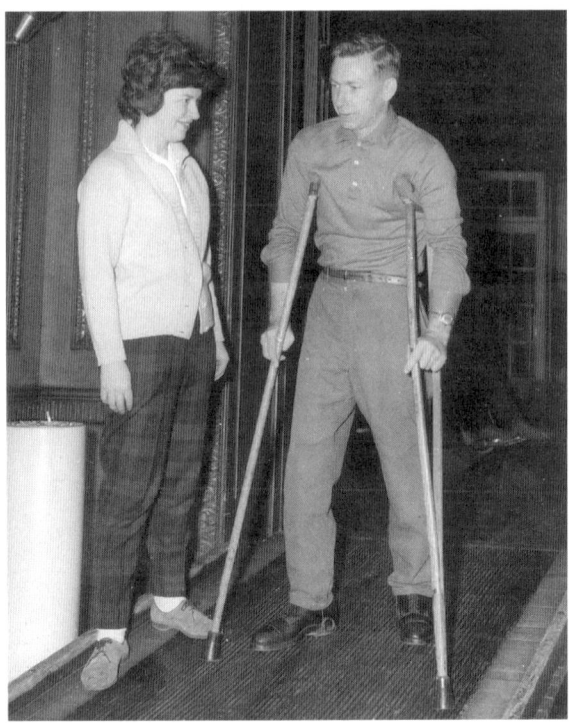

Walter Cameron, who injured his spine working as a logger in 1956, during a return visit to Lyndhurst in early 1964. At this time he was working with his father on a farm. Barbara Gilleland is the student physiotherapist with him. First published in the *Workmen's Compensation Board News Bulletin*, March 1964. Photo courtesy of Loma Stone.

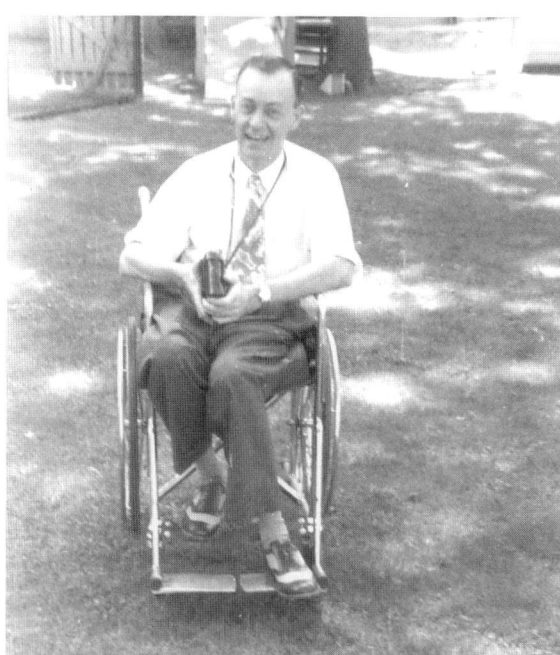

Ken Langford at
Lyndhurst Lodge,
circa 1960. Photo
courtesy of Ken
Langford.

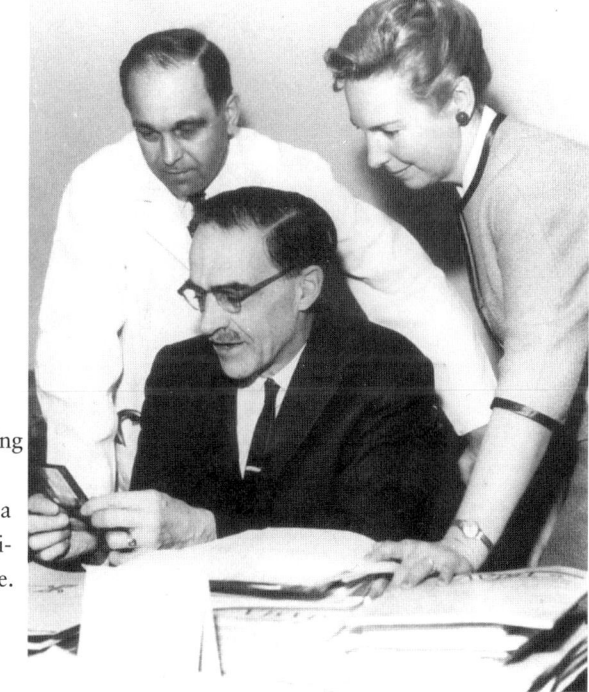

Doctors William
Geisler and Megan
Wynne-Jones standing
behind A.T. Jousse.
Undated photo, circa
1960, from the origi-
nal Lyndhurst Lodge.
Photo courtesy of
Eileen Jousse
Woloshyn.

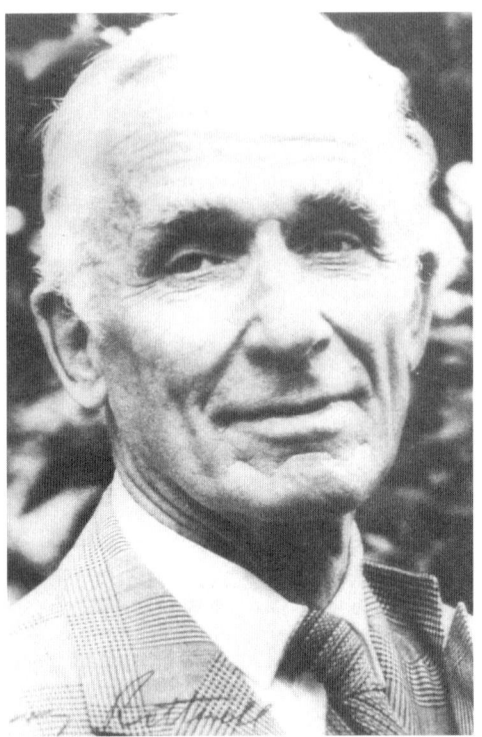

Dr E.H. Botterell in later life. Photo courtesy of William Geisler.

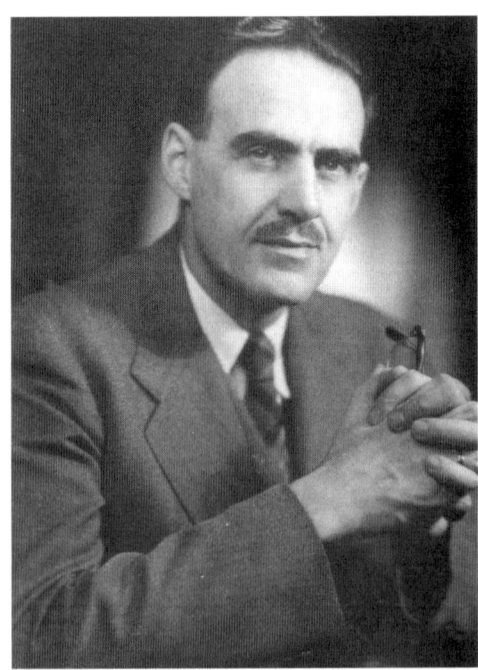

A.T. Jousse (undated). Photo courtesy of Ken Langford.

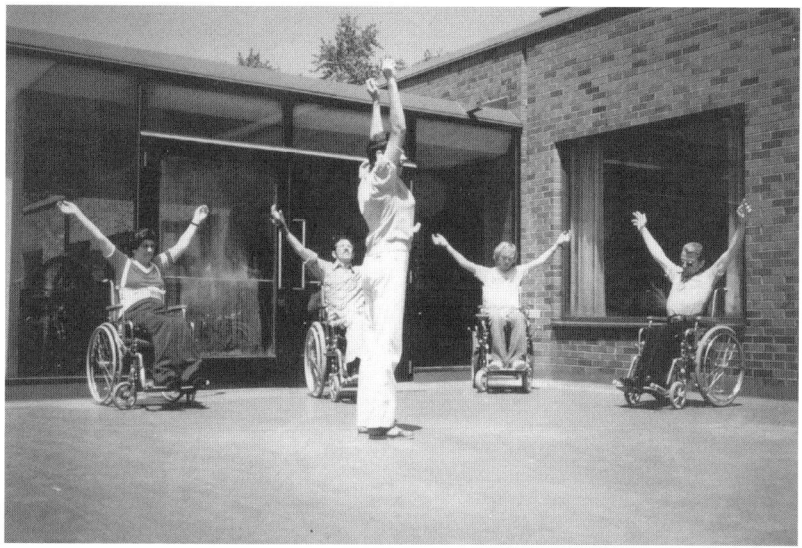

Outdoor physiotherapy chair class at the new Lyndhurst Hospital on
Sutherland Drive, mid to late 1970s. Photo courtesy of William Geisler.

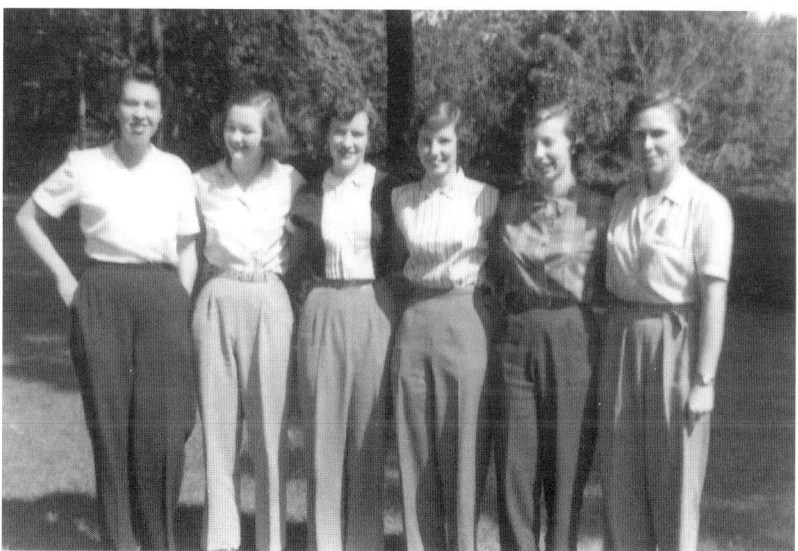

Barbara Duffin, head physiotherapist (far left), with physiotherapy staff,
Lyndhurst Lodge, circa 1960. Photo courtesy of Ken Langford.

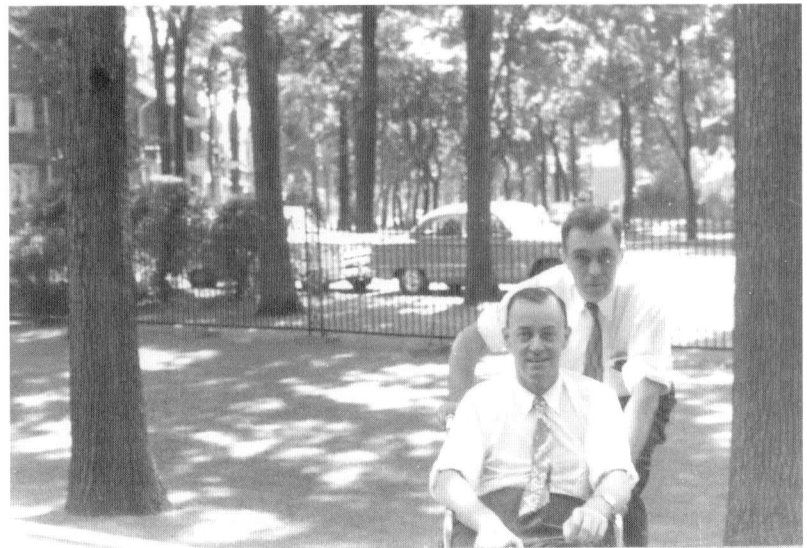

Ken Langford and Dr William Geisler on the grounds of Lyndhurst Lodge.
Undated photo, likely circa 1960. Photo courtesy of William Geisler.

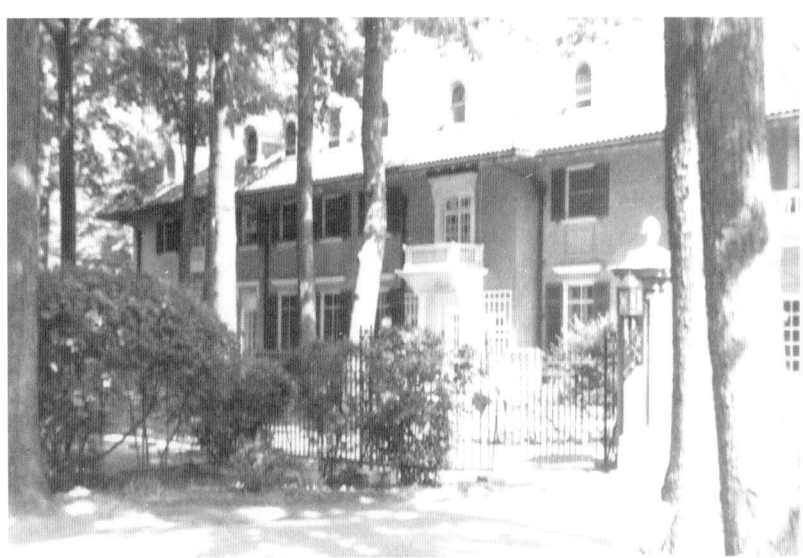

Lyndhurst Lodge, circa 1960. Photo courtesy of William Geisler.

3

A Reputation for Rehabilitation:
Lyndhurst Lodge, 1950–64

"They treated you like a person and not a number."[1] After almost being left for dead following an accident that left him quadriplegic, Myrll Jackson found the three years that he lived in Lyndhurst Lodge gave him a new lease on life. His experiences reflect the significant changes that continued to be felt by people with spinal cord injuries who found themselves at the old mansion. It was also felt by people with various other types of disabilities, notably polio survivors, who made up the next largest group of patients. In the 1950s and early 1960s Lyndhurst's reputation for rehabilitation grew apace in Canada and elsewhere. As this chapter shows, it took a good deal of work on the part of both patients and staff to continue the momentum for change that was established during its first years under the DVA. Now a fully operational rehabilitation centre run by the CPA, Lyndhurst was treating more people like Myrll Jackson, who experienced its program first-hand.

BUILDING PROJECTS AND FUNDING SOURCES

With independence from the DVA secured, the newly enfranchised operators of Lyndhurst Lodge quickly began to expand on the services and facilities established during the previous five years. Shortly before ownership was transferred to the CPA, a committee, which was to become the de facto board of governors of the facility, was struck. Its members included Andy Clarke, John Counsell, Ian Johnston, J.S.H. Thomson, and J.D. Woods.[2] By September 1950 they had overseen the construction of a new pool for hydrotherapy at the Lyndhurst site. This ended the previous arrangement whereby people were sent by cab or motor-coach to Dividale Convalescent Hospital for treatment in a pool. The new ten-foot by twenty-foot therapeutic pool was built at the back of the sixteen-bed east wing with funding from Canadian Breweries Ltd. A few months later the garage at 153 Lyndhurst was altered to make it into an office for the CPA. CPA national headquarters thus moved from its home of five years in Maple Leaf Gardens to the property that they now owned and operated. During the first nine months of CPA control, the cost of treating people from Ontario added up to $84,752.64. To help meet these costs, a fundraising campaign was launched in the fall of 1950 to raise $30,000 for the CPA.[3]

By the first anniversary of CPA ownership, bed space had been made available for forty-one people. As well, a part-time speech therapist had been hired to help people who required assistance in this regard. Within the next few months, the Lyndhurst gym and physiotherapy department expanded by 1,100 square feet, through the financial backing of the CPA and the employment of an engineer from Canadian Breweries to oversee the work; the Breweries had helped to build the therapeutic pool, and in 1954–55 they helped to build a new west wing that housed twenty-four in-patients in rooms of either two or four beds apiece. This increased the overall total number of beds at Lyndhurst to fifty, as the older part of the building continued to house twenty-six in-patients; by 1960 overall bed space rose to fifty-two. A provincial inspector from the Department of Health, which also helped to pay for these improvements, noted in 1955 that the new washroom facilities were "of a sort which facilitates their use by seriously handicapped persons." The existing building was remodelled to improve examination rooms and make a lounge for patients and visitors. A small classroom was built in the east wing for students who took tutoring and a new dining room that seated sixty people was added. In addition to the province, a major funding source for these changes was T.G. Ferguson, a member of the CPA board and head of Canadian Breweries.[4] A new elevator to replace the ten-year-old lift that operated between the first and second floors, as well as automatic fire detectors and alarms, were installed to improve accessibility and to meet safety requirements.[5] Ken Langford, general secretary of the CPA during the 1950s, explained that fundraising for Lyndhurst was primarily undertaken by L.M. Wood (before his death in 1959) and John Counsell. Wood in particular "had a wider field of acquaintances with money and he was able to raise what amount of what money we needed for awhile."[6]

To qualify for provincial funding for building improvements, specifically for the construction of the new west wing, the status of the facility had to be changed. The CPA applied for and received approval from the Ontario government on 27 May 1954 to officially classify Lyndhurst Lodge as a convalescent hospital under the Public Hospitals Act.[7] This made future construction projects much more feasible and would pay major dividends twenty years later when the entire operation moved to a new building. In the meantime, the province helped with needed local improvements. Of course, the most important financial support from the Ontario government dated back to 1947 with the first annual grant to help defray the cost of treatment for civilian paraplegics, as discussed in chapter 2. This funding had risen from $25,000 annually in 1947 to $65,000 annually by 1956. The money was very much needed, as a provincial official found out. The difficult financial position in which patients and the CPA operators of Lyndhurst often found themselves during this period is described in a report written by J.K. Jamieson of the Ontario Hospital Services Commission.

Jamieson visited Lyndhurst on 10 August 1956 to obtain first-hand information about how the $65,000 annual provincial grant was being spent. This grant was issued to the CPA to cover treatment costs for civilians who were not covered by the DVA. By this time, the rate per patient was $12 per diem, with most municipalities paying half that amount for patients from their region. However, some indigent patients were charged entirely to the provincial grant because they came from "unorganized territory" – no fixed address. As well, small municipalities in the northern part of the province were not pursued by Lyndhurst for payment because these locales already relied on the province for debt relief. In some cases where it was thought that patients and municipalities could pay, no money was forthcoming, so the CPA had to turn to the provincial grant for reimbursement. Patients who could afford to pay and who stayed for less than a month were asked to pay the full amount of their stay. However, when a person was there longer than one month they were charged a lower rate, with the province picking up the remainder.

In addition, different insurance policies covered people from different provinces. Ontario Blue Cross, for example, did not cover patients at Lyndhurst Lodge, while Blue Cross in other provinces and the Saskatchewan Health Services did. Jamieson concluded his report by observing: "Many patients present a rather serious problem in that they arrive at Lyndhurst Lodge saddled with heavy hospital and medical bills incurred in general hospitals. Many have to be trained in new occupations and their earnings subsequent to discharge are usually limited, making it difficult for them to repay their indebtedness."[8] The need for a remedy to this problem was none too soon in coming: the Ontario Hospital Insurance Plan, or OHIP, to pay for patients' ward fees. But before describing its impact on Lyndhurst, it is important to provide additional details on how the lodge operated financially before a provincial hospital insurance system existed.

During this period the CPA guaranteed treatment expenses at Lyndhurst, a practice that began with the civilians in the late 1940s. If a patient could not pay for their treatment the CPA raised the money by collecting funds from the patient's municipality or from the province. Familiarity with the rehab facility's work helped with this task. In the early 1950s Tommy Douglas, premier of Saskatchewan, visited Lyndhurst. He had been brought to the facility by a *Globe and Mail* reporter, Lou Golden, and was "impressed" with the set-up. Not long afterward, Ken Langford was in Regina on CPA business where he met with Douglas. During this meeting, the premier told his visitor that Saskatchewan would henceforth pay for people with spinal cord injuries to go to either Lyndhurst Lodge or to Winnipeg. Langford happened to see the Saskatchewan Minister of Health after leaving Douglas, and told him of this decision, of which he had no inkling. "He was surprised."[9] Such personal contacts between government officials and Lyndhurst were crucial to getting more financial support for patient care.

Another person whose association with Lyndhurst would last for half a century began work there when doctors received much of their pay through private and non-profit health insurance companies. Dr William Geisler studied rehabilitation medicine at Lyndhurst in 1952–54 and was hired as full-time staff beginning in July 1958, after studying internal medicine in Toronto and following his return from a CPA Fellowship in Europe to visit various rehabilitation institutes.[10] He eventually became assistant medical director. Since doctors were not compensated through universal state funded medicare in Canada until 1968, there were a variety of other funding sources.[11] Physicians Services Incorporated (PSI), a doctor-sponsored insurance program that pre-dated OHIP, was one of the ways in which Lyndhurst's physicians were paid. Geisler explained that the CPA would assure him that he would get paid a certain rate, such as $8,000 a year. If PSI paid him this full amount in a given year, then the CPA would not need to pay the difference. However, when PSI paid below the assured rate of salary, the CPA would pay the extra. When PSI paid him above the amount agreed to by the CPA, it was his to keep. PSI in their turn made 10 per cent of each dollar earned by the physician whom they paid. Doctors at Lyndhurst also earned money in the course of seeing patients from the WCB and at the Toronto General Hospital. Associated Medical Services (AMS) was another medical insurance agency from whom Geisler recalled getting some income. This source proved to be not as reliable as PSI: "At the end of one year being paid by AMS, we got a letter from the AMS: 'Dr. Jousse, we want all of our money back.' And then the fellow in charge of AMS of the day whose name I am prepared to forget wrote to say that: 'The type of treatment that you are giving these patients is not medical treatment. It is not covered by AMS' ... That was a dreadful thing to happen and we had to give back all of the money. So that is where we got paid and that continued until OHIP. Obviously we were very pleased to see OHIP come in because our income appreciated but the type of care we'd give the patient didn't change one iota."[12]

The introduction of OHIP on 1 January 1959 significantly improved the financial position of Lyndhurst Lodge's patients. The CPA annual report noted: "It would be hard to over emphasize the importance of Hospital Insurance to paraplegic patients."[13] According to Ken Langford, OHIP "certainly affected the way the patient's treatment program was paid for ... You didn't have to go looking for grants and municipal help once that came in ... We were sort of out of the payment for treatment business. Our only concern throughout ... is that they get the best quality treatment."[14] The hospital at which they resided could at last be assured that the province would pick up the tab for everyone regardless of income level. The CPA directors who operated Lyndhurst reported after the first full year of OHIP that "the revenues have more closely approached the costs of operation. As a result the operating loss for the year 1959 was reduced to $5,590 as compared with $25,064 in 1958. But more significant than this is the fact that the insurance plan has removed from the patient a burden of long term hospitalization costs for which no insurance was formerly available."[15] The daily ward rate per patient went from $15.22 in 1959 to $17 in 1960, a substantial sum in those days for most people, but especially for people of limited resources.[16] By 1962 this amount had increased to $19.61 per diem and the daily rate for 1964 at Lyndhurst was $23.05 per patient.[17]

These constantly rising costs could put pressure on staff to discharge patients who were not responding to the rehabilitation program in a manner viewed as warranting continued residence at Lyndhurst Lodge. During a meeting with provincial officials in 1961 Jousse mentioned that "placement of patients classified as chronic was a serious problem for the Lodge since much needed beds were occupied for long periods by patients for whom nothing further could be done. Dr Jousse ... [hoped] that something could be done to speed up the discharge of this type of patient."[18] While no figures were given, this group was almost certainly the 5 to 6 per cent of the patient population mentioned in statistical surveys from these years as being discharged to chronic-care facilities, as will be explained shortly. A closer examination of these sources brings to light a number of issues related to the historical development of services at Lyndhurst for people with different types of disabilities.

PATIENTS AND REHABILITATION

To be a patient at Lyndhurst between 1950–64 was to be a part of a hectic drive towards rehabilitation. Personal stories and statistics give ample evidence that the place was a hive of activity. But before mentioning some names and numbers, it is important to set them in the context of the admission policies that developed during this period. As will become evident, having a spinal cord injury did not automatically guarantee that patients would end up at Lyndhurst, even if they came within the catchment area and their doctor wanted them to go there. Admission policies were based on an assessment of whether or not a person had a good chance of returning to the community, as Jousse explained to provincial inspector Dr Gordon Caudwell in March 1964. This visit was instigated by a complaint from a doctor in St Thomas, Ontario, who said a woman in her late sixties with quadriplegia had been waiting two years for admission to Lyndhurst.

Jousse informed Caudwell that it was their policy to admit, if possible, equal numbers of both paraplegics and quadriplegics who were "in the younger age group. Consequently, preference is given to those patients who offer a potential for improvement as well as a life expectancy to warrant the rehabilitative effort." Paraplegics, he said, had an average stay of seven months while quadriplegics averaged nine months. To maintain relatively equal numbers in what was then a fifty-two bed health-care facility, fewer quadriplegics were admitted at one time than were paraplegics. The latter group's beds became available more frequently because of their shorter average stay. The medical director also mentioned that people with disseminated sclerosis and cerebral palsy were seldom admitted, in the former case, because their condition "constantly shows remissions," and in the latter, because of their youth. Caudwell informed the provincial Department of Health that this admission policy explained why the elderly quadriplegic woman was not admitted to Lyndhurst as "she offered much less rehabilitative potential than a younger person." He concluded: "The work which is accomplished is second to none in spite of the rather limited physical properties of the present Lyndhurst Lodge building."[19]

These admission policies help to explain the composition of the patient population during these years, as well as why the rate of reintegration into the community was so high; many people admitted were from a group who had greater potential for living outside a health-care facility. By the early 1950s upwards of 500–600 people were being seen by medical staff either on an out-patient basis or during ward rounds at other facilities. This was a huge increase from earlier years and a sign that Lyndhurst's reputation was attracting more people to its tree-shaded doors. During the early part of the 1950s patients with "a greater degree of paralysis" than before began to come to the lodge.[20] This group – individuals with quadriplegia – would grow in numbers during the following years. By 1956 sixteen people, or 32 per cent of the total patient population, were quadriplegic, the highest it had ever been up to that time.[21] In 1958, when a total of 106 people with spinal cord injuries were in-patients at Lyndhurst, their average stay was about six months. Of course, the actual stay of many people varied significantly from the average. Some stayed for several weeks while others were there for several years, depending on their disability.[22]

One of these people was Myrll Jackson. Injured in a car accident while working as a miner near Sudbury in 1951, he became a high-level quadriplegic when he was twenty-nine years old. His chances of survival were almost immediately written off at a local mill hospital. "I was declared dead after the car accident," he recalled about his time at this small facility of about six beds and one doctor per shift twelve miles west of town. Shortly after he arrived, the staff had gone to deal with another accident. When the nurse came back, she said upon seeing Jackson, "Oh my God, I forgot to turn off the oxygen!" By this time, the doctor had already gone off shift and left for a vacation. But before he did this, he signed and sent the injured miner's death certificate, even though Jackson was still very much alive! "He didn't think I'd live more than 10 minutes." Jackson only learned about this when a friend who was present later told him about this episode. A year later when he was at Lyndhurst, staff contacted the provincial government to obtain educational funding for him. The only problem was "the government responded by saying there has been a mistake, this man has been dead for a year!" Eventually this was cleared up and he received the funding. But Jackson's experience is stark evidence of how quadriplegics were still being literally written off in the early 1950s, at a time when he said only six in every thousand high quadriplegics survived very long. Fortunately, not everyone was as fatalistic as the first doctor Jackson had contact with after his injury.

He was sent on a stretcher by train to Sunnybrook Hospital in Toronto. When he arrived, Jackson was unable to "even raise my head." His feet had turned purple because of poor blood circulation from lying down all the time. It was an enormous effort for him to even sit up for a minute or two, as blood would rush to his head and he would become completely disoriented. "I couldn't get my arms up." Eventually the nurses did have him sitting up two or three times a day "so I would get used to it again." After a year of being stabilized in Sunnybrook, he was transferred to Lyndhurst, where he lived from 1952 to 1955. Staff tied a thread through Jackson's fingernails with a door swing over his head to enable him to do lifting exercises. Because of his leg spasms, one leg had to be strapped down when orderlies helped him put his pants on, "but it didn't work as it hurt." These spasms also prevented him from being kept on a stryker frame, so he had to be flipped over in bed. "I was happy to be doing something and wasn't worried about being uncomfortable."

His meals were brought to him and he ate them with a spoon that was tied to his hand. When he was unable to eat, staff assisted him. Jackson found that relations between patients and staff at Lyndhurst were different from those at other health-care facilities he had been in. They socialized together inside and outside the lodge, whether it was out on the grounds in warmer months or going to hockey games, movies, and musicals such as "Oklahoma" with employees. Both Jousse and Geisler spoke with all the patients, and Jackson got along well with both of them. However, he remembered a difference of opinion with Botterell at the Toronto General Hospital. As with other Lyndhurst patients who required acute care he was sent to the TGH. He recalled that Botterell had transplanted "a cord from my wrist and hooked it onto my finger" in an effort to make some of his right hand move. However, the operation did not succeed. Afterwards, "I had an argument with [Botterell] as he wanted to operate on my left hand ... He told me he was the boss, but I asked to see if this operation was successful on other people and he didn't like that." So the operation did not proceed. But rehabilitation did proceed much to Jackson's satisfaction, though he hints at the stress underneath all the activity. "Even though I was there longer than expected, if I knew what you had to put up with it would have been more mentally difficult ... I have nothing but good things to say about Lyndhurst."

After his rehabilitation was completed in Toronto, Jackson moved back to Sudbury briefly before returning to live with his parents in his home-province of Saskatchewan. He eventually settled in British Columbia. He has lived in Vancouver since 1968 and has been involved in wheelchair sports, winning numerous medals. Reflecting on his foreign travels as a wheelchair athlete, fifty years after being written off as dead, Jackson's summary of his experiences speaks volumes: "I had a better life after I was in a wheelchair than before."[23]

Another quadriplegic at Lyndhurst during this period was Bev Hallam. Injured in a car accident in Parry Sound, Ontario, at the age of eighteen, he arrived at Lyndhurst Lodge in December 1961, three months later. Upon arrival in the new wing, he saw several other quadriplegics. "I thought: 'My goodness, they look in terrible shape. Good thing that I am going to recover and get out of here.' Which of course never happened. It was quite a shock!" The routine when he was there for three years in the early sixties was mat class with physiotherapist George White in the morning, in which people would "sit up and roll and sit up and all that kind of stuff." Afterwards would be chair class in which exercises were done in wheelchairs to "strengthen your upper body." These groups sessions were followed by one-on-one strengthening exercises with individual instructors. Male patients had a good deal of contact with the orderlies, who taught them self care, particularly regarding bowels and bladder. Hallam also mentioned how much he learned from other patients, such as "life skills" about "how to deal with people staring at you" in a society that "was not very friendly to wheelchairs."[24]

Just as more quadriplegics began to make their presence felt, so too the number of people with polio at Lyndhurst grew following the 1953 epidemic of poliomyelitis across Canada. People with polio arrived at Lyndhurst from as far afield as Saskatchewan and Nova Scotia. This was at the same time that the Salk vaccine to prevent polio was being tested in the United States. It was disseminated throughout the remainder of the decade, leading to the eventual eradication of polio in North America.[25] By the mid-1960s polio patients were no longer flocking to

Lyndhurst's doors. However, from 1950 to 1964 they made up the third largest group of disabled people in the lodge, after paraplegics and quadriplegics. Though people with polio formed a substantial group, Lyndhurst policy ensured that admission of polio patients did not prevent people with spinal cord injuries from finding a bed.[26]

One person with polio who did find a bed at Lyndhurst was Mabel C. Brown. Originally from Ottawa, she contracted polio at twenty-two, while studying to be a nurse in Chicago in September 1954. Mabel was sent to Lyndhurst in July 1955, where she remained for the next thirteen months. Prior to this, she recalled having lived a "very sheltered home life in Ottawa." By contrast, Lyndhurst was initially "a great shock," as she was in the "company of a lot of people, with the likes of whom I never had a lot to do with in my life." Being one of twelve female patients among forty male patients, "we were really outnumbered." She mixed with male patients in the course of her stay, such as during exercise classes. She found their behaviour upsetting as they could be "really coarse. The jokes that they would say to each other was sort of like what I call graveyard humour. It was their way of coping with their new crisis in life. Some of their jokes were just awful to have to listen to. To me it wasn't anything that I had ever experienced before. They weren't all like that but the ones that I heard were ... So I remember thinking I was in hell. That was my early impressions at Lyndhurst."

Having gone from being a nurse-in-training to a patient, Mabel Brown found herself in a very different situation from what she was used to in a health-care setting. She remembers being extremely frustrated during this early period. Staff would leave her in her room sitting in a wheelchair trying to unbutton her blouse, which she was unable to do at first. After "quite a while" she was able to complete this task on her own. Frustration and anger was used as a motivator by staff. At first she found this concept "kind of shocking" but eventually she accepted it "because if you get kind of angry with yourself you really try hard."

Within a week of her arrival, one particularly distressing event took place. Dr Geisler told Mabel that the next day they were going to see whether she could walk along the parallel bars, to determine whether she could ever walk again. "Well that was terrifying to me to be told that my whole future was at stake according to how I did tomorrow morning." It turned out to be a "disaster." Distraught at what she thought would be a "pretty bleak future" Mabel wrote her family a postcard with the message: "Come and get me. I am completely dis-couraged. Nothing great is going to happen here. I don't want to stay." However, with the support of family and friends, she decided to stay, though she experienced "a real downer" when she realized she would not walk again. Soon after this episode, Dr Jousse spoke to her. "He said, 'You know, most people sit in this world for most of their life.' They were spectators at sports, drive to work sitting in a car, sit behind a desk ... If I was determined to walk with braces and crutches, I would be using something like seven hundred percent of my strength that I had in the muscles that are still functioning ... 'Besides, your hands will be busy holding crutches and you won't be able to carry anything from A to B and bring anything back from B to A'." She found him "compas-sionate but still firm" and "very, very logical." This helped her get through her stay at Lyndhurst as "mat classes ... physiotherapy, the pool, filled our days ... I had no problem with the purpose of it all, it was very good."

Rehabilitating people with polio was described by Jousse in a 1954 article, shortly before Mabel came to Lyndhurst. He noted the impor-tance of regular physical exercises to prevent muscles from atrophying and becoming deformed. This "passive" exercising of joints in the affected limbs was ongoing from the time a person contracted polio. The timing of active exercises requiring the person to move was assessed around two weeks after the acute phase of polio had passed and the person's temperature was stable. Another two weeks of bed rest was necessary to watch out for "late paralysis." If paralysis was not significant, exercises could begin within a month of contracting polio. However, if paralysis was major "with severe systemic involve-ment," then exercises were not to commence until three to six months, perhaps longer, after the onset of polio. If there was no indication of recovery from complete paralysis after two months, Jousse said that "resting the completely paralysed limbs is without point" and exercis-ing of non-paralysed muscles was to start as soon as the person's health permitted. Eventually, exercising both normal and paralysed muscles was made routine to enhance a polio patient's physical stamina. An important part of the exercise regimen was establishing in the polio patient's mind the ultimate goal of physical independence: "The pro-gramme of physical restoration is only meaningful if it is directed toward a specific goal. Exercise simply to make a patient stronger does not hold his attention for long. It is necessary to relate it specifically to such an object as learning to walk again, or learning to get about in a wheelchair or even, if the disability is severe, of mastering the simple details of self-care."

After exercises had been initiated, the use of prosthetic aids, such as crutches or braces, was introduced. This was followed by an assessment of the person's future goals after rehabilitation was concluded. These objectives were to be based on fitting the person into society by "helping him to relinquish the goals and ambitions he held before becoming disabled, and to establish new ones which are realistic and attainable in the light of his altered capabilities." Jousse noted that, since no two people are alike in how they respond to treatment, "rigid periods of convalescence are meaningless." In concluding his article, the medical director of Lyndhurst set out his basic philosophy, which applied not only to people with polio but also to other disabled individuals: "The essence of rehabilitation is thus to assist the man to accept his disability, relinquish his previous goals and establish new ones, and to pursue the new goals with all the determination at his command." This involved a team effort from staff members involved in the person's care, the doctor overseeing the rehabilitation regimen, and "the total support" of the disabled person. When the person was unable to meet the demands of this program, Jousse wrote, "rehabilitation becomes impossible."[27]

Mabel remembered some people were discharged early because they did not accept the Lyndhurst philosophy. "I heard Dr. Jousse once speak to an older woman, really sharply. He said, 'If you don't co-operate with us you just can't be here,' which of course had to be because they had limited beds ... You really had to go along with what they wanted you to do." Eventually, Mabel became friends with other women patients and led a Bible study session every Monday night. Attendance was nearly always perfect as they studied one chapter of the Book of John each week, "twenty one chapters, so twenty one weeks roughly, some were holiday weeks." One woman was of particular importance in the way Mabel came to see herself. Originally, she thought of herself in a wheelchair as "abnormal." Some women at Lyndhurst had become so depressed over their situation that at least two of them were sent to a psychiatric hospital. Another woman, Janet H., also had polio. She was unable to hold up her head, which had to be positioned with a brace to enable her to breathe. "She was the most gracious, pleasant young woman. She was a role model for me and she gave me hope that a person with polio could be normal still, fit into the big wide world, even though there is a major change in your image. That was a very important help for me to see such a person. She was just a delightful personality ... Janet was just riding above it all. That was a very major thing for me to see that. It gave me hope."

After discharge, Mabel lived with other women friends in Toronto for ten years and picked up where she had left off at the time she contracted polio by applying to go back to nursing school. However, the University of Toronto faculty was initially less than enthusiastic. Jousse had to go in person to convince the administrator in charge that a person in a wheelchair should be allowed into the nursing program. "He was really put out that of all people that should understand disabilities and be able to help, the nursing faculty should be the most open but they are the least." After he advocated on her behalf Mabel was allowed to attend. It was agreed that she would provide her own help accessing the building which, like most places, had stairs. "That was a major thing that Lyndhurst did for me." She earned her nursing degree and eventually returned to Ottawa where she retired after working as a hospital medical librarian. Decades later when recalling her time at Lyndhurst, Mabel said, "The legacy was phenomenal. When I arrived I was able to do nothing for myself and left able to do almost everything ... I mean you wouldn't want to go back. It was not something that you would invite yourself back to. I remember back to the earliest weeks thinking I was in hell, discovering that it wasn't so terrible after all. And month by month it got more and more meaningful."[28]

The best picture obtained for the overall patient population up to near the end of this period is from data compiled in late 1963 on all discharged in-patients from Lyndhurst Lodge up to that time. As can be seen in Table 1, people with spinal cord injuries made up the largest group of in-patients – 58 per cent of the total – between 1945 and 1963. Of this group, 41 per cent had complete or partial paraplegia. Several people who helped to make up these numbers remembered what Lyndhurst was like for paraplegics during this period.

Gordon Paterson was there at the same time as Mabel Brown. On 21 May 1955 he fell from a window on the second floor of his parents' home in Whitby, Ontario, crushing three vertebrae in his back and becoming a paraplegic. He recalled "the shock of suddenly losing the sense or a feeling" in the lower part of his body. He was an in-patient at Lyndhurst from August 1955 to January 1956, followed by a year in the TGH, and then several more months at Lyndhurst. While at the TGH during the summer of 1955 Paterson met Jousse, "tall, black mustache, glasses, a limp" and off to Lyndhurst he went.

Table 1: Summary of discharged Lyndhurst Lodge patients, 1945–63

	Total	Presently Alive	Presently Domiciled	Dead
Complete Quadriplegia	122 (5%)	90 (74%)	27 (30%)	32 (26%)
Partial Quadriplegia	289 (12%)	244 (84.4%)	21 (8.6%)	45 (15.6%)
Complete Paraplegia	422 (17%)	317 (75%)	14 (4.4%)	105 (25%)
Partial Paraplegia	597 (24.3%)	507 (85%)	22 (4.3%)	90 (15%)
Hemiplegia	202 (8%)	180 (89%)	21 (11.6%)	22 (11%)
Multiple Sclerosis	122 (5%)	109 (89%)	18 (16.5%)	13 (11%)
Muscular Dystrophy	53 (2%)	49 (92.4%)	1 (2%)	4 (7.6%)
Poliomyelitis	405 (16.5%)	390 (96%)	6 (1.5%)	15 (4%)
Cerebral Palsy	31 (1%)	31 (100%)	2 (6.4%)	0
Amputees	42 (1.7%)	35 (83%)	1 (3%)	7 (17%)
Parkinson's Disease	9 (60%)	7 (78%)	0	2 (22%)
Rheumatoid Arthritis	13 (90%)	13 (100%)	0	0
Others	151 (6%)	144 (95%)	2 (1%)	7 (5%)
Total	2,458	2,116 (86%)	135 (6.4%)	342 (14%)

Note: "Presently Domiciled" refers to chronic-care facilities and nursing homes. Percentages for this category are based on comparison with the "Presently Alive" category. Percentages have been rounded off to the nearest number. Source: Archives of Ontario, RG 10–154, Hospitals and Institutions Central Files Reel Listing, Reel 280, MS 6098: A.T. Jousse to Dr R.S. Peat, Ontario Hospital Services Commission, Toronto, December 2, 1963 (attachment).

The differences between the TGH and Lyndhurst were obvious. For starters, the food was better. Whereas, in eleven weeks at the TGH he had lost fifty-five pounds, at the lodge he ate roast beef, chicken, and other hot meals with room for seconds. Most importantly, "You weren't in a hospital setting anymore, you were in a rehab setting." People were taught self-care which was never done at a general hospital. Depending on their physical condition and personal preference, some male patients would use a catheter, which had to be drained regularly by orderlies and which also caused more bladder infections. Other males used a condom attached to a leg bag to urinate. The orderly responsible for assisting with bowel movements if enemas were not working quickly enough was the subject of a rhyme among the male patients, according to Paterson: "'Lyndhurst Lodge is the place to go for quads, paras and polios and in the washroom if you should linger you will get Herbie's finger.' Because it was the digital manipulation of the bowel. Herbie was an old Englishman, skinny, bent over. He use to walk around with his rubber glove hanging out of his back pocket."

One intimate area that was never discussed with Gordon Paterson was sexuality. "I never asked the question," he recalled. But he did remember another patient who did ask about sex after injury. A married man with children insisted to Dr Jousse that he would try to have more children. The medical director responded, "I wouldn't advise staying home from work to try." As with other patients, like Mabel Brown, he learned a good deal from his fellow residents. One day, Colin, who was quadriplegic, asked Paterson why he was waiting in the genito-urinary room. When Paterson responded that he was waiting for an orderly to empty his urine-filled bag, Colin responded "Oh go tell it to the padre!" This attitude that you get on with things "has stood me in good stead all through my life."[29] After leaving Lyndhurst, Paterson worked as a draftsman for the Ontario provincial government for many years. He is now retired and lives in Toronto with his wife Nancy, with whom he raised two sons whom they adopted in the late 1960s.

A male patient who has requested anonymity also described how Lyndhurst's rehabilitation program helped him after he became a paraplegic in a diving accident at the age of seventeen. In December 1959, six months after this accident, he was admitted to Lyndhurst Lodge from a hospital in his hometown in southwestern Ontario. Unable to sit up without fainting, barely able to feed himself, he spent the initial period of residence "getting my faculties together." Since meals were not brought to their room, this new resident had to go to the dining room, "Which was a good idea in retrospect. It got my arms and shoulders functioning, which they hadn't been up until then."

This former Lyndhurst resident spoke of staff member Mary Lou Kerr as "a terrific physiotherapist." It was thanks to her that "I got as much back as I eventually did." She and her colleagues attached weights to exercise different limbs and also did work on finger and wrist function. The chair exercise class was run by George White "a gruff army guy but we knew very well that he was on your side." One class was particularly memorable. When it was nice enough outside, chair classes were held on the Lyndhurst tennis court, left over from the mansion's old days. "George had a loud army sergeant voice ... do this and do that, sounded like he was being tough on everybody." If someone was tiring, which happened naturally enough, "he would be over behind pretending to slap you over the back of the head or rubbing your shoulders. He was really a good guy. And one day he brought a whip and he was cracking it around the tennis court and all of a sudden police cars arrived ... Once the police found out what was not happening, that none of us had marks on us [they left]. A neighbour complained about somebody whipping these poor individuals in wheelchairs ... We thought it was a big joke."

He considered Lyndhurst Lodge as more like a "university residence than a hospital" with similar goals "that you were going to graduate and get yourself together." One of the steps on the way to "graduation," for the men patients on the first floor, was moving to the independent wing in the old part of Lyndhurst. There was a patients' lounge between it and the new wing for males who required "much more intervention." People were expected to dress themselves in the independent wing, make their own bed, and do daily tasks without the assistance of orderlies, who were seldom in this part of the building. This former Lyndhurst resident also spoke about people for whom there was to be no graduation, but who were discharged after not being able to meet the rehabilitation regimen there: "CPA and Lyndhurst structured the time in insisting that you either perform or go home. If you were not going to work at your therapy conscientiously, day after day after day, you went home ... I don't think many of them are around really. Alcoholism took them and pressure sore problems and pneumonia. If you get yourself in a situation like that and your health is bad ... You have to keep your circulatory system working. People who went home who didn't reach their full potential as far as rehabilitation goes wound up in bad health, no doubt."

When it came time for his own discharge in September 1961, twenty-one months after first arriving, this former Lyndhurst resident expressed concerns common to other people who were long-stay residents in facilities they had come to rely on: "I would have rather stayed." Going back into the community "was a daunting thing" in an era when wheelchairs were not as reliable as they later became. Concern about his physical condition added to his apprehension. Eventually, this man found full time employment and is now retired.[30]

Margaret Staton was perhaps the youngest paraplegic patient at Lyndhurst, arriving first as an out-patient in the late 1940s when she was three or four years old and becoming an in-patient by the time she was twelve. She was born in Baltimore and lived in Atlanta. When she was two, she developed a spinal tumour that led to partial paraplegia and to various visits to Lyndhurst as both an out-patient and in-patient until she was in her late teens. Her mother was Dr Botterell's sister and since medical help for paraplegics in Georgia was not very good until the 1970s, she became a regular visitor to Toronto throughout the 1950s and into the 1960s. She remembered older patients as well as staff who "took me under their wing" and looked after her. Her age did not stop her from doing the same exercise program as the others did. "Sometimes I did feel intimidated with adults but they also gave me a lot of slack since at that age kids don't have much of an attention span and they could also see that I was making progress."[31]

Progress was also evident among the general population whom Lyndhurst served. Whereas only a few decades earlier, 80 per cent of people with spinal cord injuries died within two years of becoming disabled, the 1945–63 figures from Lyndhurst show a compete reversal of this statistic (Table 1). Of the 1,430 quadriplegics and paraplegics discharged from this facility during this period, 1,158, or 81 per cent, were listed as "Presently Alive" by Dr Jousse. Furthermore, of this group of living ex-patients, only 6 per cent were recorded as being "Presently Domiciled," that is, they lived in a long-term care institution. Again, this was a complete reversal of earlier years when most people with spinal cord injuries who did survive for any length of time were expected to live out their lives in institutions. By the early 1960s upwards of 94 per cent of former Lyndhurst patients returned to the community. Lyndhurst's leading role in Canada in this regard was evident by 1956. The CPA estimated that each year across Canada, more than 200 people with spinal cord injuries returned to the community after treatment in a hospital or rehabilitation centre, of which more than half "graduated" from Lyndhurst Lodge.[32]

Mortality statistics provide another important perspective on these developments. Of 599 paraplegic patients treated at Lyndhurst Lodge, Sunnybrook Hospital, and the Toronto General between 1945 and 1958, ninety-four, or just over 15 per cent had died. While the survival rates of people with spinal cord injuries had vastly improved, the authors of this study made it clear that they still experienced a significantly higher death rate than did able-bodied people. Even "carefully treated paraplegics" died at three times the rate of the general population, with infection and poisoning of genito-urinary organs claiming up to half of all fatalities.[33] These statistics continued to underline the crucial importance of continuing proper urological care for those with spinal cord injuries.

Lyndhurst had by this time clearly developed a reputation for rehabilitation. Yet it was also clear that being discharged was the beginning of another struggle for inclusion in society, which was largely inaccessible for people with physical disabilities. This was especially so for some former Lyndhurst residents who had no home to return to.

Concern over the type of facility some patients were discharged to was raised by Dr Jousse in late 1959. He wrote about a male patient in his late teens who was about to be discharged to "The Sunnyside Home for the Aged" in Kitchener. Jousse felt the reason municipal authorities arranged this accommodation was to avoid "financial responsibility" for him in another, possibly more expensive location. In response, Dr R.S. Peat of the Ontario Hospital Services Commission acknowledged that Jousse "states the situation well" but then went on to write that the home was a "modern" facility which had an arts and crafts program "which would be desirable if the patient's condition suits this type of thing."[34] How this situation developed is not revealed by the sources, but it indicates the difficulty of finding proper support in the community for some people with spinal cord injuries who were not able to live on their own or with their family.

In another instance, in the fall of 1964 Jousse wrote to the Commissioner of Ontario's Hospitals, Dr B.L. Brosseau. He suggested that young females with spinal cord injuries who had nowhere to go, other than chronic-care facilities, might instead be discharged to live in a hospital's nurses' residence. There, young women with spinal cord injuries may be able to receive any necessary care from student nurses who lived in residence with them. They may also be given employment as receptionists at the residences, which Jousse noted was frequently done with older women. He argued that it would prevent such individuals from being a continued cost to the health insurance program if they were to become self-sufficient. Jousse also wrote that such an arrangement would ensure that they would continue to have assistance with proper care, when necessary, in a facility with health-care workers of their own age: "You must be aware that the complaint of the young people who, when disabled, are confined to hospitals rendering ongoing care for the disabled, is to the effect that they are surrounded by old, senile individuals and completely devoid of young companionship." Brosseau responded cautiously by writing that he did not think this idea was "entirely possible."[35] However, he agreed to meet Jousse to discuss it further. What came of this meeting is not revealed by the sources.

As far as is known, this proposal did not proceed any further, but, it indicates the desperate measures being considered to find alternatives other than a chronic-care facility for young people with spinal cord injuries when they were unable to return home. So while the lodge was successful in discharging people back into the community, the community was not always willing to receive them in a manner allowing for dignity and independence.

For Bev Hallam, getting out of Lyndhurst meant finding a boarding house near a Toronto high school, where he completed Grade 13. It was "one of the few schools in the city that had an elevator."[36] So he was able to pair up vocational and living quarters in the same area. Jousse was considered "flexible" in regard to allowing patients to stay in Lyndhurst until they had a place to stay, or to return if this was required, according to Ken Langford: "The patients came first." Rehabilitation was not finished until they had suitable living arrangements outside the facility. Unlike in later periods, no time limit was set on how long someone could remain at Lyndhurst.[37]

Finding accessible quarters was obviously essential, but locating ground level buildings was not easy by any means during the 1950s. Ken and Mary Langford found them to be "very scarce." They were able to purchase a house that had a level entry after living in a hotel for a year, then in an apartment for several years, and later in a bungalow that was relatively accessible. Similarly, John and Maida Counsell lived in Toronto's easy-to-enter Park Plaza Hotel for several years before finding a house that allowed access for a person in a wheelchair.[38] It stands to reason that there was a greater chance to find a few accessible places in larger cities where there were more buildings. However, it is interesting to note that one of the earliest studies undertaken on post-discharge life for Lyndhurst patients from 1953 revealed that a good portion of them went to live in places other than Toronto or large urban centres. Of 385 respondents, all of whom were people with quadriplegia, paraplegia, or polio, just under two-thirds lived in a town or in the countryside and 58 per cent were married. Another 55 per cent from this overall group used wheelchairs while 13 per cent used crutches. This same survey discovered that the 276 males who drove a car were almost evenly split between those who used hand controls and those who did not.[39]

Being able to drive a car was obviously an immense boost to greater independence for anyone with a disability. Learning how to get in and out of a car with a wheelchair was an important part of preparing for this post-discharge life. During the 1950s and 1960s, in doing so some Lyndhurst residents literally grabbed the nearest car they could get a hand on. Much of the time, this happened to be Ken and Mary

Langford's car. Since he was employed in the CPA head office on the lodge grounds, patients found it convenient to practice on the Langford car. It proved to be so popular that the door nearly fell off, as the cumulative weight of all those people grabbing the handle caused the door to sag to near the breaking point. Another car was eventually donated for this purpose.[40]

To make surveys like the 1953 study more comprehensive and meaningful someone had to be employed to focus on this task alone. That person was Dr Megan Wynne-Jones. Beginning in 1955 she started twenty-six years of work at Lyndhurst, compiling and analysing statistical data that would be crucial to the clinical study of spinal cord injuries. This included setting up a card system during the late 1950s that was used to categorize various types of disabilities efficiently prior to the widespread use of computers.[41]

The CPA, Manufacturer's Life Insurance Co., and a local tracking firm, Equifax, helped to find people who had been discharged. Manufacturer's Life Insurance also helped with statistical analysis, assistance that helped to bring down insurance rates for people with spinal cord injuries in years to come. The results of these studies were published both in medical journals and in the annual reports of the CPA.

One of the first examples based on this more controlled system is outlined in Table 2. A survey undertaken in 1958–59 involved questionnaires sent to former Lyndhurst patients, of whom 72 per cent responded, 63 per cent being people with spinal cord injuries. Reflecting data that was consistent with statistics compiled before and after this survey, 95 per cent of respondents were recorded as living outside a hospital. Of this group, 81 per cent lived at home, either with their spouse or with other relatives, such as their parents.

Employment status is also consistent during this period, when statistics from the 1958–59 survey are compared with a survey conducted in 1962 involving records then available at Lyndhurst Lodge (see Table 3). In both instances figures hovered just over 50 per cent, with the earlier survey being slightly higher with 54.5 per cent of former patients finding employment. This was most likely because of the inclusion of people with disabilities other than paraplegia and quadriplegia in 1958–59 unlike in the 1962 study, which focused exclusively on people with spinal cord injuries.

Dr Jousse wrote, referring to those who were not on the job market, "it is clear that very few complete quadriplegics return to work and many die [25 out of 104, or 24 per cent]." He also noted that many

Table 2: 1958–59 survey of former Lyndhurst Lodge patients

Males 545 (74%) Females 189 (26%)	
Complete Quadriplegia	34 (4.5%)
Partial Quadriplegia	82 (11%)
Complete Paraplegia	159 (21.5%)
Partial Paraplegia	186 (26%)
Polio	190 (26%)
Hemiplegia	24 (3%)
Others	59 (8%)
Living Outside Hospital	95%
Married and Living in Their Own Homes	54%
Living with Parents or Relatives	27%
Living Alone in House, Apartment, or Boarding House	14%
Living in Hospital or Nursing Home	5%
Regularly Employed	56%
Not Employed	31%
Attending School	8%
Retired (age 60 or above)	5%
Employment Rates for People with:	
Public School Education	43.5%
Secondary School Education	69%
Specialized Training	76%
Working at similar or the same work as before disability	41%
Respondents who took vocational training after disability	29%

*   Based on 734 responses out of 1,017 people contacted (72% response rate)
Source: Canadian Paraplegic Association, National Office, Ottawa: CPA 15th Annual Report, 1960, 13–15.

ex-patients were not employed full-time, still others were paid lower wages than able-bodied people doing the same type of work, and a few people earned more than they had anticipated would be possible prior to becoming disabled.[42] Employment difficulties faced by ex-Lyndhurst residents mirrored the wider barriers faced by all disabled people in society and would be a source of increasing attention in years to come. Those employed to work with disabled people at Lyndhurst are also an important part of this story, and we now turn to their experiences.

STAFF AND STUDENTS

Bev Hallam recalled seeing Dr Jousse conducting the morning rounds on the wards with "one of the nurses, maybe some physios and occa-

Table 3: Employment status of 931 Lyndhurst Lodge SCI patients, January 31, 1962

	Total	Employed	Not Employed	Status Unknown
Complete Quadriplegia	79	17 (21.5%)	45 (57%)	17 (21.5%)
Partial Quadriplegia	193	80 (41.5%)	81 (42%)	32 (16.5%)
Complete Paraplegia	252	135 (53.5%)	89 (35.5%)	28 (11%)
Partial Paraplegia	407	248 (61%)	106 (26%)	53 (13%)
Total	931	480 (51.5%)	321 (34.5%)	130 (14%)

Source: A.T. Jousse, "The Evolution of the Treatment Programme for Paraplegics in Canada," *The Journal of the Association for Physical and Mental Rehabilitation* 16:5 (September–October, 1962), 135. In this survey of employment records at Lyndhurst as of January 1962, 1,290 people with spinal cord injuries were tabulated. Out of this number, 359 were deducted as people who were not then able to obtain work, because they were deceased (236); in school or some kind of vocational training (76); or retired and over 65 years of age (47). Of the remaining 931 people who were "available for employment," their status was listed as is shown. The statistics have been corrected slightly in the percentage column from those originally published. Also, the total number of the complete survey of this entire group, before deductions of people who were not available for work, adds up to 1300 in the down column listing the four SCI categories, and 1290 for the numbers listed across different employment status columns. The 1290 figure is correct, as ten people too many were mistakenly added to the "Partial Quadriplegia" column (264 when it should be 254).

sionally with a pile of nursing students or a pile of medical residents ... I always felt that they always talked to the wrong end. The first thing when they came in was pull down the sheets and have a look at your rear end. And I said: 'No I am up here.' Because pressure sores were pretty common stuff and you had to learn how to manage those."[43] This ex-patient's perspective on a daily part of interacting with staff and students who trained at Lyndhurst brings us to the working life of the people who ran the rehabilitation programs and kept the physical plant operating.

By the second half of the 1950s, sixty-five staff were employed at 153 Lyndhurst.[44] Doctors, nurses, orderlies, physiotherapists, gardeners, maintenance workers, cleaners, dietary staff, and administrators all had responsibilities in keeping Lyndhurst operating for the benefit of the men and women who occupied the wards. Salaries ranged anywhere from just over $700 a month for the highest-paid employee to just over $100 for the lowest-paid worker.[45] According to Margaret MacDonald, the "pay was poor ... in comparison to the head nurse" at the TGH paraplegic unit.[46] Another employee during the early 1950s, Evelyn O. Paul, worked as a physiotherapist. She recalled her starting salary in 1949 was around $150 a month and had risen to $175 a month by 1953 when she left to have a family: "It was what we expected but we were never really satisfied of course. We would have liked to make more ... but that was not unheard of. We managed."[47]

A report by provincial inspector Louise Jamieson in the early 1960s helps to provide a broader picture of the overall employment at Lyndhurst Lodge. Nursing staff in early 1962 included the matron, Margaret MacDonald, ten full-time registered nurses, fifteen orderlies, and one chief orderly. The daily routine for nurses and orderlies who looked after fifty-two patients at this time was based on three basic shifts common to all health-care facilities. Six registered nurses and seven orderlies worked from 8:00 a.m. to 4:00 p.m.; one registered nurse and two orderlies worked from 3:30 p.m. to 11:30 p.m.; one registered nurse and one orderly worked from 11:30 p.m. to 8:00 a.m. This worked out to an average of "2.8 hours of nursing care per patient," according to the provincial nursing inspector, Louise Jamieson. Of these nursing staff, 58 per cent had received professional training while 42 per cent had not. By this time the matron's salary was $395 per month. The other nursing staff had a general basic salary of $305 per month with up to $50 in raises per year. Professional staff could take up to three weeks' annual vacation while non-professional staff had two weeks' vacation. In-service education at Lyndhurst Lodge at that time consisted of a weekly meeting between doctors, nurses, and orderlies at which the progress of individual patients was discussed. As personnel policies were not at that time written down, Inspector Jamieson recommended that this be rectified, with staff being provided with written policies. As well, she recommended the development of an in-service educational program including speakers, films, a library, and attendance at relevant conferences.[48]

As a follow-up to these and other recommendations, Dr Jousse wrote six months later that "we have always had an inservice education programme, although one could not call it comprehensive, and it has been for nurses and physical and occupational therapists and others who may be interested." He also noted that since the beginning of OHIP in 1959, money had been set aside for staff educational purposes, such as for ordering books and films. However, Jousse went on, Lyndhurst did not normally invite outside speakers for talks, though international visitors did meet with staff members during trips to the facility. Heads of departments were also sent regularly to relevant conferences; extending this to other staff was to be considered. Personnel policies were also written down, though there was no mention of whether they were distributed to staff.[49]

In addition to their regular work caring for patients, Lyndhurst's medical and nursing staff were also involved in training programs for students from near and far. By the early 1960s, Lyndhurst had instituted a fellowship program whereby a medical student working towards a degree became part of the staff for the school year. During this period he or she received training in treating people with spinal cord injuries. Graduate nursing also was undertaken at Lyndhurst with a graduate nurse from Australia working on staff for six months in 1963. Several male graduate nurses also spent two weeks training at the lodge. Eight undergraduate students divided into two shifts each from the Nightingale School of Nursing spent six weeks during the spring as part of their training. Another fifteen to thirty nursing students would come for a day from local universities, nursing schools, and hospitals to advance their understanding of nursing care in the field of rehabilitation medicine.[50]

Doctors in training also came to Lyndhurst as part of their studies. Between 1945 and 1957 fifteen doctors had some kind of training at Lyndhurst Lodge and were thereafter employed in six out of ten provinces across Canada.[51] As well, visiting clinicians came to Lyndhurst each year and took back to other parts of Canada and the wider world their impressions of what they learned there. In 1953–54, for example, doctors from eleven countries visited.[52]

In 1962 an agreement was reached with the University of Toronto whereby medical appointments to Lyndhurst Lodge would be made by a joint CPA-University of Toronto committee. This allowed the rehabilitation centre to formalize its teaching affiliation with the local university for medical, physiotherapy, and nursing students, a practice that had started in the fall of 1945.[53] This affiliation with the U of T, as well as the affiliation with the Nightingale School of Nursing by 1964, increased teaching obligations for Lyndhurst's staff. According to the CPA annual report for that year, these increased teaching demands "required great patience on [the staff's] part due to their almost complete lack of teaching space or facilities in the present buildings."[54] Another report from the early 1960s by a provincial inspector noted that the director of nursing, Margaret MacDonald, had "considerable teaching responsibility" for both staff and visiting nurses. It was also noted that while male nursing staff were desired for certain duties, none was available, so male orderlies were relied upon instead. Some of them were considered "excellent" and others "are not very adequate."[55]

Throughout this period, all of these employees at Lyndhurst Lodge were paid by the CPA. In practice, the relationship between the lodge and the association was inseparable, though technically the staff of each was separate. Ken Langford, who worked for the CPA head office on the grounds of the lodge during this entire period, mentioned that medical rehabilitation treatment staff were the responsibility of Dr Jousse. The CPA handled the financial operation of Lyndhurst and employed vocational counsellors, such as Jim Bartlett. Both Lyndhurst and CPA staff worked together as a team in regard to patients.[56]

In addition to dealing with employees' salaries, employees' separation had to be addressed. After fifteen years of existence, Lyndhurst Lodge and the CPA began to deal with the issue of retirement of employees. It was decided that the hospital committee would review the list of people over sixty-five each year to decide on who should and who should not be kept on the payroll.[57] The same year that this was decided, John Counsell stepped down as managing director of the CPA effective 1 October 1960, though he continued on as president until 1965. Ken Langford officially took over the managing director's position and Andy Clarke became assistant managing director.[58] In this way, John Counsell, though still very much a presence in the facility he did so much to create and operate since 1945, became less involved in the daily operations of Lyndhurst Lodge. Counsell continued to maintain an "active interest." However, he had gradually retired during the 1950s and left more of the running of the CPA up to Langford in the years prior to his official retirement.[59] His proteges would continue his work so that Counsell's influence continued to be felt for years afterwards.

Margaret MacDonald's influence at Lyndhurst was also felt for many years, especially after she became director of nursing in 1957. Her work day began at eight o'clock in the morning when nursing staff changed shifts. With each shift change, nursing staff going off duty would meet with those whose shift was just starting to discuss what had happened during the previous eight hours. Around 9 a.m. Dr Jousse would meet with Miss MacDonald to hear the report. Then, together, they would go on ward rounds. For nearly twenty years she accompanied Jousse on daily rounds, which she described as "a real privilege." Her job during rounds was to write down his orders about each individual patient on her clipboard. After rounds were over, MacDonald would return to the nurses' office, "a little spot in the old Lyndhurst," to rewrite these instructions in the order book. But just before she did this, the nursing staff, orderlies, physiotherapists, CPA counsellors, and doctors all met in the cafeteria for a cup of coffee around 10:30 each morning after rounds. Here, they had a general discussion about the patients and any concerns related to their treatment. This was an important daily practice that continued for years at the old Lyndhurst and was mentioned by other staff who worked during this period.

The nurses worked out of a small room with two French doors, according to Miss MacDonald. But this office was more than just a place to fill out reports. Any staff member, from maintenance men to the medical director, who wanted to talk about treatment-related matters could visit. "It was a free for all ... They would notice things about patients sometimes that we wouldn't know." On one occasion, an orderly was upset after having been scratched by a cat during the night when he went to turn a patient to prevent bedsores. "I thought that was quite amusing but Henry, the orderly, didn't ... I kept a straight face but when I went down to see the patient, he thought I was going to scold him. Being a cat lover I thought it was a delightful story, but [the patient] started to tell me, 'You know Miss MacDonald that cat, it was raining, he was cold and shivering and I couldn't leave him out there.' Of course, [the patient] got a good hearing because I'm a cat lover."

Joking around with the patients was also part of the daily routine. The former head of nursing recalled one individual who took a joke by other patients to heart. A Portuguese boy who was not fluent in English said upon his departure: "Thank you for all you have done for me Mother MacDonald." Some of the other patients had told him that this was in fact her name which he took to be true. "The boys at the old wing where they were rehabilitated, they were full of nonsense."[60]

Evelyn O. Paul was a physiotherapist at Lyndhurst from 1949 to 1953 and again from 1972 to 1980. She recalled the work done in this department during the early years of her employment. Exercise classes such as those where patients were in their wheelchair flexing their limbs, were held in "a huge cavernous room" that had once been a ballroom. Individual physiotherapy sessions were held in either a patient's room or some other open part of the building. One was a room where there was "a long table and the physio would sit up on the table and the patient would sit beside her and she would tie weights to his arm." People would be walking through this room "all the time," an indication of how space was utilized for treatment in cramped quarters.

Evelyn Paul also remembered that, unlike in a general hospital, patients and staff could become quite close to one another. People would sometimes confide their personal problems to staff members. Also, Lyndhurst being such a small facility, "everybody knew everybody ... In some cases some physios married their patients ... It was rare but it happened." She also mentioned that patients who had been soldiers "were more willing to take chances than the civilian population but there wasn't a great deal of difference. I think because they were service people and they had been through a lot and weren't going to put up with any nonsense about being good patients. I couldn't blame them. The civilian populations were more polite and observed the rules more." In common with other people interviewed for this book, Evelyn Paul recalled that while the medical director allowed a more relaxed environment than would have been the case in a typical general hospital, he also had very definite expectations from patients: "Dr Jousse was extremely tolerant, but not a pushover by any means. He could be very stern about the rules. I mean if you were unwell because you went out drinking the night before, tough bananas. You were in real trouble if you weren't in the classes. He ran a tight ship as far as that was concerned. He didn't mind them breaking the rules as long as he didn't know about it, as long as they were in classes the next day."

As someone who worked closely with both paraplegics and quadriplegics, Paul explained the difference in treating both groups from a physiotherapist's perspective. Since quadriplegics had very little movement below the neck, perhaps some ability to move shoulders, they required more assistance. For example, they required help moving to and from their wheelchairs in exercise classes. Improving the muscles in their shoulders was very important and if they could flex their elbows, a special spoon was made to enable them to feed themselves. Paraplegics had more ability to move and exercise their upper bodies, including their arms and backs, and so were able to get in and out of a wheelchair unassisted. "With paraplegics you aim towards them having a full life, like driving a car, being personally independent with dressing ... But a quadriplegic is not independently dressed, but has to be dressed, has to be cared for. It is very different."[61]

Betty Brooks was also employed as a physiotherapist at Lyndhurst, beginning as a student in 1960 and then on staff from 1961 to 1980. During this time she worked under head physiotherapist Barbara Duffin, whom she called "incredible. She could tell you when, where and how anybody in the place got injured. She could tell you exactly what level they were at and what they could do and what they can't do."[62] A woman who worked in the CPA office also recalled employees who made an impression on her. Elizabeth Holman worked as a secretary in the CPA head office for four or five years during the late 1950s and early 1960s. She remembers that Assistant Director Geisler "just flew up and down the stairs. That being a private home there was a big staircase. And Geisler's office was on the second floor so he would just roar up and down those stairs ... He is really a go-go guy. He never stopped. He was just on the tear the whole time." She too remembered the joking around that took place with one incident in particular sticking in her mind. Polio shots were being administered to everyone. When it was her turn, the two most well-known orderlies, Tommy and Dick, "grabbed me by the arm and literally carried me in to where Dr Jousse was. He was standing with his back to me and when he turned around he had a needle about that l-o-n-g ... At least [a foot]. So he turned around and he said to them: 'OK fellows, in the hip.'" Joking aside, she proceeded to have her shot in the arm. This episode "gave the patients something to talk about."[63] The next day, people asked her about getting a polio shot in the hip.

One employee whose name keeps cropping up in reminiscences of both former residents and employees of Lyndhurst is Art James. He was the head of the maintenance department at Lyndhurst, a post he had held since shortly after it opened in 1945 and would hold for three decades. James lived on the grounds in the coach house above the CPA office and, in 1958, paid $30 a month in rent for his small apartment, which was included in his monthly $305 salary.[64] "He was a man of all hats," according to Elizabeth Holman. "He could do anything: plumbing, electricity, anything like that. He just seemed to do everything."[65] In addition to keeping the physical plant running smoothly, James also installed and repaired various assistive devices needed for disabled people who came to Lyndhurst. This included the arched metal bars that were fitted over a person's bed. He and an assistant in the maintenance department would fashion these bars out of lead pipes purchased at the local hardware store, according to Dr Geisler: "It was this bar that the therapist and the doctors would encourage the patients to reach, to help them sit up and get mobilized to move, to sit and transfer out of the bed."[66] James would also go to people's homes and install this overhead bar after their discharge. Before and after they left Lyndhurst he would fix people's wheelchairs, canes, and crutches. A male resident of the lodge who was there from 1959 to 1961, and who has requested anonymity, said Art James "was one of the guys, a great guy around the place ... At one point [after discharge] I had a van with a lift and it needed some things fixed and I looked up Art and he did that. He was burned in an army accident or in the air force. He had one of those gray faces that he got through plastic surgery, terrific guy ... He treated people not as patients but as friends, you know."[67] People like Art James helped former patients make the transition from the lodge to the community. For all of the different experiences that people recounted, certain aspects of this history express a common bond between patients and staff and underline the challenges that people with physical disabilities faced in the rehabilitation process as well as out in the community.

OVERCOMING PHYSICAL AND MENTAL BARRIERS
INSIDE AND OUTSIDE LYNDHURST LODGE

People who went through Lyndhurst Lodge during the decade and a half covered here, either as patients or staff, remembered it as an old mansion with a good deal of character built into it and the people who lived and worked there. But because it was so hectic and involved hundreds of people coming and going from its wards and rooms every year, it would be an exaggeration to make it sound as if it were spic and span. Concerns about conditions on one ward were expressed by a visitor in the fall of 1959. A sister of a patient admitted the previous summer wrote to the Ministry of Health that "It is a very unsanitary, dirty place. There are flies and a smell of urine all over." She wrote that the Toronto Department of Health was of no assistance. "They washed the ceiling but flies and smell is still there. They have a fly paper hanging from the ceiling in my brother's ward. They also issued fly swatters to patients who have the use of their arms and hands. My brother was burned very badly and the wounds are open yet. They keep nothing on his wounds to allow air at them. Also the bar over his bed that he used to lift to train his arms is thick and sticky with dirt. Sir, this place is not a fit hospital for these poor souls. There are some men without the use of their arms and cannot chase the flies off their faces." The Minister of Health acknowledged this woman's letter and said it would be looked into, but no further information about this matter has been located.[68] This episode indicates that conditions were, at times, very unpleasant for some patients. A former paraplegic patient who was admitted only two months after this letter was written had quite different memories of the physical set-up of a place he called "the most amazing mansion. When I was first there the ceilings had big circles and alcoves in carved wood with paintings in the centre. After I was there they painted it all white with these individual oil paintings in dark wood."[69] Margaret Staton, another former paraplegic patient, recalled the "atmosphere at Lyndhurst was different at different times of year, cold as hell in the winter, though as a child I loved the snow. It was an old house that had a homey atmosphere."[70] Dr Henry Barnett was a neurologist at the TGH from 1952 to 1970 and visited Lyndhurst on numerous occasions as a medical consultant. He remembered that it "was a bustling, busy place. I don't remember it as a place that was squeaky clean and immaculate and beautifully tiled, polished floors and furniture. It was a well-used place. It wasn't dirty and it wasn't shabby."[71]

These varied perspectives on the conditions at Lyndhurst help to reveal how the built environment of such a facility could leave such vastly different impressions on patients and visitors alike. Some remembered how physical barriers within Lyndhurst were used as part of the rehabilitation program. Nowhere is this more evident than in people's recollections of one obstacle in particular. Gordon Paterson remembered "the ramp going down to the gymnasium ... was the steepest ramp that you ever laid eyes on." When a person in a wheelchair "got to the bottom of it there was a wall right there." As a twenty-year-old paraplegic, he was able to go up and down the ramp without any assistance. "But that was the challenge to the paras like, 'When can I go down that thing?' So [you] had to pop it on your back wheels and then down you would go and stop dead at the bottom and turn and drop your wheels back down. I will never forget the first time I was able to pump up the ramp without using the handrail ... I used it as a challenge. You know when you get to the top you're really pumping; you say, 'Wow! Did I do that?'"[72]

Other former paraplegic patients remembered manoeuvring the steep ramp as a goal they were expected to meet. Margaret Staton, on the other hand, said "I never saw it as a challenge and thought that if the men could do it I could do it too."[73] Marilyn Noell, a quadriplegic patient at Lyndhurst during the early 1950s was "petrified" when she first saw it.[74] Evelyn Paul recalled: "The steep ramp was just a method of taking patients from one level to the other ... It would be ... about thirty feet long and everybody who went to George [White's] classes had to go down this ramp. If they were paraplegic they were expected to take themselves down the ramp and to take themselves up the ramp. It was a part of the program of building upper body strength, but the quads you had to help up and down."[75] Paul's colleague, Betty Brooks, remembered it as "*the* steepest ramp that I have ever seen in my life and there was a wall at the end of it ... on an angle of about a forty five degrees at least, if not more. You had to wear rubber-soled shoes if you were going to take anybody down or up the ramp because they would end up in the wall ... I would say there would probably be six feet of space between the bottom of the ramp and the wall. Not even that! That was maximum. So you had to make a quick right turn or you were in serious trouble ... a few [patients] hit the wall ... I must say it kept me in shape for skiing, pushing some of those patients up that ramp. It was not easy ... A couple of times I had the wrong shoes on and literally slid down behind them. I learned my lesson very, very quickly. Wear good rubber-soled shoes."[76]

The physical environment could also be experienced in different ways by men and women patients. "I was one of the few women there during these early years," Margaret Staton recalled. "Women were on the second floor where there were twelve beds. I didn't much like the elevator to the second floor but I was able to get around by pushing my own wheelchair as I was strong and feisty ... As someone on the first floor [where the men's quarters were] became more independent they went into another wing, so there was a physical change in location for men on the first floor. For women whose quarters were on the second floor, we stayed in whichever bed we were admitted to. For women, it wasn't as clear when it came to becoming more independent, as it was for men at Lyndhurst."[77] The elevator was an essential service for all the women patients who were housed on the second floor, whereas the men patients on the first floor did not have to use it nearly as often, only when going up one floor for a meeting with a doctor. Betty Brooks recalled that "the women, God bless their souls, were upstairs and they had to take the elevator which had the heaviest door in the whole world ... To open the door to that elevator was a major feat ... because it was heavy. So if they could open that door to that elevator and get in the elevator themselves, they had really accomplished something."[78]

The physical environment also provided plenty of opportunities for male patients to indulge in perhaps the most frequently mentioned activity that involved breaking the rules: drinking beer. Officially, it was not allowed on the premises, though off premises people could do whatever they liked. Gordon Paterson recalled beer-drinking that took place when he was a patient in the second half of the 1950s when he would have "a couple of pints of beer" on the weekend. Beer was smuggled in at night through the back door when no staff were nearby.

They were placed under Paterson's cushion. Once in his room he would hide beer underneath his bed blanket. Dr Jousse walked in one morning after a bit of smuggling, sat down on the bed just inches away from the beer, and proceeded to "push them aside." Though he could not see them as they were under the blanket "he knew what the hell it was." Then he asked, "How are you doing boys?" Gordon Paterson said drinking was never "out of hand" while he was there, though tossing away the empty beer bottles into the nearby ravine had become something of a local tradition. By the mid-1950s when he was there, a decade of empty beer bottles had accumulated just off Lyndhurst's property. "Back in those days you couldn't throw a beer bottle into the ravine because it would hit another beer bottle from years gone by."[79]

Bev Hallam remembered the assistant medical director's strict approach to drinking. When Dr Jousse was on holiday Dr Geisler would come down to mat classes on Monday morning and "request that all the booze bottles be deposited at the nurses desk immediately. Always somebody would say: 'And do you want the empties too?'"[80] Margaret MacDonald remembered a somewhat more laid-back approach to dealing with casual drinking: "Oh sometimes they would like to have a drink. I didn't say anything as long as they weren't unruly. But if I saw it, of course, I had to confiscate the bottle and I said, 'Oh this hurts me more than you,' when I pour it down the sink. One of the boys said 'Miss MacDonald that sink gets spasms all night long. I couldn't sleep from the whiskey' … That was his joke, that I caused the spasms by throwing his whiskey away."[81]

Patients were not the only people to drink on the premises; staff did it too – at Christmas parties, when it would hardly have been an infraction of the rules. Evelyn Paul remembered how drinks were kept cold by "putting them in the back of the toilet. You know where the water was flushing (laughs) … bottles of wine. Months and months later we started to have problems with the toilet and we wondered what was going on and the plumber came in and opened the back of the toilet and found a couple of bottles still in it that we had forgotten about."[82] Beer bottles raining down on the nearby ravine and wine being stored in a toilet gives an idea of how people used the cramped quarters in which they lived and worked for some rather unorthodox purposes. In addition to hijinks and letting off steam, at times Lyndhurst lent itself to more sombre occasions. Peggy Hicks, Lyndhurst secretary during the 1950s, and another woman employee would stand on the front balcony, wave a flag, and salute veterans as they were transferred to long-term care in Sunnybrook Hospital.[83]

For some people, returning to the community would be an elusive dream. For others, efforts to reintegrate dealt with a barrier that architecture could not easily alleviate: social attitudes. Mabel Brown recalled she felt so "conspicuous ... terrified and embarrassed" when she first started going outside Lyndhurst in a wheelchair. The way people approached her was so distressing that she told a friend: "If you see someone coming towards me, please turn the wheelchair around and let's go in the other direction."[84]

A public occasion where people with wheelchairs were welcomed, instead of gawked at, was the annual CPA dinner. These events began during the late 1940s and continued into the 1970s at the Royal York Hotel in downtown Toronto. An inexpensive meal in the main ballroom was arranged by hotel management and the CPA arranged to pay for any Lyndhurst patient who could not afford it. Entertainers from the United States and Canada, such as comedian Dave Broadfoot, donated their services. This event became a yearly reunion for Lyndhurst alumnae. It was also a compulsory event for all new Lyndhurst inpatients. People who had been recently disabled could see other people with spinal cord injuries who had gone on in life after their time at Lyndhurst. Katie Barton, whose mother, Nanette Cassels, helped to arrange piano music for this event, recalled that people "came from everywhere" for the dinner. "Sunnybrook and all over and in different stages of health ... It worked out beautifully."[85] These dinners were thus partly relaxation and partly another way of showing the world and each other that people with disabilities were part of the community too.

Ken Langford recalled overcoming another sort of barrier when he and his wife Mary were trying to adopt a son in the early 1950s. "In my case, the Children's Aid in Toronto would have nothing to do with paraplegics adopting children ... In fact I recall there were some documents that needed to be sworn there. They had a lawyer that was upstairs in their offices and he wouldn't even come downstairs to see me ... I think why was mainly that they [thought paraplegics] couldn't teach the child to play baseball or swimming or any more or less active activities."[86]

John Yaremko, Minister in the Ontario Conservative Government of Leslie Frost, stepped in to help get some papers signed for the Langfords to adopt a baby boy. From 1951 to 1975 Yaremko was the member of provincial parliament for Lyndhurst's riding and he lived literally a few feet across the lane from Lyndhurst Lodge and the head office of the CPA. Over the years he held eight portfolios in various provincial Conservative governments, including responsibility for people with disabilities. He was an avid booster of Lyndhurst throughout this quarter-century in government. Yaremko described his house as "a sort of open house" for Lyndhurst residents. "One day I returned from work and there were several residents of the Lodge over at our house bobbing for apples in the kitchen where my wife was visiting with them."[87] Yaremko's fortuitous location gives an added dimension to how the physical location of this facility benefited the people who lived and worked there. He said that this close proximity allowed him to see paraplegics moving about in wheelchairs. It was an eye-opener for him to learn about their abilities and influenced him to promote provincial support for people with disabilities. Thus Lyndhurst had a good friend in the provincial government who lived almost literally in their own backyard.

Yet for every John Yaremko who was willing to have their eyes opened there were others who kept the barriers firmly in place. Part of this was because of many of the societal prejudices that disabled people then encountered. It was also because of plain ignorance of what the word "paraplegic" meant, as Gordon Paterson recalled. "We use to go to a show up there called the Vaughan Theatre ... I remember one of the physios took this one kid who was 13 years old or 14 years old to a show up there. He always used to get out of his chair and sit on the aisle seat and some people would come to get in and of course he couldn't stand up to let them by. A woman was giving him hell because he didn't get up out of the row. The physio would come down and say, 'He's a paraplegic!' And she said, 'I don't give a shit what religion he is, he's still a little brat.'"[88] Years of work still lay ahead to educate people like this movie-goer about what spinal cord injury meant.

In the meantime, Lyndhurst and the CPA had plenty of work to do to ensure that people who had gone through rehabilitation were able to pursue their own education. One step was to establish an in-house school classroom at the lodge in 1951. The first tutor hired was Glenn Jewett, who had been a high-school teacher before World War II. He was himself a paraplegic veteran and had been a resident of Lyndhurst in late 1945. Unlike everyone else who worked there, he was not an employee of the CPA but was hired by the Ontario Department of Education. This was crucial for his students to obtain credit for their upgrading. School hours during the mid-1950s were from 1:30 p.m. to 5 p.m., after the daily rehabilitation program was finished for the roughly eight students who used these tutorial services at a given time. From 1951 to 1955 only one teacher and one student could fit into the tiny canteen then used as a classroom. However, renovations in the mid-1950s provided more space. Various topics were taught, including math, literacy skills, and typing.[89] A quadriplegic in-patient, Bill V., who was taught by Jewett, in turn also tutored fellow residents.[90] Students who undertook schooling outside Lyndhurst, whether it was high school or post-secondary, were aided by CPA vocational counsellors. Jim Bartlett had been employed in this capacity since 1949 and in December 1962 he was joined by Ross Beggs.[91] Together, they helped people to find jobs, educational programs, and places to live in the community. Bartlett "had what he called 'the money back guarantee' ... He said to a prospective employer: 'If this chap isn't completely satisfactory as an employee, just let *me* know and I'll remove him to avoid any embarrassment on *your* part.' I think he had quite a number of employers who asked if he had any more people, but I don't think that he ever had any that were dissatisfied. Jim was pretty careful to place people where they would be helpful."[92] This point indicates the vulnerability of people with disabilities when it came to keeping their jobs over the long term.

An ex-patient who found re-employment in a former job was literally broadcasting the good news. This was especially important, as many people lost their former jobs permanently after becoming disabled. Cam Langford had been a radio announcer in the early 1950s when an auto accident left him quadriplegic. While still a Lyndhurst out-patient he returned to his old job. Among other topics, Langford aired stories about Lyndhurst Lodge and the people who lived and worked there. He also made a skeleton for display at the Canadian National Exhibition to explain anatomical features of the spinal cord with various electrodes lighting it up.[93] While Cam Langford was going out over the airwaves, another lodge graduate, William O'Connor, a paraplegic, was writing stories for newspapers in his hometown of Buffalo, New York. His articles on employment for physically disabled people led to a citation from President Eisenhower.[94] Phyllis Bent had polio and used a wheelchair to get around. After leaving Lyndhurst, she found a job in the reservations department of the forerunner of Air Canada, Trans-Canada Airlines. Eventually, she became head of their telecommunications department, which she ran until she was replaced by computers.[95] Still other Lyndhurst graduates moved in together to offer mutual support as they sought new careers. Four male ex-patients moved into living quarters in the High Park area of Toronto; three of them were attending Shaw Business School while the fourth was reported out looking for work.[96] CPA counsellors at Lyndhurst were an important bridge between the lodge and the outside community for many of these individuals.

Jim Bartlett's new colleague in the early 1960s, Ross Beggs, was considered "a bit of a godsend" by Bev Hallam. "We became fairly good buddies throughout that period. He was a real help. He helped me get my first apartment when I was ready for that after a couple of years in boarding houses. And he helped me to get into [Ryerson] university ... He was a pretty straight shooter. He didn't pull any punches ... He assessed your situation, what you were up against, what you might be able to do and what you should do and that kind of stuff ... He became kind of the leader or the head worker in that regard."[97]

Yet while people like Bev Hallam were returning to the community, finding jobs and getting on with life after leaving Lyndhurst, the place they left behind was in dire need of an overhaul. The cramped living and working quarters could be both homey and nerve-wracking, with so many people crowded into such a small space doing so many different, intensive activities. By the early 1960s the search was on to find somewhere new. Having firmly established their reputation for rehabilitation, the operators of Lyndhurst Lodge began to make plans for relocation to more spacious quarters. As will be seen in the next chapter, it was a goal that would take another ten years to realize. In the meantime, life at 153 Lyndhurst Avenue was set to continue on its already well-trodden path for another decade.

4

The Longest Decade, 1964–74

"I remember being brought in on a stretcher and looking around. I was looking up and I could see all these sort of carved ceilings, and tiles and these great big windows, decorative windows. I thought: 'This is strange. This isn't like a normal hospital.' I remember going in this rickety little elevator and going to the upstairs."[1] Kathy Drummond's earliest memories of Lyndhurst Lodge in 1968, when she was admitted to live on the second floor with other women patients, provide a window onto the last years of the old building and a patient's experience of the lodge. During the three years that she lived there, plans were being pursued to replace the increasingly "rickety" facility with a building that would be more "like a normal hospital." This was far from easy. For the ten years covered by this chapter Lyndhurst Lodge operated in a state of limbo. There was a good deal of waiting and wondering. When would a new building replace the old? While this truly was the longest decade in Lyndhurst's history, people who lived and worked there had plenty to do besides wait and wonder as 153 Lyndhurst Avenue served out its last years as a rehabilitation centre.

CRAMPED QUARTERS AND
FUTURE PLANS

Plans to improve on Lyndhurst Lodge's cramped quarters began to develop during the early 1960s. Discussion about increasing bed space picked up with a proposal in May 1961 to raise the number from fifty-two to seventy beds. The Ontario Hospital Services Commission (OHSC) had agreed to this expansion "in principle" by June 1962, though the estimated $1,500,000 (later increased to $1,750,000) needed to build this addition had to be raised before final provincial approval would be given. Unlike when the original use of the building was proposed in 1944, neighbours along Lyndhurst Avenue were supportive of this proposal eighteen years later. However, objections were soon raised in other quarters much closer to home. In November 1963 J.D. Woods noted that the large amount of money that would need to be raised for a comparatively small site was less than enticing for potential fundraisers. Most important were the concerns raised by Dr Jousse. He pointed out that it was "a great deal of money" to "restore and extend" the existing facilities with an increase of only eighteen more beds. The east wing, which was to be demolished, was "cold and drafty" in winter and its replacement was necessary to improve patient care. However, the location of a new east wing would be difficult to expand beyond the size of the old wing because of its location along the ravine, which limited where they could put the desired new pool and gymnasium. A year later a new location much closer to Sunnybrook Hospital in the northeast end of Toronto had been found: the Divadale property, close to the Divadale Convalescent Hospital. By November 1964 a consensus had emerged that the old Lyndhurst property was not suitable for future expansion. Thus, the CPA board decided to purchase the larger, almost five-acre, site (as opposed to the three acres on Lyndhurst Avenue). This would allow for more room and for a purpose-built facility, and would eliminate the frustrations caused by space limitation at the original site.[2]

So began a train of events that developed over the longest decade in Lyndhurst history – planning, waiting for, and building a completely new hospital. In 1965 the CPA annual report observed that waiting to get into Lyndhurst combined with inadequate teaching facilities made establishing a "new and larger hospital building more urgent."[3] As it turned out, this urgency would take a back seat to the exigencies of time, money, and bureaucratic sloth at the provincial Ministry of Health. It was not until October 1967 that the OHSC approved "in principle" the first stages of proceeding with plans to build a new spinal cord treatment facility, beginning with submission of a plan.[4] The CPA operators of Lyndhurst wrote that these delays "set the paraplegic or quadriplegic patient back physically and mentally and, indeed, irreparable harm may be done,"[5] showing their frustration with the glacial pace of getting the building plans to move beyond the very earliest stages of development. These delays affected the internal operation of the hospital in turn.

The physical condition of Lyndhurst during this period was a challenge to staff and especially, of course, to the patients. Reports in the
spring of 1966 offer telling evidence of why a new place was so badly
needed. A provincial auditor wrote that while the Lyndhurst accountant "does a conscientious job" she had problems because of her lack
of authority in this position. Furthermore, she worked on the third
floor of the house, which was inaccessible to her supervisors in the CPA
because of their spinal cord injuries.[6] Bringing administrative positions
together in an accessible building was therefore crucial. More importantly, the daily housekeeping standards of the hospital were judged to
be in serious need of an overhaul. Excluding the basement, 34,000
square feet required upkeep. Noting that "patients wander about in
wheelchairs until midnight," the provincial consultant wrote that
places other than bedrooms were cleaned in the early hours of the
morning when patients were in bed. The floors were reported to be in
generally poor shape after twenty-one years of continual use in a rehabilitation centre. Improving the training of cleaning staff and increasing the hours devoted to housekeeping were seen as essential to
addressing these problems.[7] The floors were still creaking away when
Ed Ratelle worked at Lyndhurst in the early 1970s. As people went
about the old building, on rounds or at any other time, the old wooden
floors creaked in some places as someone walked or wheeled over
them.[8] A co-worker of Ratelle, Gavin Shanks, was a post-graduate
trainee in rehabilitation medicine when he was a resident at Lyndhurst
Lodge. He referred to it as "a homey, somewhat run down, once grand
mansion." Too hot in the summer and too cold in the winter, "It wasn't
an ideal place. The therapy area wasn't ideal either ... But you can do
good work if you have good people."[9]

What was it like for patients who lived in these surroundings? Lucille
Fortier (later Owen) was a post-polio patient who was admitted twice
to Lyndhurst in the mid-1960s after back surgery. The first floor was
more attractive with its "lovely wood panelled reception rooms ... high
ceilings and hardwood floors." But the rest of the facility was "typi-
cally institutional" with bland furniture and fittings. Getting up to the
women's quarters meant taking an elevator which had an "old-
fashioned sliding grille door" and another heavy outside door that was
not easy to deal with. This caused difficulties for quadriplegics who
had to wait for someone to get them in and out; she said the technology
existed at that time to give quadriplegics "the same freedom of movement as the paraplegics," but it was not used for the lift. Once up on

the second floor it was "like a rabbit warren," with beds for twelve women in three inter-connected rooms. To get to the second and third rooms, a person had to go through the preceding space. Forget privacy, especially for the women in the first room. There was not much closet space either, though an ironing board was on hand. The only problem was that when it was used it blocked the entrance to another room. "I happened to be in the last room in back and when I came in late on weekends, I had to try to manoeuvre past parked wheelchairs without hitting them. Everyone knew what time I got in – it was like having eight mothers." In spite of all this, "the female patients got on very well together."[10]

A woman patient admitted several years later remembered that, like Lucille Fortier Owen, she too did not like the lack of privacy in the old building. Kathy Drummond recalled not having bed curtains when dressing, which "was a real problem and it bothered me at first. I was used to having my own room and privacy." For all of the problems with the old mansion, Drummond saw it is as having positive attributes, partly because it was far from ideal. While it "certainly wasn't all homey and fun and games" she did feel Lyndhurst operators made the most of what was available to them. Since it was not set up for wheelchairs, she felt it prepared her to deal with the world outside. "So this was very good experience for coping when you go into a standard bathroom. How do you use the tap? How do you get your hair washed? How to use the toilet? There's lots of places that aren't set up at all with the raised toilets ... and wheel under [sinks] and wheel in showers and all that. It's getting better now than then but there still are a lot of places that aren't. So I think that it was very good training for us in that way."[11]

Thus for some people, feelings were mixed about the state of the old place. But the people who ran Lyndhurst had no doubt that it was time to find better accommodations. In the meantime, they had to make do.

Part of the problem with the declining state of the facilities was due to uncertainty over when the new building would open. According to OHSC representative K.A. Torrance, "What had happened is that each year the hospital thinks will be their last in these premises, consequently things are let go."[12] To help organize the administration of the hospital more effectively, J.S.T. Rajan was hired as administrator in 1966; the previous administrator, L.B. Morrison, had held this job for fourteen years until his retirement.[13] At this time a general re-organization of administrative duties began to be implemented at the instigation of the

OHSC. The five medical doctors on staff had much less responsibility than before for administrative duties, instead focusing on patient care, while bureaucratic duties increasingly came under the jurisdiction of administrator Rajan. As well, in line with earlier recommendations, a housekeeping supervisor and another cleaning-staff member were hired in the summer of 1966.[14] Nevertheless, Lyndhurst continued to be largely run by Dr Jousse and the CPA. A report in early 1967 observed that Administrator Rajan's duties were "somewhat restricted," with a management chart only then being designed to set out who was responsible for what.[15]

With the OHSC scrutinizing Lyndhurst's costs much more than ever before, tensions were bound to arise. In one instance, Jousse wrote to the OHSC in support of increasing the salary of the gardener for 1967. With his letter he enclosed a four-page compilation of this employee's duties, one page for each season, with the percentage of time spent on each task. So we learn that the Lyndhurst gardener spent 3 per cent of his time in the spring "Painting of benches, waste-baskets, machinery, etc" and another 4 per cent on "Paper-work – Designing [flower] beds, reading up on new varieties, insecticides, fungicides, herbicides, etc." In the summer he spent 20 per cent of his time mowing the lawns and 2.5 per cent "Pinching of flowers." In the fall 35 per cent of his time was spent raking leaves and 1 per cent on "Using ant and grub killer on [flower] beds and ant hills." In the winter, 30.5 per cent of the gardener's time was spent on snow removal, 25 per cent on "Sewing gym mats," 10 cent on "Venetian-blind washing," 3 per cent "Putting up and taking down Christmas decorations" and .5 per cent on "Getting of materials, gas oil, etc." Various extra jobs were also noted, including removing "wild grapes" and doing tree surgery to cut out "rotted cavities."[16] Three months later, the OHSC agreed to Jousse's request.[17]

This detailed list in support of a salary increase for an employee well down on the pecking order tells us something about the medical director's efforts to stick up for employees whom he clearly valued. It can also be seen as a clever form of satire on Jousse's part. In effect it was a savvy response to the very specific requests for information that the province had been demanding for months prior to this; two can play at this game, Jousse seems to be saying – "You want details! I will give you details!" Differences in interpretation of what certain items were needed for could literally cost Lyndhurst money. An elevator installed in 1956 was recorded by the hospital as a depreciation cost requiring $5,755.12 in reimbursement from the OHSC. However the government insisted this cost was not to be allowed as the elevator was instead classified as "general service equipment" rather than "hospital equipment for patient care." This conclusion was arrived at even though it was explained that the elevator to the women's rooms and doctor's offices on the second floor were installed "only because all patients are paraplegic" making it essential for people, not equipment.[18]

Through all of these administrative difficulties, the composition of the hospital's wards stayed the same, with fifty-two beds divided into three wards: twelve women upstairs and forty men on the ground floor, of whom twenty-four were on the old ward and sixteen in the newer ward built in the mid-1950s. OHSC nursing inspector, Louise Jamieson, wrote in the fall of 1967 that the facilities were in poor shape, with no office space for the director of nursing, no conference room, and confusion in the organization of the hospital.[19] Such reports make it evident that until Lyndhurst was able to modernize, its reputation for rehabilitation was in danger of decline, because of the conditions in which patients and staff lived and worked. A new building could not come too soon.

The ice finally began to melt in 1968, at least for a short while, before it froze again. The new Lyndhurst Hospital was categorized in early 1968 as a Regional Rehabilitation Centre by the OHSC Planning Committee so that it would be entitled to the largest amount of provincial funding.[20] A detailed written plan was submitted to the OHSC by the CPA in June of that year. With uncharacteristic speed the Ministry responded in August requesting more information. The CPA complied, submitting another report in November 1968.[21] In February 1969 the planning committee of the OHSC approved "in principle" the new building project, but the plan remained on hold for the entire year because of budgetary constraints imposed on hospital buildings by the provincial government.[22] Not until the early 1970s did the logjam break at last and construction on a new hospital began. But before taking this part of the story to its conclusion, developments in other areas of this historic hospital need to be examined.

A SURVEY OF IN-PATIENTS AND DEVELOPMENTS IN REHABILITATION

As the owners of Lyndhurst worked towards providing a new building to better serve people with spinal cord injuries, they continued to make do with the existing facilities for the never-ending influx of patients.

Throughout the decade covered in this chapter, Lyndhurst's wards were constantly full as is indicated by the following statistical summary. While in 1965 eighty-eight people were discharged from Lyndhurst, of whom seventy had traumatic spinal cord injuries, by 1967 the number of people discharged rose by almost 60 per cent to 147; 122 of these had suffered a traumatic injury. Quadriplegics comprised nearly 30 per cent of the total, while paraplegics made up 63 per cent. Thus, by the second half of the 1960s, patients with spinal cord injuries comprised the overwhelming number of patients, at 93 per cent. Other disabilities, most obviously polio, which only a few years before had been the third highest patient group after paraplegia and quadriplegia, had significantly reduced in numbers. Lyndhurst Lodge, to a greater extent than at any time since the late 1940s, housed people from the disability group for whom it had originally been established two decades earlier. Sixty per cent of people discharged had been first-time admissions who averaged nine months stay for spinal cord injuries, though the range was anywhere from over sixteen months for complete quadriplegics to around five months for paraplegics.[23]

By the end of the decade patient population figures reveal how these trends remained consistent. Of 136 patients discharged in 1969, 97 per cent had either quadriplegia or paraplegia. For the first time since polio patients began arriving in the late 1940s, no one with this disability was among in-patient population admissions.[24] However, several post-polio patients were in-patients during the early 1970s, so their presence was not entirely at an end.[25] In 1971, unlike earlier years, the published total number of patients included people who were discharged as well as people who remained in the hospital. Of a total of 141 in-patients for the entire year, 89 per cent were people with spinal cord injuries; 50 per cent were paraplegics; and 39 per cent were quadriplegics.[26] Two years later quadriplegics made up the largest group of in-patients at 43 per cent compared to 37.5 per cent for paraplegics; the facility was as busy as always in 1974 as the old building was replaced by the new.[27] Thus during the last decade at the old building, Lyndhurst Lodge continued to be crowded with people and activity even though the building became increasingly unsuitable as a rehabilitation centre. Small wonder that so much effort was put into getting on with building a new place, when the old building, which was never intended to house such large numbers all year long, was strained to its limits.

What brought many of these people to Lyndhurst? To provide more complete answers to this question than were then available, a compre-

hensive analysis was undertaken of the causes of spinal cord injuries in
Ontario during 1969 and 1970. This study, which was eventually published in 1975, found that the largest number of spinal cord injuries
were caused by road accidents (43 per cent), followed by industrial
accidents (18 per cent) and sport injuries (17 per cent). Young men in
particular were affected, as they engaged in the sort of physical activities or risky behaviour, such as fast car driving, that could lead to a spinal cord injury. So it is not surprising that the majority of the 224
people who made up the total number of spinal cord injured in Ontario
during 1969 and 1970 were males (82 per cent); Friday and Saturday
afternoons in the summer were peak accident times. These figures
explain the consistently higher number of males who arrived at
Lyndhurst in comparison to females. By 1974 nearly half of the 15 per
cent of people who died as a result of their injuries in 1969–70 had succumbed within fourteen days of their injury. The vast majority of these
fatalities were quadriplegics (87.5 per cent), with respiratory failure
being the main cause of death.[28]

Part of the serious problems affecting both the level of injury and
mortality was that Ontario is such a large province with widely sepa-
rated spaces where treatment facilities are often a long distance away.
It was not at all uncommon for an injured person's spinal cord to be
further damaged during the process of lifting and transporting the person from the site of injury to a hospital. The authors concluded their
analysis with a call for the establishment of more comprehensive "total
management" from the first hours of injury, when speedy and safe
transferral to a hospital was deemed crucial, to "life-time follow-up"
of the injured person.[29] This "total management" concept was to include
improved bladder treatment. Dr Gavin Shanks, an intern at Lyndhurst
in 1970, recalled that "urinary problems were a big deal" when he was
there. People stayed at the lodge for a long time because of "recurring
urinary inflections, bladder infections and kidney infections." Since a
good deal of emphasis was placed on a person's difficulty in urinating,
patients would get a catheter or leg bag to empty their bladder. It
was quite common for people to develop infections from long-term
in-dwelling catheters, which sometimes led to blood poisoning and sep-
ticemia. Eventually, more effective means of voiding were found, which
reduced these serious complications.[30] In the meantime, efforts were
underway at Lyndhurst and elsewhere to address some of the short-
comings that existed in spinal cord injury treatment in the province.

Another "big deal" during this period was obtaining timely access to treatment services, as was explained by the authors of the above-cited survey. Their advocacy of a province-wide system of regional facilities for acute care of paraplegics and quadriplegics reveals something about the constantly changing role that Lyndhurst was seen as having to play. By the early to mid-1970s Lyndhurst's formerly pre-eminent place in the province for the rehabilitation of patients with spinal cord injuries was giving way to the realization that more places like it were needed, even if on a smaller scale, to improve the treatment of such individuals. Already, by the second half of the 1960s, Lyndhurst's medical staff was actively involved in helping to move this objective forward.

In early 1968 Dr Jousse reported that "a great many patients" were waiting to get into Lyndhurst, because of a lack of accommodation at the rehabilitation centre and in general hospitals, where beds for acute care were in short supply. Besides advocating a new and larger facility to replace the original Lyndhurst, Jousse promoted the development of new rehabilitation services under Dr Peter Cameron in London and under Dr David Symington in Kingston.[31] Symington had arrived in Kingston, Ontario, in 1966, taking a position to start the Department of Rehabilitation Medicine at Queen's University.

Like others, Symington remarked on Lyndhurst's situation in 1966 and how if affected people with spinal cord injuries: "The spirit of the place was really gung-ho. But I know it was always crowded. We needed many more facilities. When I came to Kingston, for instance, there was a patient there who had been waiting two years with a C6 quadriplegia to go to Lyndhurst." By the summer of 1967 the first patients with spinal cord injuries began to be admitted to an acute care ward set up for this purpose in Kingston General Hospital. The first admission was the man who had been waiting for an opening at Lyndhurst. In the process of setting up the rehabilitation program in Kingston, the advice and experience of the CPA, Lyndhurst's staff, and in particular of Dr Jousse, were very important, according to Symington. Regular meetings between the two physicians (as well as with Queen's University Dean of Medicine, Harry Botterell) from 1966 to the early 1970s were crucial in giving the younger doctor input on how to establish rehabilitation services and a related academic program in Kingston. "What Lyndhurst did was more than spinal cord injury. It was a model of rehab and you can take that model and you can use it for amputees, for head injury and so on and so forth ... There was an unselfishness ...

about Al Jousse and Lyndhurst. They didn't say, 'We want it all for ourselves!' They were willing to encourage us."[32]

Eventually this model helped to influence the establishment of rehabilitation services in Ottawa, Hamilton, and London. Some patients from these areas continued to go to Lyndhurst. The establishment of regional acute care for people with spinal cord injuries in Ontario during the late 1960s and the 1970s, though on a smaller scale than existed in Toronto, was important to providing more timely treatment for people who otherwise may have had to wait for years to get into the Lyndhurst rehabilitation program. All of this reflects how the coordinated social organization of medical care and therapy, organized by public and medical officials, could be as essential as clinical advances in influencing the long-term prospects for people with spinal cord injuries. Pressure on Lyndhurst for waiting beds was therefore somewhat alleviated by these developments.

However, certain developments related to medical services ensured that pressure on the Toronto rehabilitation facility was felt from other quarters. Sunnybrook Hospital was turned over to the University of Toronto by the DVA in October 1965, thus opening it to the wider public. Spinal cord injury services there continued as before.[33] Since this hospital opened in 1949 drugs and medical supplies had been supplied to Lyndhurst through Sunnybrook, at prices Lyndhurst found reasonable while it was a DVA hospital. However, after the University of Toronto took it over, these costs increased significantly, so much so that the CPA wrote a "vigorous protest" to the OHSC when they disallowed well over $5,000 in medical supplies for 1967. The province also wanted back another $3,000 in salaries for medical secretaries, which the OHSC had previously approved, all of which raised the ire of the CPA board of directors.[34] These financial problems could not have come at a worse time.

The financial situation at Lyndhurst had deteriorated to such an extent that the CPA lent the lodge $20,000 to help pay the bills; by the end of 1968 accounts payable were four months overdue.[35] This loan was written off as unrecoverable several months later.[36] Provincial policies contributed to these difficulties. Jousse noted the adverse effect on patient care of spending cuts in Ontario in 1970. Reductions in staff at acute care hospitals led to less attention on wards, which Jousse felt "may be the reason why recent admissions to Lyndhurst from other hospitals have had more complications such as bed sores than formerly. This increases the load on our own treatment staff and makes their task more difficult and less satisfying."[37] In early 1972 staff cutbacks at

Sunnybrook led to the cancellation of all but emergency dental care for Lyndhurst patients.[38] Prior to this, Lyndhurst patients were routinely sent to the dental clinics at both the TGH and Sunnybrook. While some disabled people had dentists in the Toronto area, steps often made their offices inaccessible, so they went to public hospital clinics; the CPA paid for these dental appointments, which were not insured.[39]

Besides providing dental treatment, the TGH played another major role in relation to Lyndhurst's services. During this period, acute care was available at the TGH paraplegic unit. Workmen's Compensation Board patients had six to eight beds there in the private patients' pavilion, which was originally set up in 1946.[40] However patients with spinal cord injuries who did not come under the auspices of the WCB were kept on public wards at first until a ward for their care was established. Dr Geisler explained that this unit was created after it was found that when Lyndhurst patients were sent to the TGH for treatment of such things as urological surgery or a heart condition, their bladder and bowel management would be "dismal." Some of these patients were returned to Lyndhurst with pressure sores. In others words, while their acute symptoms would be looked after, treatment specific to their spinal cord injury would regress. To ensure that they received total care to prevent such problems, a spinal cord injury active treatment unit was established in the private patients' pavilion with the support of Dr Botterell during the 1950s. It operated through the TGH Department of Rehabilitation and Physical Medicine under the direction of Dr W.J. Gardiner until 1968; he was succeeded by Dr Geisler in 1969. When the Toronto General was merged in 1986 with Toronto Western Hospital this arrangement ceased because of hospital restructuring.[41] Geisler was in charge of the day-to-day treatment of people on this unit, which was covered by OHIP. He recalled that eight to ten physicians would be working on a fifty-bed ward. On an average work day Geisler would be responsible for up to six patients, of whom there "might be one spinal cord injured patient." After treatment was completed at the TGH, the individual was returned to Lyndhurst.[42]

In one instance a Lyndhurst patient on the TGH acute care ward did more than lie passively in bed. Geisler recalled how a man in a room with five other patients had persuaded the nurse to provide him with a privacy screen. A few minutes later, as other patients laughed away, tell-tale moans and groans from behind the screen revealed that this man and his wife were having sex. They wanted to have a baby. Geisler informed them after they emerged from behind the screen that it was not possible for a paraplegic male at that time to father a child, so the wife of this patient did not get pregnant.[43] It would be several more decades before advances were made to fulfill this natural desire to be a biological parent, though too late for this couple. Bev Hallam recalled what it was like to be a patient on this ward up to the last time he was there in the mid-1960s: "I wound up in [the TGH] a couple of times to do a tendon transplant to make the hand a better grip. And the odd pressure sore. I broke a leg once ... The hospitals don't have any units like that now. But it was good for acute care if you had to go to a general hospital. *The* place to be."[44] But not everyone chose to go there.

Mrs B. was one Lyndhurst patient who did not want to be admitted to the TGH for an operation. Originally from Britain, she had fallen off a mountain in China and eventually made her way to the Toronto rehabilitation centre. TGH neurologist and Lyndhurst consultant Dr Henry Barnett recalled, "She declined and went home to England [where] she died totally helpless in a chronic care hospital." Dr Jousse then sent him to obtain her spinal cord. Together with medical colleagues, Jousse and Barnett learned more about the physical condition of this woman, whose death was caused by post-traumatic syringomyelia. This condition develops when a cavity forms and fills with fluid in a paraplegic patient who has suffered trauma at the fourth vertebrae or lower. Eventually, the fluid progresses up the spine; this leads to a higher level of paralysis and can cause a paraplegic to become quadriplegic. It was a rare condition during this period – among 729 paraplegics at Lyndhurst thirteen (under 2 per cent) developed it.[45] Understanding post-traumatic syringomyelia helped to increase knowledge of how paralysis progressed and it also led to an operation to treat this condition. According to Barnett, "this was a major contribution to knowledge that Al Jousse made. I was delighted to be associated with him on this because if these people are left, they were like Mrs. B ... [They] die helpless. It was not necessary."[46] Though the experiences of Mrs B. during her stay at Lyndhurst are unknown, the stories of others are known and help to shed light on what it was like to be a patient during the last years of the old lodge.

PATIENT LIFE INSIDE AND OUTSIDE
153 LYNDHURST AVENUE

While plans to develop a new hospital dominated the decade, patients who lived at Lyndhurst during the last ten years at 153 Lyndhurst continued, as before, to deal with issues that many of their peers had to deal with before them. However, as will become evident, some issues began to be talked about more openly as the decade wore on and as the world outside changed. For some, adjusting to life back in the community as a disabled person was a daunting prospect, especially when the world presented challenges both inside and outside their family home.

Therese Proietti

Therese Proietti was married with two small children, one under two years old, when she had two operations to remove a tumour on her spine at St Josesph's Hospital in Toronto. For physiotherapy, she went to Lyndhurst, where she was an in-patient for six months at the end of 1964 and the beginning of 1965. As with some of the other people interviewed for this book, she did not like Lyndhurst initially, "but you get over it. I think what made me feel good was to see many more people were worse than I ... So it made me feel a little more kind of positive." She became friends with some people with quadriplegia and would go out back and drink wine. Quadriplegics would sometimes put a glass in their shirt pocket and drink with a straw; other times, Therese held their glass and helped them out in the dining room. "What really made me feel bad was those young boys had never been married and they miss so much out of life. One day that's what he said, 'You have a family. You lived. We haven't lived.'"

Though Therese said she was never "bitter" over her experiences, some friends were very despondent. A woman from Detroit that she knew at Lyndhurst had persistent bladder problems. After her return home and operations that did not change her situation, this woman killed herself. Therese also recalled broken relationships after spinal cord injury. One woman was about to be married, but a car accident left her paralysed; the man she was engaged to abandoned her. "You see that a lot at Lyndhurst Lodge. The woman cannot cope or the man could not cope ... Lots of them don't have a home to go to when they leave."

Fortunately, Therese did have a home to return to. She went home every weekend. At first she was using braces after leaving the lodge. But she became fed up with these "ugly" heavy devices. "I said, 'No more.' I grabbed them and I just threw them away in the garbage." Paralysed below the knee, she found a wheelchair easier to use and never went back to braces. When told it was time for her to leave Lyndhurst, she was upset "because I really liked it there." She felt free of the strains of home life, where her husband was angry about what had happened to her. While her two children had not remembered her any other way, her husband at first did not want to go out with her. It was important to Therese that other people accept her as she was so she said to him: "'Are you ashamed of me?' and he said, 'No. You were rehabilitated, but I was not.' I said, 'It was your own fault. You could have asked for help instead of being miserable.'" Her husband was eventually 'rehabilitated' as time went on. "Now he doesn't even see me in the chair," according to Therese. They both worked around the house so that the earlier tensions over her disability were replaced by mutual support and understanding. "So I am lucky," she concluded.[47]

Lucille Fortier Owen

Another woman in Lyndhurst in 1964 was twenty-year-old Lucille Fortier (later Owen), who was there during the summer for physiotherapy. Dr Jousse would admit some younger patients during these months for a sort of "summer camp" of physiotherapy and assessment. "I had an interesting and enjoyable summer there." She came back a second time from the fall of 1965 to the summer of 1966. The second stay was not so pleasant. Indeed, she described a place where there was a good deal of tension under the surface. Some of the women she lived with were "far from home"; they worried about their families and wondered if they would ever return to them. They often talked among themselves about marriage breakdown among people with spinal cord injuries and their non-disabled spouses. "Although there was laughter and pranks were played, I felt there was a lot of forced cheerfulness. Looking back on that time now, I expect that cheerfulness masked some pretty serious depression. The women would talk about their fears amongst themselves or to a particular nurse. There were a few nurses who demonstrated a real concern and sensitivity in helping the women, particularly those who were quadriplegics, deal with their fears and anger."

Some people were upset after arriving at Lyndhurst with unrealistic expectations that there would be "special equipment" to teach them how to walk, only to find "only weights and parallel bars" to work with.[48] While Fortier Owen was used to signing in and out of the building, having gone to boarding schools in earlier years, other people found this to be an invasion of privacy and chafed at the regimentation. She recalled disputes between patients and staff over the time to go to bed;

9 p.m. was the standard time for people who needed assistance. This rule especially affected quadriplegics. She felt this undercut their rehabilitation program as it was "demeaning to adults" and had a negative impact on patient morale. During her stay, women patients, in particular those with quadriplegia, thought that they "didn't receive the kind of attention they needed as women from the nursing staff" in regard to personal appearance, "which certainly had an effect on their morale." They did not have anywhere to make their views heard. While a patient council existed, ostensibly to provide a forum for in-patient concerns, when she was there it was more interested in social events such as barbecues.

Although occasional picnics would be held outside, many of the women wondered why no kitchen was set up for their use, nor any washers or dryers; they wanted to prepare for going home and being independent but were unable to do so. "This was an area where I felt that Lyndhurst was so old-fashioned. Or maybe just too male-oriented. As I recall, the thinking then was that women would be going home for the weekends and they'd learn on their own what kitchen renovations they needed and one of the rehab counsellors would help them implement it." One area that she felt was especially lacking at Lyndhurst during the mid-1960s was in technology that could assist disabled people to "work smarter rather than harder."

Power chairs were becoming common in other places, but at Lyndhurst at least one doctor objected to them, claiming they would make people lazy. He blithely ignored the fact that they'd make people more efficient, productive and independent. It was a common attitude around rehab centres back then – you had to be tough in rehab because the world outside was even tougher ... [I] felt that the emphasis on "toughness" over intelligence bordered on the punitive and probably prevented people from exploring and implementing more creative and social solutions to problems presented by disability.

She also noted that "that old toughness" attitude led to quadriplegics frequently being discharged in 1964–65 to long-term care institutions, such as nursing homes, when returning to their homes did not work out. "It was as though it was just one more thing to accept and adjust to." Thus for some discharged residents, leaving Lyndhurst did not mean reintegration into the wider community but, in these instances, led to a life of institutionalization.

After leaving Lyndhurst, Lucille moved into an apartment that CPA Counsellor Ross Beggs – "a man of style and wit, warmth and kindness"

– helped her to find. For a few months she shared it with Margaret Staton, another former Lyndhurst patient whom she met and became friends with while they were both residents. She also made another friend at Lyndhurst who visited her after she left: Art James, the head of maintenance, who "could fix anything from the elevator to wheel-chairs." He would drop by to do some wheelchairs repairs, for which he would be paid. Afterwards James would stay and chat with the for-mer Lyndhurst patients about life at the lodge.[49]

Bill Owen

Lucille would come to know Bill Owen, a paraplegic, especially well after he moved into the wheelchair-accessible apartment building where she lived. Ross Beggs introduced them and eventually they mar-ried. Originally injured in Fredericton, New Brunswick, in 1966, where he first made contact with the CPA, Bill Owen eventually went to the University of Toronto in 1968 to do graduate studies in English. He later taught for twenty years at Ryerson Polytechnic. When he arrived in Toronto, the CPA provided him with a list of accessible buildings to live in. He found it "remarkable that an organization could put together a list" of this kind. Since the CPA head office was on Lyndhurst property, this was how he first came into contact with the rehabilita-tion centre. He was never an in-patient of Lyndhurst. However, Owen was an out-patient at both the old and new buildings, where he saw Dr Jousse, "who took real care in and had concern for his patients. I've always had the highest respect for him." He particularly appreciated Jousse's flexibility in his treatment practices. Though Owen had a "dif-ferent regimen" when it came to bowel and bladder care from that advocated by Jousse, the doctor let his patient stay on the treatment he had had in place since his injury in New Brunswick. Owen also found Jousse "willing to reconsider his own ideas" about patient care when the results of a particular test were not what he had expected.[50]

Kathy Drummond

Kathy Drummond also expressed respect for medical treatment at Lyndhurst. She was injured in a 1968 car accident in Kirkland Lake, Ontario, becoming a quadriplegic when she was sixteen. After spend-ing four months in traction, she was transferred to Lyndhurst Lodge, where she remained for three years until 1971. These events affected her profoundly in a number of ways. "For me it was not only becoming disabled, I also was totally relocated to a big city from a small town. I was leaving home for the first time essentially and so it was like a double whammy. It was really scary. Really, really scary." She also recalled being one of the only teenagers and one of the few females. As with others before her such as Bev Hallam, Drummond was shocked by the initial appearance of fellow residents. Having seen only "two or three people in wheelchairs" before, she thought, "Well, I can't be one of these people!" Though she felt out of place at first, "you have to kind of adjust to it." Her adjustment to Lyndhurst was aided by the staff, who were, she said, "very well trained" in their field, particularly in teaching self-care. She admired both the medical director, who was "sort of a father figure, almost, for me" and the assistant medical director, who was "more kind of dynamic and outgoing, always rush, rush, rushing around ... So the care was excellent."

She also initially heard comments from other patients about her hair, which had been shaved off after the accident. "It was like a brush cut when I arrived at Lyndhurst. So good-natured teasing. They used to call me George." One resident in particular had a major impact on how she saw herself: "I guess, one of the people that inspired me most was Lew B. ... because he was a few years older than me. He had been injured in a football accident but he was a very high level spinal cord injury, even higher than I was. So he was managing to read books with his mouth stick. He eventually got a chair that he operated with his head. He was always into researching equipment and different aids that would help him out. I was quite impressed by him. He certainly gave me confidence that you could actually do a lot for yourself."

Volunteers were there to assist her at times; one student from Upper Canada College was especially helpful with her calculus. "He was a really top-notch student." Interaction with the nursing staff helped her both physically and mentally. Physiotherapist Barbara Duffin worked with her on lifting weights to stretch her arms. While doing this, the two of them got into the routine of finding answers to the cryptic crossword puzzle in the *Globe and Mail* . "That was a good memory we have. She wanted to stimulate my mind as well as my nerves and muscles."

The nurses at Lyndhurst "were like good friends," according to Drummond. They took her Christmas shopping because she believed it was important to get out and do this. The head nurse, Margaret MacDonald, and another nurse "heaved me into the car and got the wheelchair into the back" and away they went to a local shopping district where she bought everything she wanted. "We had a lot of laughs. I remember we fell into the car because we didn't do such a good job on the transfer thing. But it was really like a very important first step before you tried it on your own or even with your family." Another nurse, who later became a nun, took her to France for a ten-day holiday in 1970. Driving around the country in a "tiny car" with her wheelchair on top, she found that all the cobblestone steps and small elevators meant that "Nothing was accessible over there ... But it was quite exciting! I am glad I did it."[51]

Since she was only sixteen at the time of her accident, Drummond needed to complete high school. The vocational prospects for quadriplegics at this time were not good. However her youth allowed her a greater chance of securing a job after discharge. A few years before, an in-depth study on the employment and educational situation of former Lyndhurst patients was published. It clearly showed the immense obstacles for people with spinal cord injuries in their attempts to reintegrate into the workforce and school system, especially for quadriplegics. Of 1,204 Lyndhurst graduates, 55 per cent of all paraplegics were known to be employed or pursuing education or training; for quadriplegics the number was 38.5 per cent. Factors influencing employment prospects, in addition to the extent of their physical disability, included their age at the onset of disability and their educational level.[52] Thus, more than six of every ten quadriplegics from Lyndhurst in the mid-1960s did not have a job, nor were they in the educational system.

Drummond re-started her school studies at Lyndhurst with instruction from teacher Glenn Jewett. Then she returned to a regular high school, beginning the next fall. Since there were few accessible schools during this period – "I think there were only three in the whole city" – she had to be bused to the eastern suburb of Scarborough each day from Lyndhurst in mid-town Toronto. As one of the youngest residents at Lyndhurst, she was teased about getting her homework done. But going back to school was not fun. Instead it was "very difficult." Drummond felt "segregated" from fellow students. Having been very involved in sports when she was in high school prior to her accident, she found it "quite unnerving" not to be a part of this activity when she returned to school. Though a couple of students assisted her by pushing her around in the wheelchair and carrying her books when needed, her experiences led to a loss of confidence in herself. "I didn't really interact," she recalled.

With the help of the CPA Kathy Drummond went to York University, where she lived in residence with an attendant. She earned a bachelor's degree in psychology and then did her master's degree at the Ontario Institute for Studies in Education before moving on to work in the provincial government supervising social workers and developing policy. She recalled people's different perceptions of what they thought she could and could not do: "You always run into people who are really helpful and can see the potential and are really quite willing to make accommodations and help you out and make you feel like your contribution is worthwhile. And then, of course you run up to people that say: 'Oh, there's no way you could possibly work! So what are you going to do with it?' Or 'You'll never be able to manage that course. So no sense signing up!' You run into both."

Kathy Drummond summarized her three years at Lyndhurst as "a very, very difficult time in my life. When I look back I can't honestly say that those were happy years because I was quite sad a lot of the time. Sad over the loss of things that I couldn't do and sad over thinking about: 'Well, what the heck am I going to do with my future?' 'Where am I going to end up?' and those types of things. I also have at the same time a lot of sort of fond memories of people and things that happened that were fun and to look back ... Thirty-three years [since the accident] and I am in great shape. So they did a good job, and teaching my first attendant how to do everything to take care of me. Teaching my family ... That was the most valuable part of Lyndhurst."[53]

Tom Bailey

Like Kathy Drummond, Tom Bailey was also new to Toronto when he arrived there the year following her departure. In October 1971 when he was twenty, Bailey had been injured in an automobile accident in his hometown of Burin, Newfoundland, that resulted in paraplegia. For the next eight months he was a patient in St John's General Hospital which "had little or no rehabilitation." A rehabilitation program in Newfoundland did not exist, as approximately six people sustained spinal cord injuries in Newfoundland every year. During the entire eight months in hospital in St John's, Tom Bailey remained in bed. He recalled seeing only one person in a wheelchair, and that was a visitor. He arrived for what turned out to be three months at Lyndhurst on 10 June 1972. Bailey was transported there lying on the floor in the back of an airplane. "I was given hope regarding rehabilitation," he recalls, with people telling him he could do things. Dr Jousse "talked to me on my level" and told him soon after arriving, "You can be here a year, you can be here until we kick you out, or until you get yourself out." He also found the attendants very patient as they "had to walk softly about some of these things as it [personal care issues] can blow someone's mind."

After a week, he was transferred to the independent ward, and like countless patients before him, he viewed going up the steep ramp as an important sign of improvement. Besides having physiotherapy, he went outside and practised archery. "The arrows were flying all over the place and it was a lot of fun." His feeling was that "any little gain at all was a big gain," with rehabilitation taking place "in small steps rather than giant steps." He shared a room with two other men with whom he had a good deal of "camaraderie" – talking with other people with disabilities helped him deal with his situation. "Paraplegics were often competing with one another to see who could get out first, so we turned it into fun." After the first few weeks he found people at Lyndhurst were "like family around a dinner table," even having a food-fight. On the other hand, people who were not doing as well had a different response. One man who was hit by a train at a car crossing and became a high quadriplegic tried to kill himself three times when Bailey was at Lyndhurst. "He would put a fist in the wall and blood would pour out and bang himself to hurt himself. He was still there when I left. When I saw things like this it had quite an impact." There were other tensions between residents. Some patients would call Tom Bailey a "Newfie" – a derogatory insult derived from the prejudice that "some people thought back then that we were stupid. I did feel this resentment among some residents who were discouraged [at their situation] and would resent someone like me getting better." At times relationships were more relaxed, as with several quadriplegics who played poker. They would ask a paraplegic, like Bailey, to deal the cards since they were unable to do so because of their paralysed hands.

His family was very supportive throughout this period. Bailey recalled one especially memorable time shortly before he left Lyndhurst when his family from Newfoundland showed up unannounced. They took him out for the weekend, which was the first time in a year that he had been out of any health-care facility without staff. The manner of his departure back to Newfoundland was also surprising, though in a different way. After showing that he could do the necessary transfers from the wheelchair to various positions, he was judged fit to leave.

Instead of being brought to the airport, as he expected, he was sent by cab and left at the airport curb, "so I realized I was on my own. It was somewhat stressful at the time but later I looked back at this episode and was pleased that I did this myself. A fellow who worked at the airport helped me to board the plane." Back in his home province, Bailey earned a bachelor's degree in sociology from Memorial University, then went on to work for the federal government and the CPA before retiring. As far as Lyndhurst was concerned, "I was challenged but I was free to do what I wanted ... Going there was the best move I ever made."[54]

LYNDHURST RESIDENTS' EXPERIENCES

For some patients who went to Lyndhurst, returning to the community meant taking up a new job in place of their previous occupation. Dr Geisler recalled a successful anaesthesiologist who became a quadriplegic after a swimming accident on his honeymoon. His new wife, whom he had met in Japan, supported him throughout his time at Lyndhurst and afterwards. This man was retrained as a radiologist with support from Geisler and the Royal College of Physicians and Surgeons while still at the lodge. Upon completing rehabilitation, he worked as a radiologist for six years at the Hospital for Sick Children in Toronto. At times, he would be admitted to Lyndhurst at his own request, and with the medical staff's consent, to give his wife a few weeks holiday. Eventually, this couple moved to Kitchener, Ontario, where he lived in long-term care.[55]

Another quadriplegic in-patient at Lyndhurst, Ronald McInnes, was a lawyer prior to admission. He continued this work afterwards. While he was still at Lyndhurst, according to physiotherapist Betty Brooks, he began to write a book on tenants' legal rights, which was published in early 1973. When professionals or well-to-do people came to Lyndhurst, they lived with individuals from all backgrounds. Brooks recalled that at the old Lyndhurst "there was no class distinction" between rich people and "ordinary folk." Everyone lived on the same wards, ate the same food, went through the rehabilitation program together. No one had a private room at Lyndhurst Lodge. As an example of this breakdown of the social hierarchy, Brooks recalled a young male patient from a wealthy Mexican family whose best friend was a male patient from an "ordinary" family in Collingwood, Ontario.[56] There was literally no space at 153 Lyndhurst Avenue for social snobbery.

TEMPER OF THE TIMES

The period that all of these people lived through – the second half of the 1960s and the early 1970s – was a time of great social and political turmoil throughout North America. Various communities were involved in the struggles for civil rights and more openness about sexuality. As is to be expected, in-patients and out-patients of Lyndhurst were affected by these developments. Some of them wanted to do something about the world around them. One such concern was addressing the issues related to physical accessibility. Bill Owen recalled how inaccessible most of Toronto was during this period: "In 1968 ... you had a built environment in Toronto and probably everywhere that didn't take the needs of the disabled into account. To travel anywhere on the sidewalk, to go grocery shopping, to the laundromat, or even between buildings at work, you had to go up and down driveways to cross the streets to the sidewalk on the other side. This meant you were often on the city roads evading cars. Or I looked for laneways and alleys. I was once stopped by a policeman who told me not to use the streets. I told him I would when the City put in ramps. There was no accessible transportation – I took cabs to work for my first five years at Ryerson – and accessible buildings of any sort were rare. This made employment as well as life in general difficult."

To improve these conditions, a Toronto-based group called the Action League for Physically Handicapped Advancement, or ALPHA, was founded in 1967. Bill Owen was chairman from 1969 to 1971. Part of the wider disability rights movement then growing across the continent, ALPHA lasted until the mid-1970s. How did this influence accessibility issues for people at Lyndhurst? By the late 1960s some ramps were installed at the University of Toronto for disabled students who needed access to buildings. Ross Beggs had helped to get these built for the use of former Lyndhurst patients. Bill Owen mentioned that the CPA was able to get ramps placed at a few corners where they considered them necessary. ALPHA advocated that curb cuts should be placed everywhere to ensure that accessibility was widespread rather than limited to selected places. Though the CPA did not support this universal approach, in June 1970 a municipal by-law was passed in Toronto, at ALPHA's instigation, to have ramps gradually replace curbs. Owen said that ALPHA chose the gradual approach because it was more likely to be approved. "That was one of the things we are proud of, that we committed the City to build ramps when the curbs were being replaced."[57]

This organization was also involved in promoting accessible public transportation.[58] Bill Owen explained the different approaches to disability issues that developed during this period. The CPA "at least in Ontario acted on the belief that its main responsibility was to assist the disabled person's re-entry to the community as quickly as possible and resume a job or position." They argued that the disabled person needed to adjust to society, rather than to call for systemic changes in society to accommodate disability.

One of the important ideas in the concept of disability rights was the development of the idea that we are part of society; therefore, we deserve to be included in the planning of society. As part of society we must be able to enjoy the services and facilities that society has available. They must be made accessible. To demand that society change was diametrically opposed to the CPA attitude that the person with a disability adapt. Obviously, the CPA came to change its position.[59]

Wheelchair sports were another area of contention. Originally organized in Britain, wheelchair sports became a major point of interest for increasing numbers of disabled people, including ex-Lyndhurst patients. The first Paraplegic Games in Canada were held in Winnipeg from 8–12 August 1967 and the following month the Centennial Paraplegic Games were held in Montreal. While CPA National "look[ed] favourably on this development" they eventually decided to not actively support it as they felt it would conflict with their own fundraising campaigns. The association felt that wheelchair athletics were not essential for rehabilitation, since most people who used wheelchairs did not get involved in team sports. However, they believed disabled people should be encouraged to participate in whatever activities interested them. The CPA emphasized the importance of helping people to learn to take care of their own daily needs as much as possible and to find appropriate educational and job opportunities in the community.[60] Lyndhurst, which was run by the CPA, had a similar viewpoint. Myrll Jackson, who was himself very active as a medal-winning athlete, recalled: "I went back to Lyndhurst to visit Dr Jousse and mentioned wheelchair sports to him and he said 'We don't mention wheelchair sports in this hospital.'"[61] Bev Hallam, known as a "super-quad" for his sporting ability, was also very active in wheelchair sports during this time. He explained that the CPA position on wheelchair sports was tied into plans that were then percolating for Lyndhurst's new building:

"They may have had their hands filled trying to get this place built. It was certainly in the planning stages at that time in the sixties. That's where their energies were diverted."[62]

The sexual revolution that was energizing the body politic during this time also affected the way disabled people at Lyndhurst were counselled. According to Bev Hallam, this changed from when he was a patient there in the early 1960s: "During rehab there was no formal discussion of sex and the paraplegic and sexual functioning and that kind of stuff. Just what you could find out from the other guys and they weren't going to say too much. By the time the seventies came around, after the pill and whatever, and the popular culture had picked up on sexuality or whatever you want to call it, it became part of the program of CPA counselling. Well, at least you talked to people about what was going on."[63] As the following chapter will show, this aspect of counselling at Lyndhurst became a normal part of treatment services in the new Lyndhurst building. But long before official sexuality counselling services existed at this rehabilitation centre, a far less public form of dealing with sex existed for some male patients. According to then Assistant Medical Superintendent William Geisler, CPA Rehabilitation Counsellor Jim Bartlett at times found a prostitute for certain male patients at Lyndhurst.[64] When he was a medical intern there in 1970, Gavin Shanks said this was allowed since "these people had been deprived of a lot of, you know, ordinary human joy ... Rumor had it that there were girls that hung out around the corner of Bathurst and St Clair, ladies of the night you might say, who volunteered services for some of the younger male patients at Lyndhurst Lodge. That was spoken of but I never saw any of it. I don't think that it happened on the premises. But that was sufficiently well known that I think it had to be something that was known and tolerated and that was the way the place ran."[65]

Just as popular attitudes were challenged and changed on a whole range of issues outside Lyndhurst, so too they influenced daily life inside the old mansion. Gavin Shanks recalled that Dr Jousse was well aware of the more permissive atmosphere that was swirling inside and outside Lyndhurst Lodge in regard to other things besides sex. Many of the patients were smoking "dope" when Shanks was there, which some of the staff objected to. "Al had, I am sure, as good a nose as anybody and he was very aware of the world. And I am sure that he knew if there were one of two people in that room that was full of that unmistakable odor what they had been up to. But it didn't bother him. I mean that was part of life. That was part of growing up, part of dealing with your disability and that never seemed to be an issue."[66]

Perhaps the simplest act of rebellion uncovered during these years of ferment centred on the pay-phone that patients could use in the building. It was reported in 1966 that some patients had found a way around paying for long-distance and local phone calls. They had "discovered a method whereby the money spent for a call would be recovered through telephone mechanics." Bell Telephone then "stationed an observer who discovered the method used." Changes to the telephone were made, but recovering costs for previous calls was not possible "because the patients are alert to any mechanical weaknesses of the telephone."[67] While Lyndhurst's owners made plans to move out of the old premises, patients ensured that the last years in the original building were far from routine or regimented. As people interviewed for this book have made clear, Jousse did not like a lot of rules. This laid-back atmosphere was felt on the wards and in the daily lives of the people who lived and worked there. To further probe this side of the story, we now turn to the work lives of staff to see how the changing times affected them.

SALARIES AND STAFF

One area of frequent change during the decade under discussion related to staff pay and benefits. This was a particularly pressing item among one segment of the staff that the hospital feared losing to other facilities. Concerns over salary levels for Lyndhurst orderlies led Jousse to write to the OHSC in the spring of 1965. He claimed that higher wages for this position at several other chronic-care facilities were luring away experienced staff. This "threatened our treatment services," according to Jousse. He wrote that Lyndhurst had provided training for years for orderlies who worked at chronic care hospitals in the Toronto area "and as far afield as Nova Scotia and Saskatchewan." The Victorian Order of Nurses also sent male nurses to train at Lyndhurst "in order that they may render more adequate care to male patients, particularly the paraplegic patients living in the community." Of the fifteen to sixteen orderlies regularly employed at Lyndhurst, three had worked there for more than fifteen years and two had been there for twenty years in 1965: Basil Thomas and Richard Martindale, Tommy and Dick as they were known to countless patients and staff. The staff that Jousse wrote were leaving solely for economic reasons had been employed at Lyndhurst for over five years. Jousse made Lyndhurst's dependence on this group of workers clear: "I am writing to point out that if we lost orderlies, it may well be necessary to close down our operation because the care of these patients is dependent on first-rate nursing and orderly service. Furthermore, if we lose our present experienced group of orderlies, it will not be easy to replace them and, in fact, years of experience are essential to the development of a first-rate orderly."[68]

Four orderlies left Lyndhurst for higher wages elsewhere at the time that this letter was written. As this represented a quarter of the orderly staff, Jousse's concerns were obviously well founded. Effective 1 May 1965 wages for Lyndhurst's orderlies went up from a starting salary of $250 per month to $262 with an increase from $315 to $327 per month for orderlies with five years seniority; the top three orderlies made between $335 and $420 a month. This was still lower than what Lyndhurst had requested. Nevertheless, their pay scale inched closer to pay scales at places like Riverdale Convalescent Hospital, where salaries for orderlies averaged $11 to $30 higher per pay grade.[69] Four months later it was reported that Lyndhurst was short one orderly, indicating that three out of the four positions left open had been filled. Nurses also had a slight wage increase of 1 per cent in comparison to the average increase that year of 3.5 to 4.5 per cent for orderlies.[70] This figure improved a few years later. Salary levels for 1968 were passed, subject to OHSC approval, with overall increases averaging 12 per cent, from 10 per cent for nurses to 19 per cent for physiotherapists.[71] Physiotherapists, though on the low end of the pay scale, were extremely busy. In 1967 the physiotherapy department provided 17,543 in-patient treatments and 1,740 out-patient treatments.[72] There were thirty-two nursing staff positions in 1967, with a little more than half of the personnel being classified as "non-professional."[73]

During the late 1960s and early 1970s, employee benefits improved at Lyndhurst in a number of areas. Vacation time for staff in 1966 was set at four weeks after the first year of employment for the medical director, hospital administrator, and director of nursing; three weeks for all other staff after one year of employment; and four weeks after fifteen years of employment. Sick time for all staff, after three months employment, was set at an annual total of twenty-one days.[74] However, by early 1968 these sick days were revised in light of the prolonged recovery required for "a diligent, reliable orderly" of ten years service, Joe Norvaisza, who was recovering from a heart attack. Subject to final approval from Dr

Jousse and the OHSC, sick days were increased to seventy to ninety working days from twenty-one, which was similar to other hospitals at that time.[75] In 1970 the hospital administration wrote an employee's manual that outlined employment conditions and benefits.[76]

A year later, the hospital board reaffirmed a mandatory retirement policy for employees who turned sixty-five. However, they also noted that an employee could request, on the medical director's recommendation, a deferment of their retirement for "one year at a time," with the ultimate approval resting with the Lyndhurst hospital board. This option was used and granted for several employees, such as Rehabilitation Counsellor James Bartlett. Notice of pending retirement was given three months prior to the actual date.[77] Other staff opted to leave after many years of service. George White, physical therapy instructor at Lyndhurst since September 1945, retired in January 1972. He died shortly thereafter.[78] As with employment positions anywhere else, staff members who were derelict in their duty could lose their jobs. Jousse reported to the hospital board a documented case of one orderly who was "known to maliciously tease patients and mildly abuse them [and] had on a recent occasion prior to Christmas refused to assist an ill patient because the orderly was having his tea." He then did not show up for work on Christmas Day and called in sick the next day. He submitted his resignation after it was asked for upon his return from three days off.[79] Another employee who enjoyed tea, but who also conscientiously did her job, was a woman Lucille Owen remembered as Zohra. She was a non-medical worker who organized refreshments and was a "warm, maternal and helpful presence" among the women patients, particularly when they were depressed and longing for home.[80]

The Service Employees International Union (SEIU), Local 204, was certified to represent people like Zohra – orderlies, kitchen and maintenance staff – beginning on 4 December 1971. During the early 1970s, the bargaining unit at Lyndhurst represented forty employees. However, many people remained outside the bargaining unit, including "professional nursing staff, physiotherapists, occupational therapists, rehabilitation counsellors, supervisors or foremen or persons above that rank, office staff, persons regularly employed for not more than 24 hours per week and students employed during the school vacation period." A few months before Local 204 was certified at Lyndhurst, this union had negotiated a two-year contract for employees at seven other Toronto hospitals, so it was very well established in local healthcare facilities.[81]

The first contract was negotiated and approved by both sides in the spring of 1972. Two years later, in June 1974, after months of negotiations and arbitration, a contract was settled in which all employees represented by SEIU earned salary hikes of $1,200 to $1,500 above the previous contract, which ended in December 1973; an additional wage increase in 1975 gave another $1,183 per year for each person covered under the contract.[82] In 1972 Evelyn Paul returned to work at Lyndhurst as a physiotherapist, which was then a non-unionized position. She recalled, "I made the princely sum of $7,200 dollars a year. I thought I had died and gone to heaven."[83] Paul also returned to a facility where different jobs had been created since she had last worked there in 1953.

Several people who began to work at Lyndhurst during this period took on new areas of responsibility. Dorothy Waddell began her job as director of volunteers in April 1969. The volunteers developed into an "integral part" of Lyndhurst by involving members of the community with in-patients.[84] In 1972 Ross Beggs was appointed as the national liaison representative for the CPA, providing advice on how to improve services in the various CPA divisions across the country. This was to take no more than three months a year; the rest of his time would be spent working with people at Lyndhurst.[85] Two close colleagues of Waddell and Beggs were also hired at this time. In 1970 two new re-establishment counsellors were hired by the CPA to work out of Lyndhurst: Edmund Ratelle, who started work on 4 May 1970; and Charlie Saso, who began on 14 September 1970.[86] Both worked at Lyndhurst throughout the 1970s and remember what the people and place were like during these tumultuous times.

Charlie Saso, who spoke in the highest terms about the patients he worked with and his colleagues from Dr Jousse down, recalled how working at Lyndhurst as a CPA counsellor involved more than staying on the hospital grounds. Instead, after discharge "we followed [ex-patients] out into Toronto, Thunder Bay, Ottawa, wherever they happened to be throughout Ontario." Far from saying, '"Good-bye. Good luck and that's it.' It was: 'We'll be there for you, perhaps in a more limited capacity, but we will be there for you as well.'" An important part of this work was to enable a person to make connections with support services in their local community, whether it be medical assistance, mental health counselling, legal aid, financial help, employment, or educational agencies. Saso said that his professional work "was multidimensional. It was holistic in its approach. From the social work perspective, we dealt with the whole person. Psychosocially, medically, paramedically, spiritually." Sometimes, his job led to unexpected places. Two ex-Lyndhurst patients whom he worked with ended up in Toronto's fortress-like Don Jail, where Saso visited them. He felt guilty about this situation, since he was working with them at the time; however, Saso emphasized, he was not judgmental about their being in trouble with the law. Eventually they got out of jail and went "on with their lives."

Back at the old Lyndhurst during the early years of his work there, Saso remembered what he called the "family atmosphere" and how it lent itself to his job. Working as a team with "doctors, nurses, physios and later on OTS ... orderlies, the cleaning staff, the dietary staff" was a "big thing." During rounds with Jousse and Geisler, Saso said staff would talk with the patients in a "give-and-take," to try to understand what they felt about their situation. It was a multidisciplinary approach to treatment. Saso said that while the final decision about patient care was up to the doctors, they consulted the staff and listened "very carefully and very closely" to the patients.[87]

In an interview several years before Saso was hired at Lyndhurst, Jousse spoke about some "terrible clashes between staff and patient, clashes that go on for weeks and months." Noting that the staff have "strong opinions," he said that employees told him if they thought he was treating a patient "too soft or too hard ... People who can't stomach that kind of give-and-take soon leave."[88] While some patients interviewed for this book spoke of not wanting to leave, others wanted to depart before the staff believed they should. Saso said no one was forced to stay at Lyndhurst if they wanted to be discharged earlier than expected. "That was always a topic that people were interested in knowing ... I can hear them to this day, saying ... 'How long, doctor, do you think I am going to be here?'... And they'd give them their opinion and then they would say: 'Well, what do you think?'"

When people did leave, the ever-present obstacles for disabled people outside the lodge quickly revealed themselves. Saso recalled how he and Ross Beggs had to help a quadriplegic board a bus when this man returned to Ottawa. The bus driver would not do it so they lifted this person aboard. In other instances, attitudinal barriers posed problems for someone wanting to get on with life outside institutions. One man with quadriplegia who came to Lyndhurst was described to Saso as "hell on wheels" by the hospital that sent him there. Saso became his social worker and found this person was "the exact opposite" of the characterization he had been given. Instead, he found him to be "a wonderful fellow" who wanted to return to his home in eastern Ontario. The hellish part was the attitude of people who did not want to accept him! Saso recalled going to a meeting in this man's community. Almost everybody at the meeting demanded to know: "Well, how come you're discharging this guy? How come he is coming back here?" The CPA counsellor's response was "Well, by the way, this just happened to be his home and this is what he wanted. And he is not going to be at our hospital." After having to deal with "that kind of an attitude" the story "did have a happy ending." Though his situation "wasn't ideal," this man did return home to live with people who supported him as a member of the community. "See here is another guy that was not going to be put into a long-term care facility for chronic care, as good as they are, as necessary as they are. He would have no part of that ... That usually happened. I mean sometimes people were not able to do what it was they wanted to do for whatever the reasons were, but our role was to try and help them to be wherever it was they wanted to be."[89]

Saso's colleague Ed Ratelle also worked as a CPA rehabilitation counsellor at Lyndhurst from 1970 to 1980. He mentioned that socializing with people they worked with outside of the hospital, though before they were discharged, was part of the job. Going to a bar or to eat at a restaurant was a good way to get people out of "their safe cocoon in the hospital." At times an accessible washroom was not available for someone who needed to relieve themselves after drinking too much so they had to empty a leg bag on the nearest street. Some passers-by wondered "What the heck we were doing."

The ward rounds had a "pecking order," with staff following along according to rank and seniority, according to Ratelle. For the patients, "some of the poor folks there had a hard time" having to expose their buttocks "to this little military parade of medical personnel and we would all examine to see how their pressure sores were. It wasn't a fun time. Some of them would be very putrid things. But they came to Lyndhurst because it was the one place that we can get them healed up and other places didn't know about it and sometimes people died." The smell in the early morning was also pronounced, as routines dealing with bowel and bladder care were carried out, though this smell changed as the day went on.[90]

Loma Stone, a nurse who worked at Lyndhurst for twenty years, beginning in 1959, recalled that orderlies and nurses both started their routine at the same time when turning patients to prevent pressure sores. "Turning a patient is a big job ... We both started at the same time, the nurses would go to the females and orderlies would do the males. We had our independence unit that you turned to when you get the patients to a certain amount of independence. The patients, before they became independent, they had to learn to turn in the bed and some of the ways we did it would be considered cruel. But you're half asleep and you could go in the night time and [we] pull the blankets off of them. 'Come on turn.' And there [are] four patients in a room. So the first fellow, he's turning while you are doing the second one that can't turn." Stone noted that Dr Jousse did not want any private rooms, so that all patients would be together with several others in a room "when they would look across and see a patient in another bed, he might see a quad that's learning to turn over and here's a new quad that can't even sit up." Thus seeing their roommates in these situations, "they'd know that it's possible for you to accomplish this and to see other patients do it made the difference." In another instance, she recalled a young woman in her teens who had become quadriplegic after a car accident; she went from taking forty-five minutes when putting on one sock to getting dressed in fifteen minutes.[91] The physical and emotional distress of having to re-learn life's daily habits can only be guessed at by all but those who experienced it.

Two staff members who were most involved in assisting with these personal-care needs were orderlies Richard Martindale and Basil Thomas, known as Dick and Tom. By this time they were "old timers." Their decades of experience since Lyndhurst's first days were highly valued by intern Gavin Shanks, particularly when it came to their treatment of male patients' bowels and bladders. "If you didn't learn as a physician to take the advice of someone like experienced orderly staff you were in big trouble because they knew when things were going bad with patients and when they were having medical emergencies. So they were really a key part of the team even though from some points of view they were low men on the totem pole of the health-care hierarchy. But everybody knew them and they were absolutely integral to the operation of the place."

The influence of Dr Jousse was also integral to the development of this young doctor in training. The medical director did "a spectacularly good job of doing first-class work, providing first-class medical care in some pretty austere medical surroundings." Jousse was also able to deal with personality and territorial differences among staff, as well as "patients' frustrations better than anybody I have ever seen." Shanks learned a good deal about being "more humane" during his internship at Lyndhurst. Listening to people was an essential part of this learning experience. Shanks recalled how in 1970, with student activism in the air and on the streets, Jousse responded to activists among medical interns who made their way not only to Lyndhurst Lodge, but right into the medical director's office. In addition to being in charge of Lyndhurst, Jousse was head of the department of rehabilitation medicine at the University of Toronto. Medical residents were becoming organized at this time into an advocacy group called the Professional Association of Interns and Residents of Ontario which was "trying to enforce some rules and regulations." The U of T rehabilitation residents from this group met in Jousse's office and "he was always very receptive. I don't remember him ever thinking that anything that we asked for was entirely unreasonable. His answer would usually be: 'Well, if we can find the money.'"[92]

Canadian-born medical students, like Gavin Shanks, were joined by people from other countries who came to Lyndhurst to study rehabilitation medicine. Two women doctors from Thailand arrived for postgraduate training at Lyndhurst as well as at other facilities; one arrived in July 1966 and the other in March 1967. They worked in Canada for two to four years.[93] In 1970 Dr Tran, a South Vietnamese physician, trained at Lyndhurst for nine months, after which he returned to his native country to lead a rehabilitation centre there.[94] Nimmi Bharatwal, originally from India, first met Dr Jousse when he was chairman of the department of rehabilitation medicine at the University of Toronto, where she was a post-graduate student in 1969. Several years later, in 1973, she spent six months as a resident at Lyndhurst and remembered being "really impressed with the type of work that he was doing." She recalled working with physicians, such as Dr Noptanya, who came to Lyndhurst from Thailand. Bharatwal, like Shanks when he was a resident there a few years earlier, also attended conferences each Friday with the rest of the staff to discuss patients. She noted that this weekly conference indicated that "the interdisciplinary team was always there. It wasn't called so ... We talked about all of the new admissions, discussed progress and all the things that concern these patients while they were with us and planned for their discharge. So the interdisciplinary approach was always there. This new terminology has been introduced now but the philosophy didn't change."[95] One thing that was about to change, at long last, was the place where all this activity occurred.

THE NEW BUILDING TAKES SHAPE
1970–74

Interminable bureaucratic delays in getting the new building underway served as a backdrop to Dr Jousse's remarks at the twenty-fifth CPA Annual Meeting in April 1970. He told people that the lodge was filled to capacity, with a long waiting list. This "emphasized the need to get on with the development of the new and larger hospital."[96] Though they were planning for a future move, the past was also marked. A plaque was unveiled on 1 May 1970 by Deputy Minister of Veterans Affairs John Hodgson to mark the twenty-fifth anniversary of the founding of Lyndhurst Lodge by the DVA. As they reflected on past accomplishments, everyone present knew that the plaque unveiled that day was marking the beginning of the end of one building as they made plans for a new hospital. More than five years after originally contacting the Ministry of Health about building a new place, the OHSC finally gave approval in 1970 to go ahead with plans to build a 106-bed hospital. Autumn 1972 was the prospective start date for construction.[97] Sketch plans were submitted and revised throughout 1971 with input from staff, architects, and OHSC planning committee members.[98]

In May 1970 the CPA board of directors approved the firm of Mathers and Haldenby to be the architects for the new building.[99] This led to some acrimony, as architect Charles Meek, who had been consulted for about eight years prior to this by the CPA board, was rejected; he submitted an unexpected hefty bill soon afterwards. T.G. Ferguson, a long-time CPA board member, resigned over the choice of architects.[100] In spite of these rumbles, the project moved forward. By the end of 1970 an additional one and a half acres of land next to the Divadale property were secured from the University of Toronto for $1.[101] This allowed more room for the future hospital. By early 1971 the architect had "worked through the Physiotherapy Department" to come up with suitable designs for this area.[102] But problems continued. The CPA board minutes make clear how fed up the operators of Lyndhurst were with the constant delays and indecision by provincial government officials when noting "our frustrations in dealing with the Hospital Planning Committee of the OHSC. Since November 23rd 1970 [four and a half months earlier] the kitchen in our hospital plans has been relocated at the direction of the OHSC consultants from the main floor to the basement, back to the main floor and then back to the basement again."[103]

By July 1971 some progress had been made when CPA assistant managing director, Andy Clarke, reported that differences with the province over the designs ended when the "OHSC has abandoned its former fixation that we should have a split-level design hospital with a rectangular nursing wing and CPA offices in the basement."[104] Instead, a triangular nursing wing and four bedrooms for patients were agreed upon under block schematic plans. In November 1971 Clarke reported on "seemingly innumerable and often interminable meetings" between Lyndhurst representatives, the architects, and OHSC planners, though "substantial agreement" was achieved on the design.[105] These problems were worked through and by the end of 1972 the designs had been completed, contractors were hired, and the provincial Ministry of Health had guaranteed funding. However work on construction was held up yet again by factors outside the control of Lyndhurst's owners. This time it was the turn of objections filed before the Ontario Municipal Board hearings and the committee of adjustment.[106] After overcoming appeals about setting up shop on the Divadale property, on 30 March 1973 the CPA was finally able to secure ownership from the University of Toronto of all the land they wanted for the new building.[107]

Finally, on 18 April 1973, excavations began for the new 106-bed hospital on the Divadale site in North York.[108] The cost of the new building, excluding the new office space to be paid for by the CPA, was estimated to be $5,721,495.[109] The CPA estimated that they would spend between $250,000 and $300,000 for their part of the building.[110] An ad hoc committee of Dr Botterell, Dr Jousse, Ken Langford, Andy Clarke, and John Counsell recommended that the new building be called "Lyndhurst Hospital," which was approved by the CPA on 10 April 1973.[111] To maintain continuity with its past history and name-recognition, the CPA board agreed that the Lyndhurst name would be maintained on the new site on Sutherland Drive.[112] The CPA also decided in June 1973 that the new hospital would have a laboratory-workshop for spinal cord research, something that Dr Botterell was particularly prominent in advancing.[113] Ken Langford remembered how the design for the new building was developed. "I worked for about a year with [the architects] designing the place. Working with the various department heads and Dr Jousse, as to what their requirements were and trying to explain that to the architects until they came up with what I think was a *very good* plan for a hospital. For instance, one of the things that I was most insistent about is that I didn't want these long, narrow corridors with rooms off each side. It's a little too institutional. So the architect said: 'Well would you mind a triangular hospital?' I said: 'Fine.' So they designed all of the [patients'] rooms on the outside perimeter of a triangle and all of the other facilities of the hospital that were needed for support facilities were on the inside of the triangle. So all the rooms were fresh and bright and all of the corridors were short."[114]

Physiotherapist Betty Brooks said, "Ken and Andy were open to any suggestions that any staff member had, nursing staff, physio staff." They regularly went over to the CPA office to look at the plans as they developed. The head of physiotherapy, Barb Duffin, suggested one particularly important change to the design. The toilets in the plan were all originally designed so that it was only possible to sit on them from one direction – right to left. Duffin recognized this as a serious flaw, as some patients are stronger when transferring from left to right. After she pointed this out to the planners, the necessary changes were made to accommodate people who needed to get on the toilet from one side or the other, depending on their abilities.[115]

Walter Gordon had offered to help raise money for whatever building costs were not covered by the OHSC; however the CPA and the sale of 153 Lyndhurst made such a campaign unnecessary.[116] Finally, after more than a decade of pushing the project forward, delays, and starting up again, the new building was completed. The move from the old premises to the new two-storey building in the eastern suburbs of Toronto on Sutherland Drive was completed during one weekend in mid-July 1974. The administrators moved on 19 July and the following Monday, 22 July 1974, the treatment staff and patients were transferred to their new quarters. In August 1974 a few weeks after moving into the building, Dr Jousse said that the general response to the new hospital "has been one of pleased amazement, that the building is both utilitarian and pleasing to the eye." Jousse praised Ken Langford and Andy Clarke, both former patients of the old lodge, for guiding the building project from beginning to end over many difficult years.[117]

The views of former patients and staff about the move from the old to the new are perhaps best encapsulated by the two following quotes. Kathy Drummond reflected a view expressed by some other people interviewed for this book when she observed: "You didn't really feel like you were in a hospital. So ... to me that's what was positive about the old place before they moved up to ... the new hospital that was built. Mind you, it has much nicer facilities: lots of room, proper accessibility, big washrooms, and all that stuff. But the old place was more like a home and you didn't mind staying there a bit longer ... When I go to the new place now, I think: 'Boy! It's a lonely place.' You know, big empty hallways, very much a sterile kind of setting."[118]

Rehabilitation counsellor Charlie Saso spoke for still other people when he remembered that the old place "wasn't logistically and professionally" suitable for a rehabilitation site. While "a lot of tears were probably shed" over leaving the original building, there was also the attitude "Let's get on with it. Obviously it was necessary. It had to change. The old building was too antiquated. It wasn't adequate any longer. We were crowded, crammed in there. People had to wait for the elevator to get up and down. And you lived in cramped quarters upstairs at the old one, so ... that couldn't continue ... And then the moving day was a big one too. When we moved into the new place, they had a special ceremony ... and that was a great link from the old because all of the people that were from the old place were at the new one ... And so the services continued."[119]

History is multi-dimensional, like the buildings people remember in such different ways. One thing was certain – the longest decade of delays and uncertainty over future building plans had at last come to an end. The Ontario Minister of Health, Frank Miller, officially opened the new Lyndhurst Hospital on 13 November 1974.[120] As people gathered for the official ceremonies, former patients and staff mingled with people who were currently residing or employed there. A new era was beginning. The next few years would see changes to the internal operation of the hospital that would be every bit as significant as the move from Lyndhurst Avenue to Sutherland Drive.

Lyndhurst on Sutherland: From Autonomy to Amalgamation, 1974–98

"I remember being on the stretcher and seeing the beautiful walls and the art on the walls and the windows and natural light. You know, just open space. It was not a typical hospital setting."[1] Barbara Turnbull's recollection of first entering Lyndhurst Hospital on Sutherland Drive in 1984 indicates how much the physical atmosphere had changed. Other changes were also felt during this period, not a few of which caused great controversy among residents and staff. Broader societal and political changes outside the hospital had a significant impact on developments inside the rehabilitation centre. Ultimately, some of these outside pressures for change led to the end of Lyndhurst as an autonomous facility owned by the CPA for the treatment of people with spinal cord injuries. As will become evident, the re-making of Lyndhurst Hospital from what it was before was perhaps its most consistent feature during its last quarter century of existence as an independent facility.

CHANGING OF THE GUARD AND THE END OF LYNDHURST'S "OLD CONCEPT"

Though Lyndhurst now operated out of a new building, some old problems continued. In the first months of operation on Sutherland Drive only fifty-three beds were open, just one more than at the old building when it was closed. Obviously, this was not what people had been hoping for. The distress of having to wait for a bed opening was aggravated by the knowledge that bureaucratic foot-dragging was delaying the funding of more space for patients at the new building. A woman who was quadriplegic dictated a letter in April 1975 about the impact of this delay on her life:

Because of a car accident last year I have become totally disabled in both my legs and naturally need total care now for the rest of my life. Since the time of the accident some minimal movement has returned to my arms. My doctors tell me that I could get some very good physiotherapy at Lynhurst Hospital in Toronto that might help me to train my muscles in my arms to operate [or] at least perhaps to be able to feed myself.

I have been waiting for a bed for several months now and I am told that there are beds available and that I am one of the people on the waiting list, but that it is you people that are stopping the hospital from opening up the new beds. You cannot image how difficult it is to keep waiting week after week to hear news from the hospital that I am able to be flown down from Thunder Bay because there is a bed available. You do not require that someone look after your every want and need, no matter how small and, therefore, your need or the department's need is not great. Mine is.

I respectfully request that on behalf of the other people who are waiting as well as myself that you consider what our position is and that you have some understanding and compassion and cut through what ever bureaucratic red tape is holding this opening up.[2] [Original writing]

A standard response was sent to this person promising to look into the matter. It is not known when she was admitted. Pressure from such people did eventually have a positive effect. In late 1975 the provincial Ministry of Health approved the opening of fifty-three more beds at Lyndhurst commencing in 1976, theoretically doubling the total number to 106, which is what the new hospital had been designed to accommodate in four units. However, this did not happen. Instead twenty-seven more beds were opened as scheduled, increasing the total to eighty. Eventually ninety-five bed spaces were approved in 1979, though the actual number of funded beds soon fell back to seventy-nine to eighty within several years and was reduced to seventy by the mid-1990s because of provincial cuts.[3] These oscillating numbers underscore a central part of Lyndhurst's history that never seemed to be too far away – uncertainty about the level of services that were to be provided.

This uncertainty affected the type of treatment that people received and that others were employed to provide. Lyndhurst Hospital during the late 1970s and early 1980s was undergoing a sea-change in its staff composition and rehabilitative direction. Because of the far-reaching impact this would have on the way in which the hospital operated and on the people who resided and worked there, it is necessary to look at how this came about.

Some of these changes went according to plan and were marked with retirement parties and tributes to departing pillars of the hospital. The most obvious changes took place at the top. After thirty years as medical director, Dr Jousse retired in June 1975. He continued to see patients and to serve on the board and on various committees until he resigned from these voluntary positions in 1980 because of differences over the direction the hospital was taking. Jousse was succeeded by his long-time assistant, Dr William O. Geisler, who held this position for four years.[4] In 1977 Ken Langford retired as managing director of the CPA, having served in this capacity since 1961 and on senior staff of the association since 1946.[5] Together, Jousse and Langford had run the medical and administrative aspects of the hospital for years. While this changing of the guard was voluntary, other changes that caused great tumult during this period led to some involuntary departures. Most significant was the implementation of a different direction in the hospital's long-term stay policy.

The board decided to commission two studies about the state of Lyndhurst Hospital in the late 1970s. Long-time CPA board member Helen Phelan and retired medical director, Dr Jousse, issued a report on the operation of the hospital in July 1978. While no serious problems in patient care were reported, serious problems were found to exist in internal staff relationships and between patients and staff. They noted that there was no "effective feedback system" for patients to voice their views of the treatment program and that "cultural changes and the changes in the expectations" of patients had a marked influence on Lyndhurst's atmosphere.[6] They also recommended that an expert in paraplegia be brought in from outside to examine services at the facility. Accordingly, Dr Alain Rossier of the Harvard Medical School, who was himself a paraplegic, interviewed staff and patients in the fall of 1978. One of the most important recommendations from these reports was that a full-time psychologist was needed at Lyndhurst. This position, which was filled in the summer of 1979,[7] was important because of the depression often experienced by people who had acquired a physical disability for the first time. The shift from being able-bodied to being physically disabled could seriously affect a person's mental health, because of finding oneself restricted as never before, in a world now experienced as full of physical and attitudinal barriers against people with disabilities.

Rossier's report expressed concern that services for patients with spinal cord injuries were being developed by other local hospitals, because of the long waiting periods for admission to Lyndhurst. He was also concerned that too many patients (fifteen to twenty people) remained in Lyndhurst after their treatment program was finished. He argued that they received "essentially nursing home care." According to Rossier, this "gives the impression that Lyndhurst is reversing the rehabilitation purpose for which it was designed." In response, Geisler mentioned that the Queen Elizabeth Hospital had a twenty-five-bed chronic-care unit, while Mount Sinai Hospital had a sixty to seventy-bed rehabilitation wing, as did St. Michael's Hospital, where a smaller unit was established. Patients with spinal cord injuries were being referred to these facilities, though they had a maximum in-patient stay of seventy days, after which patients were discharged to their homes or to long-term care. Lyndhurst had a much longer in-stay policy. The two major sources of referral for Lyndhurst patients in Toronto at this time were Toronto General and Sunnybrook. An indication of why patients remained in Lyndhurst for longer periods than an outside observer such as Rossier felt was necessary can be found in a reference a few months later to the province not allowing seriously disabled people to be discharged until bed space could be found for them elsewhere.[8]

Before, during, and after these studies, new procedures began to be put in place that transformed the rehabilitation centre in a way that made many who had worked there for some time very uncomfortable. Betty Brooks, who worked as a physiotherapist at Lyndhurst from 1961 to 1980, recalled that during her last few years there the University of Toronto "got far more involved than they had been and started calling the shots." What followed shocked some long-time employees like Brooks. In the late 1970s she recalled that "anybody that had been at Lyndhurst for any length of time was dumped." She remembered joking with another employee about when it would be their turn to be fired. "They just wanted to get rid of anybody that had the old concept of what Lyndhurst should be." The "old concept" meant that people with spinal cord injuries were allowed to stay at Lyndhurst for as long as it was deemed necessary for their rehabilitation. Now, recalled Betty Brooks, under the changed ideas in the late 1970s and early 1980s, as soon as a patient was admitted, he or she was given a discharge date. "You can't do that with people like that. It takes some [patients] six months to adjust, it takes some [patients] a year and a half to adjust. You can't just say this guy was hurt in June so he is out of here in December. That was the concept that they were going with when I left ... They let Barb Duffin go so I was acting head for thirteen months."[9]

It was no surprise that some employees organized to protect their jobs in the wake of these developments. In the spring of 1977 the Ontario Nurses Association won 55 per cent of the vote among nurses at Lyndhurst to be their bargaining representative.[10] Some non-unionized employees were also quite active in making their views known regarding the need for improvement in certain areas of their jobs. At the same time, Lyndhurst's physiotherapists were also organizing around workplace issues.[11] Two years later nearly all physiotherapists signed a letter to the board asking for equal wages with the nurses. In response, approval was given to increase wages for all non-unionized staff by a total of 8 per cent by 1 October 1979.[12] Betty Brooks applied for the head physiotherapist position but was not hired. She left for rehabilitation work at another local hospital in September 1980. Within the next six months "at least ten to twelve" physiotherapists departed. Brooks remembers this period at Lyndhurst as "quite devastating, very demoralizing, like you didn't know from day to day where you stood ... I think the thing that was kind of scary was everybody that was let go were all people from the old concept, you know the old school."[13]

Andy Clarke noted that with all of these changes there was a temporary decline in experienced staff.[14] The "family atmosphere" that Charlie Saso spoke of at the old building had vanished with many of those who had worked as social workers, nurses, and physiotherapists at the original Lyndhurst Lodge.[15] In its place was a new direction with decreased time limits as to how long a person could stay in rehabilitation. This is reflected in statistics. In 1974 the average stay for first-time admissions had been seven and a half months. In 1982–83 the average length of stay had been reduced to four and a half months for new patients.[16] Thus, less than a decade after it opened, Lyndhurst on Sutherland had been transformed from a rehabilitation centre where time limits on patients' stay were open-ended, based on a doctor's overall perception of how self-sufficient a patient was and whether there were accessible living arrangements in the community, to one in which residency at the hospital was more circumscribed. While some long-term patients did stay longer than the average, the limited average length of stay signalled a break with the more flexible procedures of the past.

DOCTORS AND INTERNS

If some long-time employees found these changes too much to bear, attracting people to Lyndhurst also posed problems. During much of the 1970s and 1980s, the Lyndhurst Hospital board minutes indicate serious problems in hiring and keeping doctors of physical medicine – physiatrists – on staff. Part of the reason was the low level of pay for this job. In early 1975 Dr Geisler suggested to the board that to attract more physicians to Lyndhurst, doctors would have to be offered at least between forty and forty-five thousand dollars.[17] This figure soon shot upwards. In November 1977 Geisler pointed out that the most a doctor of physical medicine could make at Lyndhurst was approximately $30,000 per year. To attract more people to this position an annual salary of $65,000 was required. While some physicians were hired during this period, the board noted in early 1978 the "extreme difficulty" of securing the employment of physiatrists at Lyndhurst.[18]

All of these problems meant that during the early 1980s getting medical students to become residents at Lyndhurst was very difficult. The hospital board was told that within the academic community "Lyndhurst has the reputation of being old fashioned," though they were also told that all areas of medicine were short of residents.[19] These challenges were exacerbated by disputes with the region's main post-secondary institution. The University of Toronto told the hospital that they would not allow Lyndhurst to arrange a new affiliation agreement, to replace the previous one from 1972, until connections with the CPA were severed. This was not a simple thing to do since the CPA owned the building. The university held this position because they believed that the CPA interfered in Lyndhurst's operation. Therefore, the U of T would not consent to a new agreement until Lyndhurst was a free-standing corporation by itself (which never happened). The province, on the other hand, told the hospital that Lyndhurst had more important things to worry about, such as finding a medical director and obtaining more space for patients. Shortly thereafter, one of these objectives was met. Dr P. Tepperman was hired as the new medical director in the fall of 1986; he served in this capacity for five years. This appointment in turn led to the hospital having more leeway to conduct negotiations with the University of Toronto. Even though the link to the CPA was not severed, the university and the hospital reached an affiliation agreement towards the end of 1986.[20]

Throughout these difficult years, medical professionals outside Lyndhurst continued to work with their colleagues on the rehabilitation centre's staff. In addition to part-time medical personnel, a good number of medical specialists served on the Lyndhurst medical advisory committee or were consultants at the hospital. Their expertise was critical in the treatment of spinal cord injuries. In 1976 two highly regarded neurosurgeons, Dr Charles Tator and Dr Ron Tasker, were appointed as Lyndhurst consultants. That same year, Dr E. Peter McDougall, a plastic surgeon, was also made a consultant.[21] In 1985, after eleven years at Sunnybrook Hospital where he established an acute spinal cord injury unit with Dr Jousse's assistance, Tator moved to Toronto Western Hospital. There he set up "several large laboratories" that focused on spinal cord injury research, one of the largest operations of its kind in Canada. Tator also worked closely over the years with the CPA and former Lyndhurst patient Barbara Turnbull to raise funds for spinal cord injury research. This work led to the creation of the Canadian Paraplegic Association Spinal Cord Injury Research Laboratory at Toronto Western Hospital.[22] Fellow neurosurgeon Ron Tasker, working out of the Toronto General Hospital since 1961, specialized in the relief of pain; he was one of the world's preeminent doctors in this field. Many of the people he saw had been patients at the old lodge and others were patients at the new hospital.[23]

The most extensive clinical surveys of Lyndhurst patients completed during this period were two studies on life expectancy among people with spinal cord injuries published in 1977 and 1983, which followed up two earlier studies from 1961 and 1968. Doctors Geisler, Jousse, and Wynne-Jones of Lyndhurst and Dr Breithaupt, medical director of Manufacturers Life Insurance Company were the co-authors.[24] A total of 1,938 paraplegic and quadriplegic patients who had been discharged from Lyndhurst between 15 January 1945 and 31 December 1980 were followed in the last complete study, which was published in 1983. Of this final group, who were tracked from December 1973 to December 1980, after deaths and the just over 2 per cent who could not be found, 1,478 were located alive, of whom 1,252 (85 per cent) were male and 226 (15 per cent) were female. It was found that the death rate was a little over two and a half times higher than the provincial average, with both male and female statistics being similar. Within these figures, complete quadriplegics died at a rate 7.67 times higher than the average non-disabled provincial population; for complete paraplegics the rate was 3.18 times above average; partial quadriplegics died just over two times above average; mortality for partial paraplegics was just under two times higher than normal.

It was also found that peak incidence of injury occurred among people in their twenties (just over 40 per cent of the total), while people injured when they were ten to nineteen or in their thirties made up almost 19 per cent each of the total number of people surveyed. In other words, just over three quarters of spinal cord injuries were found to have occurred between the ages of ten to thirty-nine. The causes of death for people who died up to 1973 and mortality for those in the years between the end of that year and 1980 revealed some startling figures. Death rates due to renal disease were cut in half, from nearly 31 per cent – the highest cause of death up to the early 1970s – to just over 15 per cent by 1980. However, suicide rates more than doubled and deaths due to alcoholism and liver diseases nearly tripled during this same period, 1973–80. The reasons for this are not detailed in this publication; however, the reminiscences of patients like Tom Bailey (see chapter 4), clearly show that the psychological and physical impact of going from able-bodied to physically disabled, in a world that was less than hospitable in dealing with such life changes, led to enormous distress, leading to suicidal tendencies and addiction problems.

In others areas, such as cardiovascular, respiratory, and neoplastic diseases, death rates remained relatively stable. Deaths due to respiratory disease and suicide were "alarmingly" above average when compared with the general population. Though survival rates were definitely improving, these long-term studies indicated that people died because of the complications – both physical and emotional – that arose due to their spinal cord injuries – rather than because of the injury itself. Depression and despair at the barriers they faced could and did drive some people with spinal cord injuries over the edge to their deaths, indicating the crucial importance of mental health support for people living with disabilities. This reaffirms the crucial importance of a well-organized system of health care and service provision to a person's prospects following spinal cord injury, as was noted in the preceding chapter when referring to the creation of regional acute-care facilities in Ontario in the late 1960s and 1970s.

While the death rates for people in this overall disabled group were higher than for the general population, the 1983 study found that for people at the ages of twenty, thirty, forty, and fifty years of age in three of the four groups of spinal cord injuries, life expectancy increased between 1973 and 1980, except for partial paraplegics, for whom life-expectancy figures were relatively stable. This ranged from an average increase of eight more years (survival lasting from thirty-two to forty years after injury) for a twenty-year-old complete paraplegic to an increase of nine years life expectancy (survival lasting from twenty to thirty years after injury) for a twenty-year-old complete quadriplegic.

Since intermittent catheterization was not used in treatment in most instances, the authors speculated that advancements in antibiotics, renal dialysis, medical knowledge, and educating disabled people and their caregivers out in the community about preventing complications contributed to the generally positive picture that came out of these findings. Both Dr Geisler and Dr Bharatwal noted that since the late 1970s they had not seen any paraplegics or quadriplegics on renal dialysis, "a tremendous improvement" from the past, according to Bharatwal.[25]

Some past developments that stayed constant rebounded to the benefit of the hospital and the professionals who trained there. As in previous decades, foreign medical students and practitioners came to study at Lyndhurst, one example among many being the visit in the late 1980s of a urologist from China, who came to learn specialized treatment of the neurogenic bladder.[26]

Dr Bharatwal, who had been on the medical staff at Lyndhurst since May 1975 and who was also medical director for two years during the early 1980s, said that visitors were interested not only in the rehabilitation method but also in the architectural design of Lyndhurst.

They were all interested in the layout, such as bedside set-up, the room sizes, the washrooms, the toilets, etc. But they were also interested in the equipment. We have a lot of equipment that many people have not seen before and couldn't afford in some of the developing countries. They were also interested in the teaching of the patients and their families, our philosophy and details about clinical programs we ran.[27]

How nursing staff and therapists dealt with changes during this latter period at Lyndhurst Hospital reveals how the break with the past was felt slowly but surely among one group of employees in particular.

THERAPISTS, NURSES, AND ORDERLIES

During the first decade on Sutherland Drive more positions were available in the new hospital than had been in the old. However, this did not mean all of these jobs were filled as needed. With additional beds being opened (albeit temporarily as it turned out) more staff were hired.[28] The establishment in 1976 of an OT department with three employees (this grew to eight by 1981) was particularly notable. The primary focus of OT staff was to educate both quadriplegics and paraplegics;

they offered advice on self-care and on how a person with quadriplegia can use their upper body. The province had effectively told Lyndhurst that they must establish an OT departmnent, something noted with some resentment by Lyndhurst staff.[29] It was another indication that, as the hospital came under increasing accountability to the Ministry of Health, the ability of the treatment staff to "go their own way" was increasingly circumscribed.

By late 1985 more female patients were being admitted to Lyndhurst. At this time nursing care at the hospital had been adversely affected after outside temporary nursing help was eliminated. To remedy the pressure on staff, the nursing department was allowed to go over budget by $40,000 to hire the extra staff that they needed.[30] A few months later an outside report on Lyndhurst's staffing needs indicated that, in comparison to other similarly sized facilities, the hospital was understaffed in several areas but was not overstaffed in any department.[31] It took almost three more years, until fall 1988, before both the nursing and physiotherapy departments were fully staffed.[32]

Though the Lyndhurst board minutes state that primary nursing was introduced to Lyndhurst in May 1986 and was in use throughout the facility within a year, Dr Geisler recalled that this concept was not new. He remembers that the practice of having one nurse assigned to educate five specific patients on self-care was first introduced in 1957–58 under Dr Jousse. The new approach in the latter part of the 1980s had more to do with nurses having to spend less time with a patient and more time writing up documentation.[33]

Bill Brown worked at Lyndhurst for several months in 1987, the only male nurse in the facility at that time. He recalled that primary care was based on the theory of a nurse developing with a patient a "plan of care" that was to be effective for twenty-four hours with each nurse who came on shift. But, at times, theory and reality clashed. "I remember they assigned me to a very difficult [patient] ... who didn't really want to work with me ... It was very hard to establish a therapeutic rapport because I think maybe he rightly felt that he had been passed from nurse to nurse to nurse ... That was part of the difficulty with the primary nursing model." Bill Brown also recalled the day-to-day working regimen during which he worked all three eight-hour shifts. The night shift was "very, very busy" because of the need to watch for any medical emergency and to turn patients to prevent pressure sores. Days were more stressful than afternoons, as he found the mornings were "regimented" when it came to getting people up early and through the routine of bladder and bowel care as well as breakfast. There were "a lot of complaints" from patients who "didn't feel that their call bell was answered quick enough." Brown also recalled being well-trained by other Lyndhurst staff, including an orderly on the verge of retirement who was a "delightful man." This orderly taught nurses how to do an intermittent catheterization for a patient.[34] As will become evident, this catheterization procedure was to change soon afterwards.

Unlike nurses, whose collective qualifications were not called into question, orderlies occupied a much more tenuous position. The men who held these jobs found that their qualifications were often questioned. Though these exclusively male staff positions had co-existed alongside their predominantly female counterparts among the nursing and physiotherapy staff since Lyndhurst opened in 1945, the changes that had earlier affected so many of the so-called "old guard" would eventually catch up with orderlies as well. The difference was that when the "old guard" were replaced their departments were not eliminated. Things turned out differently for this group of male employees.

In 1987 Lyndhurst's orderlies were told that, to keep their jobs, their status had to be raised to Registered Nursing Assistants (RNA) by 1990, meaning that existing employees would have to enroll in RNA programs to upgrade their credentials.[35] The Service Employees International Union (SEIU), which represented orderlies, agreed that the RNA staff should all be males.[36] It was also agreed in 1987 that the male-female nursing staff ratio was to be kept at fifty-fifty.[37]

An orderly who worked at Lyndhurst throughout the entire period covered by this chapter remembered how the work-life of orderlies was affected by these various changes. Lloyd Charles was employed to work with male patients at Lyndhurst from 1972 to 2001. He recalled applying for the job at the old Lyndhurst by going through the telephone book and calling them up. "When I started working there I thought they [people with spinal cord injuries] were just sick and they were going to be getting up in two months and running around. I basically had no views, because I don't think that I met anybody with a spinal cord injury before I started working at Lyndhurst. I'd seen people in wheelchairs but never thought of it." New orderlies were taught on the job. For twenty-six out of twenty-nine years' employment he worked the afternoon shift. Assisting male patients with transfers and emptying their bladders and bowels were part of the daily routine for attendants. At times he was questioned about this part of his work by the people he worked with:

You know my motto at Lyndhurst has always been: "I treat the patients with dignity and respect and I expect the same from them." So we got along fine. There was the odd person, you know, that was difficult but you learned to handle this kind of person as you go along ... I enjoyed working with people. I guess it is sort of different than most people because the patients would ask me over the years: "How could you do this job? ..." From when I started until I left. My answer to them would be: "What's wrong with helping another human being?" Like the actual, I call it the dirty part of the job, you sort of looked beyond it and moved on. The patients would ask: "How could you? How could you do it?" They were sort of very short sighted. All they could see is the dirty things: "How could you do that?" Right, without looking at the whole picture. Personally I've always looked at the whole picture.

Charles recalled that while he did not socialize a great deal with in-patients outside the hospital, he and another attendant took one young male from Bermuda, with no family or friends in Toronto, "under our wings" and brought him to a Bob Marley concert and a few other shows. "He had a wild time."

The one major change in orderlies' duties during his nearly three decades' employment dealt with catheterization. Up to the mid-1980s orderlies changed intermittent catheters for male patients. However, around 1987, this policy changed to using Foley catheters, which were "indwelling catheters" that stay in place for four to six weeks, unlike the intermittent catheters, which were changed every six hours. "The nurses were the only ones who were allowed to do Foleys. They claimed that the orderlies were not professional, whatever that means. I personally did it for I think fifteen years myself and then you turn around and they say: 'You are not a professional.' So what can I say? ... So that's why they switched to the nurses."[38]

Since it was illegal for health-care employees to strike, as they were deemed an essential service, any labour disputes had to be settled through negotiations or arbitration. Charles was chief steward at Lyndhurst for the SEIU local, which represented orderlies. "We had problems that we worked out ... People just don't go to union meetings except when you've got a contract. Everybody wants to know how much raise they are going to get ... People were satisfied." Perhaps the most significant gradual change that took place during his employment at Lyndhurst was in the ratio of orderlies to nurses. Originally, when it came to male patients the nurses "never touched the guys with a ten foot pole. Orderlies did that." Over time, nurses started to physically assist with male patients "because sometimes it got really unbearable. It was hard work." With fewer orderlies employed and more nurses taking their place "they just had to pitch in. For example, say I was working the weekend and somebody called in sick and there is just a nurse to call, it was a no choice situation ... Night [shift] was one on one, one orderly and one nurse. Afternoons were two nurses and two orderlies. And days were, I think, two orderlies and probably six nurses. That was at the end [in 2001]. At some point it used to be a base of four – four until the orderly population started dwindling. Then it was three [orderlies and five nurses per day shift], then the last count was two [orderlies per day shift]."

He estimated that the orderly staff went from a high of thirty-five during the 1970s to seventeen in 2001. The decline in orderlies, he suggests, was a management decision to hire fewer of them and more nurses. After twenty-nine years' employment at Lyndhurst, "we all got canned. All the orderlies. Well, again they said that we were doing things that we weren't supposed to do because we were not professionals, so they replaced us with registered nurses." Charles then established his own attendant care business in Toronto. Referring to his own situation after Lyndhurst as "a blessing" he summed up his three decades there in the following words: "I had a good time. How to describe it ... I had a blast because I enjoy working with people. I had a lot of laughs ... It was not just about work but interacting with people."[39]

A few years before the attendants were all fired, former Lyndhurst resident Michael O'Brien was a patient under their care in 1998–99. "I thought that the *esprit d'corps* was really very much the result of a number of extremely competent attendants that had been there at Lyndhurst for a number of years. They had been there, many of them, for years. They came generally from the Philippines and from the Caribbean and they were great fellows. They could handle the bladder and bowel care, get you in and out of bed quickly and efficiently and much better than the nurses that were there. Much to my shock, and I think as a result of the amalgamation and budget cutting, all these people have been let go and it's just a shame, a shame. They were *really* good. They were good for morale and they had been there for years. They knew more about how to do things. You could gain more information from these people than anybody else. So I don't look upon that very kindly."[40]

Perhaps one of the most controversial episodes in Lyndhurst's labour relations history occurred in the final years of its existence as a stand-alone facility. In 1993 P. Au, who had worked at Lyndhurst for four and a half years began sexual harassment and racial discrimination proceedings against a male employee. This process lasted four years and involved the hospital as a defendant in a widely reported legal case in which the former employee brought a "precedent setting claim of [sexual] harassment as a workplace hazard." The episode became especially controversial after she lost her job in November 1993. Lyndhurst management stated that the termination of her job "was not linked in any way to [sexual harassment] allegations" but was part of wider lay-offs during that period. Eventually, the Ontario Labour Relations Board ruled in favour of Lyndhurst in 1997.[41]As will be seen in the pages that follow, patient life at Lyndhurst also had its share of controversy, mixed in as always with the daily routine of life at a rehabilitation centre.

PATIENT LIFE AT LYNDHURST

The new hospital had no difficulty filling up those beds that were available during the two and a half decades covered by this chapter. During the second half of the 1970s, people with paraplegia or quadriplegia made up between 80 to 90 per cent of all first-time admissions.[42] By the second half of the 1980s, this group made up three-quarters of first-time admissions, most of whom came from hospitals in the Toronto area.[43] While people continued to arrive at Lyndhurst from elsewhere in the province, by and large, the spread of rehabilitation services to other areas of Ontario and elsewhere in the country meant that Lyndhurst had gone from being a national and international facility during its early years, to a provincial rehabilitation centre in middle age, to one that primarily served people who lived in the Toronto area by the end of the twentieth century. However, one aspect of its history remained consistent throughout these changes – waiting lists to get in. Long waiting lists put a particularly onerous strain on the constant demand for bed space during the last decade of Lyndhurst's existence before amalgamation. In the fall of 1994 as many as forty people were waiting at acute-care hospitals for up to six months to get into Lyndhurst's rehabilitation program.[44]

The causes of spinal cord injuries for people who came to Lyndhurst that were recorded in 1996 continued to reflect many of the same causes that had been around since the days of the original lodge: 50 per cent were due to motor vehicle accidents; 14 per cent were caused by falls; 12 per cent were the result of sporting activity, especially diving; 10 per cent were due to tumours; 7 per cent were from being injured on the job; and another 7 per cent were recorded as "other."[45] Twenty years earlier, one of the people whose cause of injury would have come under the "other" category found himself at the new hospital two years after it opened.

Kirby Rowe

In the summer of 1976 twenty-eight-year-old Kirby Rowe was injured when the small plane he was in for a sightseeing trip in northern Ontario landed with a "thump." His spine and legs were fractured and he became a paraplegic. After receiving very good care from Dr Dave Hoffman at Port Arthur General Hospital in Thunder Bay, Rowe was transferred to Sunnybrook Hospital in Toronto. Like many people with spinal cord injuries before him, he was put on a stryker frame while undergoing acute care. The main purpose of the stryker frame was to allow one staff member to turn the patient without unduly moving the fractured spine.[46] Rowe's description of this frame is perhaps the most vivid: "Some people would call it a torture device. It is essentially a metal frame of two identical pieces ... They put you on one and strap the other one on top of you like a sandwich. Then they will spin you over, like from your back to your chest and vice versa, the idea being to prevent pressure sores from developing from being in one place all of the time. And also to afford a much more rigid ... piece of stability to make sure that your spine healed properly. They don't use them anymore."

After about fifteen weeks of acute hospital care, Rowe was sent for rehabilitation to Lyndhurst, where he remained from November 1976 to May 1978. He remembers being "pretty timid at first, because everybody was in wheelchairs. It was kind of frightening you know." After thinking for a few days that being at Lyndhurst was "the end of the road," where he would stay forever, he got over what he felt was like a "bad dream ... Once I got up and around and I met some nice people and everybody was so positive and enthusiastic. I am talking about the staff primarily at that point. I mean, reassuring me that: 'Jeez, I was lucky!'" Since his injury was low down in his spine – an incomplete paraplegia – Rowe was able to move his legs somewhat. His first roommates "were all C–4 quadriplegics. You know, *completely* dependent and all younger than me." As with other people before him, discussed in earlier chapters, Rowe's sense of his own disability was greatly influenced by his interaction with other disabled people, particularly quadriplegics who had far less physical mobility than an incomplete paraplegic like himself.

Rehabilitation was a "good experience." In addition to mat and chair classes, he also had individual physiotherapy sessions with Brenda Rotenberg, whom Rowe described as "wonderful." She encouraged him with "a little pep talk" when he felt "blue." This taught him to combine "enthusiasm" about his rehabilitation with a "dose of reality" about how much he could do physically. Initially his rehabilitation included the use of braces and walking with crutches. Nobody said that he would not be able to walk again. Instead, he was told: "'We're not sure. It could take two years before we know what kind of return you are going get.' So, I sort of had to discipline myself to say: 'Okay. In the meantime, work hard at getting back in shape again, your upper body and what not. And, see what happens.' So that's basically what happened." Though he continued to use crutches after he left Lyndhurst, he found it was "exhausting" and "precarious" so he eventually switched to a wheelchair.

The atmosphere in the building was laid-back. Many staff wore casual clothes, and Rowe found the surroundings physically accessible inside and beautiful on the grounds outside. Having come from the massive Sunnybrook complex, he found that the new Lyndhurst building did not have the institutional feeling he was used to. Since it was a "small community," Rowe recalled seeing the same people each day, some of whom became friends. Many of them were teenagers or in their early twenties. At this time, the building had two patient wings on the main floor and one active patient wing on the second floor. The active second floor wing was used as an independent ward for residents who were not in need of as much assistance as people on the first floor. Since there were fewer staff on this floor than on the first floor, Rowe recalled that some of the younger patients had some "pretty wild parties" at night, some of which "would get a bit out of hand." People at these parties would be admonished the following day. In some instances, party-goers had too much to drink and slept until noon. While some people became upset when this happened, others said "Look. The guy broke his back. He is eighteen years old. You know, he is just trying to get through it."

While partying on the independent ward was one way of socializing, another popular venue was the nearby Laird Tavern, which had a level entrance. It was several long blocks away from Lyndhurst Hospital, on the nearest main thoroughfare, Eglinton Avenue. During the warmer weather it was well patronized by Lyndhurst residents, some of whom had "running tabs" with the bar operators. "It was great ... a first introduction to society, if you will, getting back into the community." Using familiar places like this to ease the transition out of the hospital was important, since the thought of returning to the "cold, cruel world" was worrisome to Rowe and some of the other people he knew. Lyndhurst was "like a security blanket and is one of the dangers of long-term rehab."[47] Their concerns about prospects in the wider world were justified. While three-quarters of those who were first-time admissions in 1977 returned to their own homes or that of a relative or friend, another quarter had no such luck. Instead general hospitals or long-term care facilities were their destination. As well, just under one-third of this overall group of 119 people had been able to find employment or had returned to school; two-thirds were neither employed nor in school.[48] Plenty of barriers remained in place. Fortunately Rowe was able to find employment. He eventually became an employee of the CPA in British Columbia and was head of the new Ontario Division from 1980 to 1989. His involvement in advocacy work mirrored the activism inside the new Lyndhurst building where he had been a patient.

Patients' Councils at Lyndhurst Hospital

One of the more obvious examples of how patients dealt with life at the new facility was the committees they set up to air their views. In March 1975 members of the Patients' Representative Committee asked to establish liaison with the hospital board to discuss their concerns. This was agreed to by the board who "acknowledged that since patients in Lyndhurst tend to be long stay and are physically dependent, they are in a weak position viz a viz the staff."[49] Three representatives of the committee met with Dr Geisler and Ken Langford to discuss several complaints about certain staff members. One complaint was withdrawn due to lack of substantiation, while they said that "substantial improvement" was observed in the conduct of the other staff members they were concerned about. Board chairman Jack Blain said there was "some substance" to the patients' concerns and noted that they went to great lengths to bring their views to the attention of the board. The board decided that in future treatment issues raised by the Patients' Representative Committee would be dealt with by the medical director while the hospital administrator would address other issues.[50] Later that year the newly hired administrator, Douglas Perkins, reported to the board that he had held "constructive" talks with committee and "was able to do something about their recommendations in the administration area but those in the treatment area meet with a cold reception from the 'old guard.'"[51]

These efforts by current and former patients of Lyndhurst to have more input into the conditions and treatment that affected their lives took place during a period of increased activism by disabled people in Canada, the United States, and elsewhere.[52] Perhaps the most obvious example of heightened international awareness was when the United Nations declared 1981 to be the International Year of Disabled Persons. The following year, when the new Canadian Charter of Rights and Freedoms was signed into law, Section 15 specified protection of any person from discrimination on the basis of physical or mental disability. This particular legal victory did not come without a struggle, as the CPA and numerous other organizations had to fight long and hard to have the human rights of people with disabilities included in the new charter.[53] All of these developments quite naturally encouraged people with disabilities to be more outspoken at the local level when it came to advancing their place in society. This was felt at Lyndhurst Hospital, as in so many other communities, in the early 1980s.

In February 1980 the Lyndhurst Hospital Patients Transportation Corporation was incorporated. Operated entirely by patients, with no involvement from the hospital, this non-profit provincial corporation was set up mainly to provide transportation for Lyndhurst patients in and around the local community. It also made their views known about other issues affecting "the said patients with regard to their education, culture, recreation, comfort, rehabilitation and convenience."[54] In early 1980 the Kiwanis Club donated a van for the recreational use of in-patients, who took charge of it under the auspices of the Lyndhurst Hospital Patients Transportation charitable organization. Besides being used for drives, the van was used for parties held in the hospital parking lot and had liquor stored in it, causing the board some concern. Perhaps in response to this unorthodox using of the hospital parking lot, a new leaflet outlining rules for patients was printed in the summer of 1980. It stated that patients could be discharged if they were found to have consumed or be in possession of "unauthorized drugs or other behaviour modifying substances."[55] The old informal system of looking the other way or dealing with consumption of drugs and alcohol on an individual basis was now changed to a stricter policy.

No one was looking the other way when one particularly contentious issue arose two years later. Catheterization of male patients was a major issue for both patients and staff. In early 1982 two trained orderlies were responsible for this job among male patients. When the hospital proposed that female staff also do this task, some nurses objected and so too did many male patients. The argument by the Medical Advisory Committee was that catheterization practices needed to be improved to prevent infections. This topic was soon talked about well beyond the grounds of Lyndhurst Hospital.[56]

One way of raising awareness and money for the activities of the Lyndhurst Hospital Patients Transportation Corporation was selling cartoons to get their point across. Apparently, a complaint was received from the College of Nurses of Ontario about the selling of these cartoons. Though the precise nature of the complaint is not specified, it referred to patients taking a "vocal" stand in regard to wanting their catheterizations done by same sex staff – presumably, this is what the cartoons were concerned with. Administrator Randy Swan informed the college in February 1983 that "the majority of these patients in this hospital have made it clear that their concerns on this issue will be heard. Although we may not all agree with the methods of their expression, nevertheless we must hear their concerns."[57]

In September and October 1982 two different surveys were done by the Lyndhurst Patients Transportation Corporation, supervised by former Lyndhurst patients and the Kiwanis Club. In the first survey, eight anonymous former patients, who ranged in age from their teens to their mid-forties, were asked their opinions about having "residuals," that is emptying of bladder and bowels, done by male or female staff. Six quadriplegics and two paraplegics made up this first survey group. The seven males and one female expressed the desire to have this personal care done by someone of the same sex. They also made a number of comments that reveal how patients experienced this treatment. One former male patient who was quadriplegic mentioned that he felt he was "nothing more than a piece of meat in the General Hospital. I would not want that to happen at Lyndhurst, it would be a disaster ... The first thing I noticed in Lyndhurst was that males did the males and females did the females and I thought that was right on." A former female patient who was quadriplegic said: "The paralysis and hospitalization destroys your sexual image. When Rehab staff considers your feelings enough to provide someone of the same sex to take care of your personal needs, then you gain some of your sexuality and self-respect back."

Some of the males interviewed also said that their privacy was not respected, as nurses would come in when an orderly was doing their residuals. Rapport between a patient and staff who did their residuals was particularly important. A quadriplegic former male patient stated that this function was done in "almost a locker room fashion ... a jocular way which helped to shift the mind of one's awareness from the inability to do it yourself." While some spoke very highly of the care they received in Lyndhurst, others interviewed were very critical. Comments about a depressed atmosphere among the patients and slow response by some staff to requests for assistance were mentioned. One paraplegic former patient bluntly stated: "Lyndhurst was like a hell on earth." The person who compiled this information said some of the people with spinal cord injuries that he had met "over the years" at Lyndhurst had called themselves "inmates rather than patients." One in-patient at Lyndhurst who was interviewed outside the above surveyed group, said he felt "stripped of all your dignity here ... and there is nothing you can do about it." Nurses interviewed for this first survey said they "instinctively felt that there was something wrong in them doing male catheterization on a regular basis." The nurses also said that they had never been asked for their opinions on this topic, "only that they are expected to do it." The person who sent this report to hospital and provincial health officials insisted that practices "that degrade the populace" of hospitals like Lyndhurst need to be changed at once.[58]

With such strong feelings on this issue a more detailed confidential survey, with only the gender identified, was held on 18 October 1982. This time, current in-patients were canvassed for their opinion. As with the first survey, it was initiated by the Lyndhurst Hospital Patients Transportation Corporation and overseen by Kiwanis Club members and former Lyndhurst patients. The survey question asked: "While in Lyndhurst Hospital who would you prefer to look after your personal care needs on a regular basis?" Of nine female patients surveyed, eight were recorded as "Pro Female" and one was "Pro Male." Of forty-nine male patient surveyed, three were "Pro Female," twenty-six were "Pro Male" and twenty were tabulated as "Makes No Difference." The person who reported on this survey noted that one young male patient said that at first he was embarrassed when a female did this job, "then I got used to it so it doesn't matter any more." According to the individual who contacted Ontario's Minister of Health, Larry Grossman, about this survey, "When one is told over and over by the people involved about the humiliation of having someone of the opposite sex perform these functions ... then I think anyone would feel charged with the responsibility to do something about the problem."[59]

To add further weight to their views, on 1 November 1982 thirty Lyndhurst patients, twenty-seven men and three women, signed a witnessed statement "advising that they do not want and will not consent to anyone of the opposite sex performing any function as it pertains to their personal care needs." However, this signed statement was not presented to the hospital. The administrator, Randy Swan, requested that it not be presented after he indicated that feelings about patient dignity would be seriously considered, because it "could cause unnecessary problems between some of the patients and Lyndhurst Hospital." This was agreed to by the patients' representatives. Arguing against the notion that people who disliked this aspect of their treatment "will get used to it" the person who contacted Health Minister Grossman stated that such a view "obviously never took the patients' feelings into consideration."[60] Finally, on 20 January 1983, four months after first being contacted about this matter, Ontario's Health Minister responded by noting that rules at Lyndhurst Hospital had been changed in light of the controversy: "Patients who require personal care procedures of an intimate nature will now be able to select the gender of the health care worker who performs the procedures, whenever such a person is available."[61] Patients views were heard loud and clear on this occasion and were listened to. Training more male orderlies as genito-urinary technicians was the solution settled on for this issue; women patients were catheterized by female nurses.[62] However, as discussed earlier in this chapter, this policy was again changed before the end of the decade, when orderlies were prohibited from doing this procedure.

A few weeks after the resolution of this episode, a Patient Council was started in April 1983 to allow for more input by patients into various aspects of hospital life. It was open to all patients and had an elected executive. In less than a year they had held fourteen meetings, with an average in-patient attendance of thirty people per meeting. They were involved in setting up educational events and inviting guest speakers, such as former Lyndhurst patient and CPA staff member Kirby Rowe. Patient Council members also participated in various hospital committees, established a computer room for patient use, and addressed other issues about quality of life.[63] Several years later, in 1988, it was reported that the Patients Council "has assumed an advocacy role for patients" and was involved in fundraising to purchase "recreational equipment for patients." They were also involved in the PARTY Program – Prevention of Alcohol-Related Trauma in Youth – which was started in 1986. It was designed to educate young people about avoiding the sort of mishaps that lead to spinal cord injuries. Twice a week para-medical students at Sunnybrook and Lyndhurst were shown the various stages of treatment of a person with a spinal cord injury, from initial injury to returning to the community. People who taught this course included individuals with spinal cord injuries, "some still in acute care, others in rehabilitation, and some who have returned home."[64]

Perhaps reflecting the increased activism among patients at Lyndhurst, as well as wider developments in society, formal guidelines were drawn up to address care and treatment issues that were being aired at that time. In 1984 a human rights policy focusing on the dignity of patients was approved by the Lyndhurst Hospital board.[65] The following year, in early 1985, it was agreed that patient complaints about violations of their privacy and dignity should be reported to the director of nursing or the administrator.[66] A policy on Acquired Immune Deficiency Syndrome (AIDS) was also developed beginning in late 1987 respecting the rights of both patients and staff.[67] Lyndhurst's patients' rights policy was updated in 1994 to include the "requirement that patients must immediately disclose information pertaining to assault, abuse or misconduct by staff."[68] In line with new provincial legislation, all patients were to be informed about their rights to consent to treatment, advocacy, substitute decision makers, and legal protections.[69] In 1996 a document written up by the Community Advisory Committee entitled "Rights and Responsibilities of Patients" was posted around the hospital.[70]

Throughout these developments, the Patient Council waxed and waned between the late 1980s and early 1990s. By 1996 it was reported to be "functioning well" with the purchase of a fax machine for patients' use.[71] However, it soon became inactive again. In the summer of 1998, just as Lyndhurst was about to amalgamate with two other health-care facilities, the Patient Council was reactivated. Among their concerns was the need to fix uneven pavement around the building and to provide more exercise time. Prior to the council becoming active again, patient concerns were reported to have been "regularly canvassed and problems dealt with directly on the units."[72] In the last reference to the Patient Council in the Lyndhurst board minutes before amalgamation took effect, it was noted in September 1998 that the patient library needed to be watched so that it was used only by patients and their families.[73]

In March 1998 Michael O'Brien, a fifty-six-year-old lawyer, had a skiing accident that caused him to become quadriplegic. During his year in Lyndhurst, 1998–99, he helped to re-start the Patient Council and became its leader during the last days before amalgamation. O'Brien said that the Patient Council was "effective" and "welcomed" by hospital officials. Members discussed their concerns with the chief nurse and the hospital administrator. He also felt that it helped to "diffuse situations," since patients felt "that they were finally getting someone to listen to them and to bring their concerns to the powers that be."

One of their concerns was the "dreadful" state of the sidewalks. Cracks and uneven pavement made them unsafe for people in wheelchairs. After O'Brien had fallen forward in his wheelchair and required assistance from a physiotherapist to sit up again, he "became teed off about the condition of the grounds." As a result, the sidewalks on the grounds and a nearby fire road were all re-paved. Other improvements included getting wheelchair accessible public phones. New sliding boards were purchased for transfers in the hospital; the charitable Lyndhurst Foundation purchased these boards. Recognizing that "squeaky wheels get grease," O'Brien said the Patient Council also approached the hospital about getting sliding doors installed for the back entrance onto the grounds. That way, people in wheelchairs who did not smoke could go outside without having to pass through the haze of smokers who gathered by the front entrance where the only sliding doors were then in place. Since this was done, O'Brien noted, the smokers congregate out back where a new patio and gazebo have been built.[74]

Barbara Turnbull

In addition to the activities of the Patient Council over the years, the daily life of the hospital continued; each person experienced it differently. Barbara Turnbull had been in Lyndhurst for a few weeks in January 1984 and again from April to September of that year. In September 1983, when she was eighteen, Turnbull had been shot by a robber at the convenience store where she worked. This left her a complete C–4 quadriplegic. After arriving from Sunnybrook, she initially remained in bed for several days. When staff put her in a wheelchair for the first time she passed out since she had been lying down for so long. Turnbull found this aspect of Lyndhurst "one of the biggest differences" in contrast to a general hospital. Wheelchairs at Lyndhurst did not recline, unlike those she had been used to. "What they would do when we were dizzy would be to tip the whole chair back and then you would sort of come to and get your equilibrium a little bit more, and then they wanted to be up again. So it was not easy at all."

At Sunnybrook, Turnbull had placed small towel rolls beneath her pillow on both sides of her head as a "cradle" after having been in traction so long. When she asked the nurse who admitted her to Lyndhurst, Glenna Boston – "everyone's favourite nurse" – if she could have these rolls placed under her pillow, the response was "'We don't do little things like that here.' They didn't have time for fussy little things that one individual might like ... There was an attitude that you were going to get on with things, and they hit you over the head with it. I don't say that in a bad way, they weren't unkind, they were just matter of fact with what you had to do."

On the other hand, Turnbull also felt that there "were times when I felt people could have been a little more sympathetic." When she was learning how to use her head-controlled wheelchair, nurses at first would place it next to her bed at night after turning off the clutches. Then a night nurse told her to "park it yourself" which she proceeded to do. "I think that there was a good balance of mollycoddling people to a certain extent, but then it would get to a point that it wouldn't go on too long, and then you would have to do it yourself."

One part of the daily routine that was particularly unpopular with patients was the morning rounds, when staff came by as a team to check on them. In retrospect, she was surprised "that we didn't rebel" at the rounds, which took place at seven every morning. "I heard that they formed a Patient Council not too long after and that was one of the things they first voted on, abolishing the morning rounds ... We didn't have to get up at that point so we just went back to sleep." During her rehabilitation, she spent the morning in physiotherapy and the afternoon in occupational therapy. This included learning how to type and to use a mouse stick with which to manipulate objects, to enable her to read a book on a stand or to change cassette tapes on the stereo. Her physiotherapist, Marlene Weaves, helped to teach Turnbull how to do a "one person transfer" to and from her wheelchair. This was "one of the best things" she learned at Lyndhurst and has used ever since. Turnbull expressed particularly high regard for Dr Bharatwal, whom she called "an amazing woman ... She is sympathetic, supportive, and encouraging."

Life among patients was "like everywhere else – you find your group of people." In her case, she became good friends with another woman resident and two men. They all ate their meals together and socialized while watching television in the evening. "We were the straighter crowd." She remembers other people who went out to the parking lot to "smoke dope" far removed "from the eyes of the staff," who would not have allowed this. "There was one quad that would get paraplegics to separate the lines of coke for him. They weren't people I hung out with." Among people she did know, they would joke about getting one bath or shower a week, "whether you need it or not ... They didn't have the staff to do that; otherwise we would get a bed bath or sponging down." The lack of privacy common to most hospital wards was felt here too, though they did have curtains around their beds, unlike women in the old Lyndhurst. Turnbull completed her high school studies while at Lyndhurst. She went on to write a book about her experiences, became a journalist for the *Toronto Star*, established a foundation for spinal cord research, and raised a great deal of money for the CPA's work in this area.[75] "The only thing that makes me very angry was if anyone ever referred to me as a patient now. If I could have seen my doctor in a doctor-patient setting then I might be a patient, okay. I remember after I left Lyndhurst I was ... going back and getting a hydraulic-type lift, which I never ended up using. The guy there [a technologist] was sort of trying it out on me and the guy kept referring to me as a patient. I refused to buy that equipment from him just for that reason. I told him too a couple of times that I don't live here anymore, I am not a patient anymore, I am living back in the real world. He was blind to it. As far as he was concerned anybody with a disability was a patient."[76]

Carmen Mobbs

Less than two years after Barbara Turnbull left Lyndhurst, Carmen Mobbs arrived for a five-month stay, from June to October 1986. She was a thirty-eight-year-old nurse and married mother with two children. Mobbs was four months pregnant with a third child at the time of her injury, which occurred when she fell down a staircase. After treatment at York County Hospital in Newmarket she was sent to the TGH, where she was classified as an incomplete quadriplegic. While there she was told that she would never walk again. "I tuned them out and thought: 'No, it will happen. I don't care what they say. I have a baby coming and I am going to look after this child, nobody else is.'" Dr Geisler came to see her at the TGH to assess her possible residency at Lyndhurst. "Terrified" at first by a doctor who "seemed so strict," after he examined her and explained what the place was about she thought "Oh gee, he's not so bad after all."

Mobbs arrived at Lyndhurst just as some feeling was returning to her arms, which she could move, though her legs remained paralysed. She understood that she was the first female patient to be pregnant while a resident at Lyndhurst. Prior to this, pregnant women with spinal cord injuries would have their baby first and come to Lyndhurst afterwards. Geisler took her "under his wing" and was careful about what she could and could not do in rehabilitation. At times she would get angry with him for not allowing her to do certain things. While they would have "arguments back and forth" they each "had great respect for each other." Since she was pregnant there was uncertainty about what kind of treatment she should get. It was not possible for her to have an x-ray while pregnant so they were not sure of the extent of her spinal injuries, which an otherwise standard x-ray would have revealed. This was "frustrating for both staff and myself. For example, with physio, was I allowed to stand up and try and do some walking? Was that too difficult? Did that put too much strain with being pregnant on the joints and everything like that? A lot of things were trial and error. However, everyone was so, so supportive and kind and also excited because they had never had somebody pregnant there. It was sort of exciting for them too because it was different. They could follow along each month to see how I got bigger."

The patients were also very supportive as the "younger people just thought it was wonderful having somebody there that was pregnant. It was like a little family." In addition to talking about her expectant condition, they would sit outside during the summer "sometimes ten of us in a row in a wheelchair" and discuss each others personal concerns. She also felt "comradeship" from other nurses at Lyndhurst while she was a patient there. Since Mobbs was a nurse prior to her injury, other nurses at the rehabilitation centre trusted her to self-administer heparin, a shot she had to have every day. They also discussed her medical treatment with her and asked her opinion: "What do you think? Should you be doing this? Should you not be doing this? Do you need anything else to eat as far as extra for the baby? They knew that I wasn't going to be stupid and do things that were going to harm myself and the baby even though I wanted to get going and do things faster than anybody else ... In some aspects I was given a little bit more leeway than some other patients because of my medical history."

After leaving Lyndhurst to have her baby son, who was born "very healthy," she returned home and went for rehabilitation to a hospital in Newmarket, not far from Toronto. Carmen Mobbs maintained regular contact with Lyndhurst and Dr Geisler during this time and went there for check-ups. Her children, husband and mother were all very supportive of her during a period of immense stress. Their house also had to be made more accessible to accommodate her. During her stay at Lyndhurst she went home on weekends, which she called "the best mental health" treatment possible. The year following her return home, she became pregnant with her fourth child, a daughter who was born in 1987. Carmen Mobbs used a wheelchair for two-and-a-half years after leaving Lyndhurst. Then she gradually transferred to walking with a cane, which she now uses along with a brace for her left leg.

After back surgery she required bed rest, and so was admitted to Lyndhurst for a second time for six weeks in 1992. Some things, notably the meals were the same: "Monday, for example, was fish and chips. Tuesday was chicken ... It got to be very boring." In summer there was more variety. However, there were some notable changes between her two stays, six years apart. When she was in physiotherapy during her 1986 stay, Mobbs said everyone "worked together" in a large room, which helped to foster friendships. Different people did different types of therapy, during which people encouraged each other. She noted that if someone "put one foot forward a half an inch" staff and patients alike would clap and say "Yes you did it! ... That was a big step." However, this atmosphere was changed in 1992. People came and went from physiotherapy at different times, so that it was not possible to get to know people. As well, during her first time at Lyndhurst people were called immediately if they were not at therapy, whereas the second time it took longer for staff to call the person, as the patient load was greater. One significant improvement between these two periods was that technology was better in 1992. Electrodes were being used more effectively to promote muscle stimulation, which allowed for greater wrist flexion among quadriplegics. Speaker phones, which were important assistive devices for those with spinal cord injuries, were also available. One thing that had not changed was the difficulty that people experienced during the evenings. Since many Lyndhurst patients did not have relatives in the Toronto area, they found this time of day quite difficult, particularly from six to nine at night. "I think it was the time for people to vent their feelings, whether it was frustration, anger, sadness, or happiness. It was a venting time but it was also a lonely time because if you were married or had kids, you missed your family."

The support of her husband, when so many other people with spinal cord injuries saw their relationships fall apart, was a particular source of strength for Carmen Mobbs. Her husband remembered Lyndhurst in a unique way, quite unlike anyone else interviewed for this book, as his wife recalled: "My husband and I were talking yesterday morning about Lyndhurst. I was saying so much of it I put in my subconscious. I don't want to remember because it was a part of my life that was stressful. Anyway, he mentioned that he will never ever forget the smell of Lyndhurst. It has a unique smell, not a foul smell. Just a unique Lyndhurst smell. He would say: 'Every Friday night when I would come home, when I would come in the house, you could smell this Lyndhurst smell' ... Because you know I had the same wheelchair all week. I would come home with the wheelchair and my clothes. It is just a unique ... institutional smell, Lyndhurst institutional smell. Yes. He said that he'll never forget that."[77]

Just as the support of family and friends was crucial for anyone with a spinal cord injury, other areas of support provided by Lyndhurst Hospital during these two-and-a-half decades were also very important, as is discussed in the next section.

SERVICES FOR IN-PATIENTS AND FORMER PATIENTS OF LYNDHURST

After the teaching of the necessary skills for self-care and self-sufficiency at Lyndhurst, one of the most essential services available for younger in-patients was providing an academic education. Schooling was often interrupted at the time of a person's injury. Education had been a part of the Lyndhurst's program since the 1950s. During the period covered by this chapter, the secondary school education department was funded by the Ministry of Education for patients at Lyndhurst who were twenty-one or under. It had two special education teachers. As was explained in a report in 1986–87, when there were seventeen students enrolled, students were met by teachers on a "one-to-one basis in the classroom for one hour at a time." Classes were held between 9 a.m. and noon and from 1 to 3 p.m. The academic programs were designed on the basis of individual needs. When it came time for students to return to the community, Lyndhurst teachers were in contact with their home school to provide the necessary support for their post-hospital schooling. Some students graduated while at Lyndhurst, as did a Grade 12 student – a "graduation tea was held in her honour with friends, teachers, staff and school officials in attendance."[78] The primary fields of study were math, English, and computers.[79]

Other practical areas of instruction were open to anyone who had a driver's licence. Teaching patients to transfer between wheelchair and car was taught to all those who could make use of such techniques; learning this transfer technique was aided in 1988 when General Motors (Canada) donated a car body for this purpose.[80]

Reintegrating people into the community had always been a priority of both the CPA and Lyndhurst. However, this job was not made any easier by the fiscal restraint that characterized these decades. Provincial cutbacks jeopardized Lyndhurst's ability to provide recently discharged patients with enough medical supplies and medications as they adjusted to life in the community. The Ministry of Health felt this was an unnecessary expense. Lyndhurst argued that it saved the province money in the long-run by providing a smoother transition, resulting in fewer re-admissions.[81] By early 1977 Lyndhurst had established a policy whereby various categories of patients had access to a "limited" amount of "medical-surgical supply needs," though it was understood that they would eventually have to find their own provisions after discharge.[82]

A group of Lyndhurst patients asked for assistance from the board to help set up housing for them after discharge, though no decision was forthcoming at the time of the initial request. However, by May 1983 the Nucleus Housing project was established to accommodate eleven quadriplegics who, up to then, had lived at Lyndhurst.[83] Lise Desrochers, who worked as director of development for CPA Ontario from 1982 to 1991, recalled that one day while walking through Lyndhurst she was approached by Darryl M., "an amazing guy," who had been there for eighteen months. A high level quadriplegic, he had no home to return to. Desrochers did a "big media blitz" to publicize this issue. Over the next two years, five volunteers met to plan Nucleus Housing, "the first attendant care facility for high level quadriplegics." Nucleus Housing

II followed. The people who lived there organized the operation of the buildings so that it became "a really successful model" for people with high-level quadriplegia living in the community.[84] Kirby Rowe, CPA Ontario executive director from 1980–89, was also involved in establishing Nucleus Housing in 1982–83. He recalled that this group of long-stay high quadriplegics at Lyndhurst "had nowhere to go where they could have an accessible home and attendant care on site." Provincial officials in the Ministry of Community and Social Services (COMSOC) were just beginning to fund this type of housing. "We helped this group sort of organize themselves. Got the Minister of COMSOC to come … They were all around the table. It was compelling. It was unbelievable. You know, you talk about your activism and advocacy and all that stuff. It was great. So we had names and faces and guys that really had needs. So it came to be."[85]

Ten years later a Transitional Living Program was initiated at Lyndhurst. Its aim was to prepare in-patients for their post-hospital life by "directing one's own care, booking attendants" and similar confidence-building measures. Nine beds in Lyndhurst were designated for this program. That same year, 1993, also saw the re-emergence of a Cottage Program funded by a local Rotary Club. This program had originally existed in the 1950s.[86] It allowed four in-patients to spend two days and nights in an accessible cottage outside the city. It was operated by the recreation therapy and leisure services department and included three staff members on each trip.[87]

Providing an avenue for former Lyndhurst residents to have some say in hospital affairs was also a concern. In 1993 the Community Advisory Committee (CAC) was established by the hospital to enable former patients and family members of patients to "have direct input into hospital programs and planning."[88] However, while its goals were laudable, it fell short of its function according to one former patient. Board member Lucille Owen observed in 1997 that the CAC, which was responsible for writing up human rights policies for the board, did not have many members who were people with disabilities. A few months later it was noted that two former Lyndhurst patients were invited to join the CAC; Barbara Turnbull, who was also on this committee, was asked to speak to in-patients.[89]

One particularly intimate area of life was the focus of work by Dr Murray Moffat, who was appointed in 1978 as a consultant to discuss sexuality with patients at Lyndhurst.[90] A decade later an entire clinic that focused on this topic was opened. On 31 October 1988 the

Robson Urology Clinic began operations. It was named after the late Charles Robson, a urologist who had been a Lyndhurst medical consultant. Its purpose was to help people with spinal cord injuries inside and outside Lyndhurst deal with matters relating to urology, sexuality, and reproduction. An average of forty-seven people a month were using the services of this clinic a year after it was set up; within two years this had risen to eighty-four people a month. By 1993 Dr R. MacMillan reported that the Robson Clinic had about 200 new clients a year. The birth of twins fathered by a paraplegic in January 1993 helped to promote this clinic around Canada.[91] By 1997 it was reported that six children "came to be" thanks to the Robson Clinic fertility program, and more pregnancies were on the way.[92]

Other clinical services were also initiated. Alcoholism had been a serious problem at Lyndhurst since the earliest days of its existence. Since the 1960s illicit drug use had been an issue as well. Thus it was long overdue when in 1985 Dr Sally Saunders of the Addiction Research Foundation was appointed to help people deal with addiction-related problems at Lyndhurst.[93] Addiction problems reflected the stresses that have always existed for people with physical disabilities. They have to deal with a world geared towards the able-bodied, a world to which many of them had once belonged but, because of a variety of circumstances detailed throughout this book, they found that their personal relations and employment prospects were drastically altered by a society that more often than not devalued people who could not walk unaided, or who could not walk at all. This systemic societal discrimination, coupled with the historical culture of machismo among males in particular dating back to the earliest years at Lyndhurst, led some people to find escape in alcoholism and drugs from the emotional pain of rejection and the enormous physical and psychological changes in self-perception that came about as a result of a spinal cord injury.

Perhaps the most unconventional service, and one of the most innovative introduced in this latter period of Lyndhurst's history, was its first acupuncture clinic, opened in 1992. Three staff members were assigned to this clinic, which, during its first year, "exceeded expectations," according to the board report.[94] Its primary focus was on pain management. At the same time an electronic music program became part of the therapeutic regimen. A special computer system was set up that recognized arm and hand motions as musical notes. The program was designed to encourage rehabilitation through music: "Several exercise devices are connected to the computer system, which enables participants to play musical notes by moving the devices in specific patterns. Up to four patients can play in the program at once. Different groups of participants meet each week to form bands or practise songs together."[95] Determining how technology could better serve people with disabilities and investigating issues dealing with access to community living, quality of life, and health care were all part of the work done by Lyndhurst's research department during the 1990s.[96]

Employment of people with disabilities was a major issue for people both outside and inside the hospital. As late as 1990 Lyndhurst did not have any policy on employing disabled people. In response to concerns about this deficiency, a human rights policy was approved in 1991. During discussions leading to its approval, there was debate over Lyndhurst's employment equity policy, part of the human rights policy in which "the Board came to the conclusion that since we are in the rehabilitation business, we should be a leader in hiring disabled persons, but do so without having a quota system." Instead, the board recommended contacting the CPA employment counsellor when positions became available, to inform people with spinal cord injuries of hiring possibilities at Lyndhurst.[97] All of this reflected the increasing influence of "clients" on the policies that affected their chances of finding work and being accepted as capable members of society. When the Fiftieth Anniversary Symposium marking the founding of Lyndhurst and the CPA was held in November 1995 "a consumer driven system with collaboration between CPA and Lyndhurst" was recommended.[98] A year later a "patient driven approach" to spinal cord injury treatment was also pointed out to the accreditation surveyor.[99]

Michael O'Brien, who was an in-patient at Lyndhurst in 1998–99, shortly after this objective was announced, recalled that the facilities and staff were "excellent." His rehabilitation doctor, Alborz Oshidari, strongly encouraged O'Brien to return to his career as a lawyer. "I am not so sure that I believed him at that point but here we are being interviewed in a law office. Although my practice isn't the same as it was before, I feel that I am doing reasonably well considering the circumstances." However, he felt that rehabilitation at Lyndhurst needed to go farther than it did when he was there. While patients are informed about personal care issues, such as pressure sores and bladder infections, O'Brien said that the impact of aging on the body needs to be addressed in rehabilitation treatment. How to prevent problems with bodily functions should be given more attention. A good example, he pointed out, is "the integrity of one's shoulders." Pain in this area can drastically affect the ability to do transfers and this in return would greatly limit a person's independence. He also said that Lyndhurst's rehabilitation program should educate people about the importance of physical fitness and the need for a proper diet to avoid weight gain. As well, their social workers need to direct people to services that can let them lead more independent lives. A provincial Direct Funding Program that would allow a disabled person to live at home was brought to O'Brien's attention by a friend rather than by Lyndhurst social workers. "It was just absolutely mind-boggling to me that this wasn't something that was automatic. As a result of my friend seeing the article, I immediately applied for and got Direct Funding, which permitted me to live on my own instead of in a subsidized apartment facility that provides attendant care."[100]

Efforts to make such services more accessible are evident in the last major initiative that the two founding partners established prior to amalgamation. A new Employment Resource Centre was opened on 15 October 1997 as a joint venture between the CPA and Lyndhurst at the Sutherland Drive facility.[101] Its purpose was to mitigate the high unemployment rate for people with spinal cord injuries through on-site counselling, advice, and information. This centre was a continuation of work done by CPA employees over the preceding fifty years: James Bartlett, Ross Beggs, Charlie Saso, Ed Ratelle, and others who helped Lyndhurst graduates find jobs. Not long after the opening of this centre, the hospital would undergo yet another transformation, one that signalled a break with its past history far more than anything that had happened before.

FROM CPA TO TRI – AMALGAMATION

The path that led to amalgamation stemmed from the corporate make-up of Lyndhurst and, most decisively, from the conservative political winds that blew across the province in the decade prior to the end of this story. By the late 1980s and well into the 1990s it was apparent that requests for more provincial funding were going nowhere. This was a time of fiscal restraints, cutbacks, and downsizing across the health-care system in Ontario, as successive Liberal, New Democrat, and Conservative governments said a loud "No" to any significant budget increase for various health-care facilities, including Lyndhurst Hospital.[102]

In early 1988 the provincial Ministry of Health said Lyndhurst would not receive any additional funding until the issue of who owned the hospital was settled – the CPA, which had been owner since 1950, or the hospital itself, which is what the University of Toronto had been demanding for some time, whilst negotiating a new teaching agreement with the rehabilitation centre.[103] Throughout the 1980s the CPA and Lyndhurst made various attempts to separate amicably. On 24 June 1981 the hospital became incorporated as a provincial corporation; this was intended to be part of the process on the way to full independence of Lyndhurst from the CPA. The association and hospital even had serious negotiations in 1989 to arrange a twenty-one-year lease. However, this was never finalized.[104]

During the 1990s the significant gains made during the preceding decade in employee benefits and wages had come to a screeching halt.[105] Cutting the provincial deficit was *the* major fiscal priority of provincial governments headed by the New Democrats (1990–95) and especially under the Conservatives who succeeded them. This affected Lyndhurst and many other health-care facilities in Ontario – it was a tumultuous period.[106] The funding cutbacks that characterized many of Ontario's fiscal policies during the 1990s made themselves felt at Lyndhurst in very stark numbers: between 1990 and 1997 the equivalent of thirty-six full time staffing positions were lost and nine beds were closed, thus reducing the occupancy rate to seventy.[107] By the end of the decade, the external forces that had been cutting away at Lyndhurst's beds and budget would soon do away with its autonomy altogether.

Provincial policies of cost-cutting, merging, and "downsizing" of public-sector services reached a crescendo in Ontario during the second half of the 1990s after the June 1995 election of the Conservatives under Mike Harris. The provincial government proceeded to close or amalgamate health-care facilities across Ontario. Two years after the Conservatives were elected this agenda reached Sutherland Drive like a ticking time bomb. The end of an era in Lyndhurst's history was fast approaching.

In June 1997 the board approved Lyndhurst's becoming a part of the Metro Integrated Health Delivery Network.[108] A month later, on July 23, the provincial Health Services Restructuring Commission Report was released. It called for the amalgamation of Lyndhurst Hospital with the Rehabilitation Institute of Toronto (RIT) and the Toronto Rehabilitation Centre (TRC). The board decided to accept in principle the intent to amalgamate, with a number of conditions, including: preserving Lyndhurst's rehabilitation program, research purpose, physical site, medical training programs, equality of representation in regard to how the facility is run at the board level, and recognition of the long-standing relationship between Lyndhurst and the CPA.[109] They also requested the funding of ten more beds at Lyndhurst.[110]

To deal with all of these issues, the board set up a Strategic Directions Committee. It was decided that "a patient's perspective would be a significant asset" to this committee and so one person who had been through Lyndhurst's rehabilitation program was asked to participate. People with spinal cord injuries were also asked to be involved in the search committees for the new CEO of the amalgamated body and for the chief physiatrist. Board member Lucille Owen, who was also an ex-patient of the hospital, was asked to chair a committee to review Lyndhurst's mission statement before amalgamation talks commenced.[111] This committee decided that the "two main points to be included in the Vision Statement were: (1) Lyndhurst's partnership with CPA; and (2) its unique site as being integral to achieving Lyndhurst Hospital's goals." The term "client" was also used instead of "patient" or "consumer," to indicate people with spinal cord injuries who used Lyndhurst's services.[112] This was accepted and posted about the hospital. One important part of these negotiations with the province was to ensure that the policy positions of the CPA and Lyndhurst coincided, so that a united front was presented. This was "seen as essential to preserving the integrity of Lyndhurst's spinal cord rehabilitation program."[113]

Thus the new amalgamated board included permanent representation from the CPA and participation from people with spinal cord injuries, which was what the CPA had asked for and was pleased with, according to their Ontario director, Bill Adair. There was also equal representation on the board from each of the three amalgamating facilities. The Lyndhurst site and program were also maintained. While it was to come under a new corporate name the facility on Sutherland Drive would continue to bear the historic designation, "Lyndhurst."[114]

The uncertainty that amalgamation heralded also raised concerns among staff for their jobs; a newsletter was issued by the hospital to update them on negotiations.[115] One area in which amalgamation affected the staff, even before the process was complete, was wages: non-union staff had their wages increased by 2 per cent retroactive to 1 April 1997 to align their salaries with those of RIT and TRC.[116] The official amalgamation took place on 20 October 1998 when the last board meeting of Lyndhurst Hospital was held. They approved the transfer of the property and assets from the CPA, which had owned it since 1950, to the new Tri-Hospital Rehabilitation Corporation, which henceforth came to be called the Toronto Rehabilitation Institute (TRI).[117] With the approval of amalgamation, the fifty-three-year history of Lyndhurst as a stand-alone, independent facility had come to an end.

6

Conclusion:
Lyndhurst's Legacy

Of course, Lyndhurst's history did not end in October 1998. It entered into another era under a reconstituted corporate entity. But that is another story whose pages are yet to be written.

As far as the history of the period recounted in this book is concerned, the most important point to remember is the extent to which Lyndhurst's rehabilitation philosophy was geared towards returning people to the community from which they came rather than leaving them institutionalized for the rest of their lives following spinal cord injury. As the foregoing pages indicate, this did not always happen. Some lacked the necessary support in the community and others were stymied by the wider barriers that prevent people with disabilities from taking their rightful place in society. However, Lyndhurst did improve access for many people with disabilities through their various educational and employment programs and in so doing provided an important pathway for others to follow.

The original pathway was developed by people who didn't live to see the end of Lyndhurst's independence. The year before Lyndhurst was amalgamated, Dr Botterell died.[1] The facility that Botterell had helped to create left behind a significant legacy that became a model for supporting the integration of people with disabilities into the community and moving away from the forlorn idea of "hopeless cases" who would spend the rest of their lives in institutions. Botterell and John Counsell, who died in 1976 and whose advocacy on behalf of people with spinal cord injuries helped to create both Lyndhurst Lodge and the CPA, received various honours during their lifetime, including the Order of Canada.[2] Dr Jousse, who died in 1993, and his colleague, Dr Geisler, also both received the Order of Canada for their research and work at

Lyndhurst.[3] Without any doubt the greatest award Lyndhurst received was from the many people with disabilities who went through its doors and who spoke of the help they received from staff and support workers, and from fellow residents, in negotiating the world as a person with a disability. At the same time, as has been noted in this book, some people complained about aspects of life at Lyndhurst and problems encountered while in the rehabilitation program and in the facility itself, something that is also very much part of its history. The evidence compiled for this book, and provided by people with disabilities who know it best, indicates that Lyndhurst Lodge, whatever its faults, made significant and long-lasting contributions that benefited people with disabilities in Canada and abroad. People with spinal cord injuries are better off today because of the work done at Lyndhurst since 1945.

The combined working careers at Lyndhurst of Dr Jousse, and Dr Geisler, who has continued his clinical work after retiring from the hospital in 1998, encompassed the entire history of Lyndhurst as an independent facility from 1945–98. This history saw the facility develop from a new concept in treatment services that few people anywhere knew anything about into a leading spinal cord injury rehabilitation centre at both national and international levels. The legacy of Lyndhurst can most easily be found in its significant research contribution in the field of spinal cord injury rehabilitation and, most importantly, in the large numbers of people with disabilities who benefited from their treatment at this facility. It is particularly significant that people who were veterans with spinal cord injuries were so deeply involved in both creating and running Lyndhurst: John Counsell, Andy Clarke, and Ken Langford. They helped to develop services for themselves and the wider community of people with disabilities.

As the early pages of this book indicate, a high death rate (80 per cent) within two years of injury was the common factor for paraplegics and quadriplegics up to the 1930s and early 1940s. Doctors, like everyone else, held out little or no hope for the long-term survival of people who had this physical disability, to say nothing of their chances of ever living a life outside an institutional setting. But changes, astounding ones, were on the way.

Medical innovations in the immediate and long-term care of spinal cord injury by physicians in the United States, Britain, and, most notably for the purposes of this history, in Canada by Dr Botterell paved the way for a significant reversal of this death rate. Studies on long-term prospects for people who went through the program reflected the effectiveness of the new treatment regime: of nearly 2,500 patients who had been discharged during the first eighteen years of Lyndhurst's existence, 86 per cent were alive in late 1963; 81 per cent of these living ex-patients were people with spinal cord injuries. This was a remarkable statistical turnaround from the early twentieth century. Botterell's work at the Toronto General Hospital in improving the treatment of people with spinal cord injuries between 1936 and 1939 complemented developments in the United States and Great Britain. Reports of these advances helped to begin the long process of changing attitudes and policies for paraplegics and quadriplegics. As higher survival rates were realized among wounded World War II veterans and the emphasis on post-war reintegration picked up steam, finding a place to house and rehabilitate them became a priority. The advocacy efforts of Dr Botterell, Dieppe veteran John Counsell, and businessman LM Wood during the war led to the creation of the facility that became Lyndhurst Lodge in 1945. With the hiring of Dr Jousse in late February 1945 as the first director, its organization into a top-ranked rehabilitation centre was soon achieved; so rapidly, in fact, that the lodge almost put itself out of business within eighteen months of opening. The discharge rate was so high that staff feared that the DVA would close its doors as the veterans rapidly moved back into the community, leaving behind empty beds. Thanks to the support of the veterans themselves, through the organization that several of them had founded – the CPA – and pressure from Botterell and Jousse, among others, Lyndhurst began to admit civilians by late 1946. Opening the doors to a wider population of disabled people secured its continued survival for decades to come.

By the 1950s, when the CPA took over the building from the DVA, Lyndhurst had gained an international reputation as a centre for the treatment of people with spinal cord injuries and related disabilities (most notably polio up to the 1960s). Significant studies indicated the efficacy of work at the lodge. From the late 1940s onwards, staff at Lyndhurst had been speaking and writing about the philosophy and application of their rehabilitation program, such as proper exercise techniques used in physiotherapy and the use of prosthetic aids for people with physical disabilities. By the latter part of the 1950s research by the CPA showed that Lyndhurst Lodge accounted for more than half of all people with spinal cord injuries in Canada who returned to the community following rehabilitation.

The challenges people with disabilities faced in securing employment after discharge from Lyndhurst were evident throughout the five decades covered by this study. A 1962 CPA survey reflected this: just over 50 per cent of people with spinal cord injuries were known to be employed. The role played by CPA vocational staff at Lyndhurst in finding jobs, educational opportunities, and accessible living quarters in the community for people with disabilities was an essential part of the rehabilitation program that developed during these early decades and was carried on throughout its history. Yet, the wider, systemic discrimination experienced by people with disabilities beyond the confines of Lyndhurst Lodge also meant that accessible places to live, to go to school, and to work were often very hard to locate and sustain. People with disabilities who resided at Lyndhurst, along with staff who worked there, did an enormous amount to challenge these barriers. While not always successful, these efforts provided great social dividends: now accessible living quarters, schools, and work places are more readily available, though much remains to be done. Lyndhurst patients and staff, along with many other people in the wider disability community, fought hard for these changes over the decades discussed here.

Lyndhurst's legacy can also be seen in the clinical study undertaken on the causes of spinal cord injuries in Ontario in 1969 and 1970, which was published in 1975. In this study, which included significant involvement from Lyndhurst's medical staff, the authors pointed out that the level of spinal cord injury could be made more serious by incorrect physical intervention in the first hours after an accident. Improving the lifting and transporting of an injured person to a geographically accessible treatment centre in various parts of the province was deemed essential to enhancing the prospects for disabled people during and after rehabilitation. One of the most important parts of this report was recommending less geographically dispersed treatment centres in such a large province. The sooner an injured person could get to a nearby rehabilitation centre with staff trained in proper treatment procedures, the better would be their prospects for recovery. Lyndhurst had helped to show the way, not only with their already well-established program but also by working with other places, such as Kingston, to set up regional rehabilitation services to put these ideas into practice. Thus, Lyndhurst's legacy was felt far beyond the confines of the walls and the people who actually worked and lived there for a time – people who were never patients at Lyndhurst benefited from its work, which was used as a model for treatment elsewhere in the province. It also provided a lesson in the importance of the social organization of disability services, whereby the model developed by Lyndhurst was copied and used effectively in a way that was as important for a person's long-term prospects as was any medical breakthrough in clinical care for people with spinal cord injuries.

The long-term studies on causes of death and life expectancy rates for people with spinal cord injuries were the most important medical research conducted by staff at Lyndhurst. These four studies followed one another between first publication in 1961 and the final report in 1983. Doctors Geisler, Jousse, Wynne-Jones, and their colleague from Manufacturers Life Insurance Company, Dr Breithaupt, did pathological studies that compared people with and without spinal cord injuries. Their research indicated that most people did not die because of spinal cord injuries, per se. Instead, they most often died from the consequences of their injuries: kidney disease, infections from pressure sores, and other complications. Depression leading to suicide was one of these causes, indicating the devastating impact on some people of living in a society with widespread systemic barriers that daily face people with disabilities. The importance of improving treatment in all of these areas was shown to be of paramount significance. This work was cited for years thereafter in the medical literature where long-term survival and mortality rates of this population group were studied, thus becoming one of Lyndhurst's major contributions to understanding life and death among paraplegics and quadriplegics.[4]

During Dr Jousse's thirty-year tenure as director and afterwards, this research reputation was sustained and built on, such as through the Robson Urology Clinic and the help it offered people in regard to urological, sexual, and reproductive abilities. Rehabilitation specialists, clinicians, and students-in-training traipsed through the halls and took back to their respective communities the skills that were developed among doctors, nurses, attendants, physiotherapists, occupational therapists, and social workers who worked in this field. Most importantly, many of the people who made up the patient population from the end of World War II to the end of the twentieth century – Jack Higman, Gordon Paterson, Bev Hallam, Kathy Drummond, Carmen Mobbs, and numerous others – showed how people were able to live outside an institutional setting with a disability that a few decades earlier had been considered "hopeless." Lyndhurst had played a leading role, particularly in its early years, in helping people with spinal cord injuries to improve their prospects in society.

But many challenges, barriers, and problems persisted within the operation of Lyndhurst itself. Not least of these was the need for better quarters in the original converted residential building, which everyone agreed was deteriorating after several decades of use by thousands of patients, staff, and visitors. After years of cajoling government bureaucracies, planning with architects and contractors, and waiting for various levels of approval, the new building on Sutherland Avenue was at last opened in 1974, ending one era and beginning another. The next nearly quarter-century witnessed further changes through internal staffing reorganization, including cutbacks that caused great distress among both patients and staff. Efforts to deal with ever-looming funding cutbacks that affected the entire health-care system by the late 1980s and throughout the 1990s cast a perennial shadow on Lyndhurst's operation throughout this latter period. As the twentieth century came to an end, so too did the independence of Lyndhurst. But not before the facility ensured that certain fundamental principles were established for its future operation.

In 1997 six principles were established to "guide research at Lyndhurst" in the years to come: maintenance of a focus on rehabilitation; practical application of "results-oriented" research; improvement of clinical treatments; "holistic and interdisciplinary" research to support all aspects of a person's progress through rehabilitation; involvement of patients in this research so that feedback on its efficacy is obtained; research "driven by consumers needs, interests and priorities."[5] To what extent these principles have been realized during the years following this history will be for another study to determine. For now, it is enough to say that these principles indicate the direction Lyndhurst wanted to take as it was on the verge of amalgamating. Its last independent operators strove to maintain their historical emphasis on spinal cord rehabilitation and research and made it clear they wanted to continue to do so after joining with bigger entities. Past precedent and future prospects were thus linked together in an attempt to ensure that the historically continuous goal of spinal cord rehabilitation was maintained.

An early theme in Lyndhurst's history was innovative treatment for spinal cord injuries, as their entire rehabilitation program was quite novel at first. This historical tradition has continued, even if on a smaller scale. As just one example, the acupuncture therapy introduced at Lyndhurst in 1992 had, by 2002, become "the therapy most often requested by patients" at the new Toronto Rehabilitation Institute.[6] Therapies that had once seemed unconventional when introduced eventually became part of the mainstream. Here again we can see continuity with the past – after all, Lyndhurst, when it was opened and becoming established in 1945, was anything but conventional. The philosophy and practices that went into this new rehabilitation centre challenged a good deal of received wisdom up to that point. Many thought these new ideas about how to treat people with spinal cord injuries would not amount to much. But these ideas and practices did prove themselves, and the rest, as they say, is history.

While a historical account of the post–1998 period would be premature, not least because it is too soon to draw meaningful historical conclusions about an ongoing process of change in a new institution, the state of rehabilitation in the early twenty-first century requires a few words regarding Lyndhurst's direction in the new century. According to Dr Geisler, a Lyndhurst staff member for forty years, further studies are needed on bladder emptying, particularly in regard to women patients, who become infected through intermittent catheterization at a higher rate than men. Much more work needs to be done to prevent and treat complications and to better understand depression among people with spinal cord injury. Spinal cord regeneration is an area that Lyndhurst should not be involved in because of the lack of expertise in this field, which is particularly contentious among people who are paraplegic and quadriplegic.[7]

Many people are very knowledgeable about Lyndhurst's reason for existence: all those who experienced its rehabilitation program as paraplegics and quadriplegics. Michael O'Brien, who was an in-patient at Lyndhurst when the amalgamation took place, offered this perspective on its most recent and ongoing history:

"Lyndhurst, as it was when I was there, was a very fine operation. You knew who was in charge and you knew who you could consult with in respect to various matters. Patients and staff were organized so that it almost felt like one was part of a large family. You only get that when you have people who have been there for years and are very experienced in what they are doing. Expertise and caring attitude was demonstrated at all levels of staff, professional and non-professional. There was an esprit de corps that I hope will not be lost with amalgamation."[8]

Part of the esprit de corps that Michael O'Brien referred to relates to the philosophy that infused Lyndhurst's approach from its earliest days – supporting people with spinal cord injuries in returning to the community, finding jobs, and engaging in social pursuits like anyone else, able-bodied or disabled, among friends and family members. Its entire history was geared towards reintegrating people into the community, at a time when barriers for people with disabilities were, and remain, everywhere in sight. Whether Lyndhurst's long-standing philosophy will ever change is something only the future can tell.

Notes

INTRODUCTION

1 Heaman, *St Mary's*.
2 Neilsen, *The Mental Health Centre Penetanguishene*.
3 McDonald, *For the Least of My Brethren*.
4 Silver, *History of the Treatment of Spinal Injuries*. See pages 135–44 for his discussion of developments in Canada, which is based primarily on research done by Mary Tremblay, McMaster University, Hamilton.
5 Tremblay, "Living with Disability: The Early Pioneers"; "The Canadian Revolution in the Management of Spinal Cord Injury"; "Going Back to Civvy Street"; "Going Back to Main Street"; "Lieutenant John Counsell and the Development of Medical Rehabilitation and Disability Policy"; Tremblay et al. "When elevators were for pianos."
6 Two recent Canadian examples are McPherson, *Bedside Matters*, and Reaume, *Remembrance of Patients Past*.
7 Burch, *Signs of Resistance*; Husson, *Reflections*; Kudlick, "Disability History"; Longmore and Umansky, eds, *The New Disability History*; Longmore, *Why I Burned My Book*.
8 Rioux and Bach, eds, *Disability Is Not Measles*; Hockenberry, *Moving Violations*; Barton, ed., *Disability and Society*; Oliver, *Understanding Disability*; Linton, *Claiming Disability*; Russell, *Beyond Ramps*; Michalko, *The Difference That Disability Makes*; Titchkosky, *Disability, Self, and Society*.
9 Gerber, ed., *Disabled Veterans in History*.

CHAPTER ONE

1 A.T. Jousse Appreciation Foundation, Toronto [hereafter ATJ], A.C. Clarke, 17 February 1977 talk at Lyndhurst Hospital.

2 Guttmann, *Spinal Cord Injuries*, 1.

3 Ibid., 2.

4 Walker, "Ureters and Their Orifices." He stated that the mortality rate was initially almost 30 per cent for 369 paraplegic soldiers wounded in 1916–17 but that this had increased and "is very moderately stated at 80 per cent."

5 Guttmann, *Spinal Cord Injuries*, 5; Bors, *Veterans Administration Technical Bulletin TB10–503*, 2–3.

6 Kidd, "The Treatment of the Bladder in Gunshot Injuries of the Spinal Cord."

7 Guttmann, *Spinal Cord Injuries*, 5.

8 Breithaupt et al. "Late Causes of Death and Life Expectancy in Paraplegia," 73.

9 Queen's University Archives, Kingston, Ontario (hereafter QA): Edmund Henry ("Harry") Botterell fonds, 1927–97, Box 4, Folder 4 – Paraplegia, 1945–49: William P., Bruce Mines, Ontario, to Dr A.T. Jousse, Toronto, 20 May 1948.

10 National Archives, Ottawa (hereafter NA) RG 38, Prosthetic Services – Sub-Committee Specially Handicapped, vol. 1, memorandum, Ross Millar, Ottawa to Walter Woods, Ottawa, 15 May 1944; Morton and Wright, *Winning the Second Battle*, 27, 93, 97.

11 Archives for Veterans Affairs Canada, Charlottetown, Prince Edward Island (hereafter VAC), File 31–54, vol. 1, Prosthetic Services – Reports and Record, March, 1919–March 1937: The Orthopaedic and Surgical Appliances Branch, March 1919; Growth and Development of the Orthopaedic and Surgical Appliances Branch, undated, circa 1919. The March 1919 report noted (9) that 62 per cent of the limb-fitting staff were discharged soldiers.

12 NA, RG 38, Prosthetic Services – Sub-Committee Specially Handicapped, vol. 1, memorandum, Vocational Guidance, Training, Placement and Aftercare Service, The War Amputations of Canada, 20 December 1940, 1–2.

13 VAC: File 31–54, vol. 1, Prosthetic Services, J.L. Melville, memorandum, Orthopaedic and Surgical Appliances Branch, 10 April 1930, 4; The Use of Orthopaedic and Prosthetic Appliances in the Late Treatment of War Disabilities, undated but 15/9/32 handwritten across first page. See 1–3 re nerve and spinal injuries.

14 NA, RG 38, Prosthetic Services – Sub-Committee Specially Handicapped, vol. 1, Ross Millar, Ottawa to Walter Woods, Ottawa, 15 May 1944.

15 Ibid.

16 ATJ: James Burke, Scarborough, Ontario, Interview with author, 27 September 2001.

17 Munro, "The Treatment of the Urinary Bladder"; Munro, "Care of the Back Following Spinal-Cord Injuries." I am indebted to Mary Tremblay's work, cited elsewhere in this chapter, for these sources.

18 QA: Botterell fonds, Box 5, Folder 34, E.H. Botterell, "Memories of the Care of Patients with Spinal Cord Injuries. 1936–1962" (undated manuscript, circa 1986), 5; McKenzie, "Fracture, Dislocation, and Fracture Dislocation of Spine."

19 McKenzie, "Fracture, Dislocation, and Fracture Dislocation of Spine," 265. McKenzie presented this paper in June 1934 at the Canadian Medical Association meeting in Calgary. Munro is not cited, so it is not clear whether McKenzie developed his ideas about the importance of regular turning to prevent pressure sores independently.

20 QA: Botterell fonds, Box 5, Folder 34, "Memories," 5.

21 For biographical information on Botterell, see QA: Botterell fonds, Box 2, Folder 14 – Curriculum Vitae and Bibliography; Tremblay, *Living with Disability*, 77–81; Schatz, et al., "E. Harry Botterell."

22 Interview with Dr E.H. Botterell by Valerie Schatzker, 26 April 1979, Kingston, for University of Toronto and Hannah Institute for the History of Medicine (hereafter "Botterell interview, 1979"), 20; QA: Botterell fonds, Box 5, Folder 34, "Memories," 5–6. The 1936 date is not mentioned specifically in either of these sources, but it is clear from his 1939 lecture, cited below, that this is the starting date for his work in this field.

23 Botterell interview, 1979, 21.

24 ATJ: Wilfrid Bigelow, Toronto, Interview with author, 1 December 2001.

25 Botterell interview, 1979, 21.

26 QA: Botterell fonds, Box 4, Folder 16 – Spines – "Recovery Following Severe Injury of Spinal Cord and of Cauda Equina – Lecture (194?)." Two people listed in this source have been crossed out by Botterell and so are not included in the total number of sixteen patients with spinal cord injuries. This speech is undated, but "Movie script" is written across the front page in Botterell's handwriting, a reference to the films he made of several patients in the late 1930s, for which this was the narration. The "Record of Broken Back Cases" that Botterell compiled is attached to the script in this file, along with the text that accompanied his presentations with slides. The latest date in this script refers to a person injured in April 1939, so it was almost certainly used at his presentation to the Canadian Medical Association in June 1939.

27 Wilfrid Bigelow recalled that: "Most of them [TGH doctors around 1939] didn't quite understand what he [Botterell] was doing but they realized that he was being well accepted abroad among neurosurgeons. He was stimulating

younger people like myself. They were happy to have him." ATJ: Bigelow interview, 2001. Dr Botterell's daughter, Jocelyn Botterell Allen, when referring to his pre-war interest in spinal cord injury, mentioned: "I remember him remarking that many of his colleagues were skeptical about this project at the time." ATJ: Jocelyn Botterell Allen, Toronto, Interview with author, 6 November 2001.

28 Tremblay, "The Canadian Revolution in the Management of Spinal Cord Injury." Botterell's films from the late 1930s are preserved on tape: QA, Video, E.H. Botterell and A.T. Jousse, "Evolution of the Care of Spinal Cord Injuries in Ontario, 1936–1970" (Hannah Chair for the History of Medicine and Queen's University Archives, 1989). In the opening sequence of this film, Botterell said the correct word was "revolution" rather than "evolution" to describe these developments.

29 QA: Botterell fonds, Box 4, Folder 16 – Spines – "Recovery Following Severe Injury," 3 and 6 (page 3 is not numbered); Box 5, Folder 34, E.H. Botterell, "Memories," 9.

30 QA: Botterell fonds, Box 4, Folder 16 – Spines – "Recovery Following Severe Injury," 4. This document gives two dates for Frank's injury, April and May 1937. Box 5, Folder 34, E.H. Botterell, "Memories," 7. What happened to Frank after he left the TGH in 1939 is not mentioned in the sources.

31 Quote is from QA: Botterell fonds, Box 4, Folder 16 – Spines – "Recovery Following Severe Injury," 2. See also QA: Botterell fonds, Folder 49 – "Fracture Dislocation of the Spine" – Lecture to Academy, 1939, 8–9. Because of problems turning paralysed patients with the tongs developed by Dr McKenzie, Botterell began to use Crutchfield tongs in early 1938 after seeking advice from the designer of this instrument, Dr W.G. Crutchfield of Richmond, Virginia. QA: Botterell fonds, Folder 55 – Technique, 1938–40, E.H. Botterell, Toronto, to Dr G.W. Crutchfield, Richmond, Virginia, 10 February 1938; Dr Crutchfield to Dr Botterell, 16 February 1938; Dr Botterell to Dr Crutchfield, 21 February 1938.

32 QA: Botterell fonds, Box 5, Folder 34, E.H. Botterell, "Memories," 8, referring to an update in 1986.

33 QA: Botterell fonds, Box 4, Folder 16 – Spines – "Recovery Following Severe Injury," 4–6 (quote is on 6). Forty years later, Botterell recalled that this Drinker respirator was a "big iron lung, an old fashioned kind." Botterell interview, 1979, 22.

34 Botterell interview, 1979, 22.

35 Ibid., last handwritten page is not numbered, titled "Conclusions regarding treatment"; QA: Botterell fonds, Box 5, Folder 34, E.H. Botterell, "Memories," 10.

36 *Toronto Daily Star,* 23 June 1939, found in QA: Box 1, Botterell fonds, Folder 49 – "Fracture Dislocation of the Spine."

37 Ibid.

38 Ibid.

39 Botterell interview, 1979, 21.

40 Ibid., 22.

41 Botterell said in 1979 that the June 1939 talk was "the last thing I did before I went overseas." Ibid., 22.

42 Ibid., 24–5.

43 ATJ: Jack Higman, Mississauga, Ontario, Interview with author, 15 September 2001. Biographical information on Mr. Higman (1923–2002) can be found in his obituary, *The Globe and Mail,* 19 January 2002.

44 QA: Botterell fonds, Box 5, Folder 34, E.H. Botterell, "Memories," 11.

45 Ibid., 12.

46 Ibid., 13–15 (quote is on 15).

47 For information on John Counsell's background and family, see VAC: Lyndhurst Lodge, File 1–30, vol. 1: Civil Service of Canada [Job] Application Form, 4 pages, signed John Counsell, 16 November 1944; Tremblay, "Lieutenant John Counsell," 325; Botterell interview, 1979, 30–1; ATJ: Jane Glassco, Toronto, Interview with author, 1 February 2002. Reference to Botterell's attendance at Ridley College School can be found in: QA: Botterell fonds, Box 2, Folder 14 – Curriculum Vitae and Bibliography. It is not known whether Counsell and Botterell ever met while at Ridley College.

48 Robertson, *The Shame and the Glory: Dieppe,* 334; Holleman, *From Darkness Into Light,* 4. Of 6,000 Allied soldiers who participated in the nine-hour Dieppe raid, 5,000 were Canadians. 1,137 Allied soldiers were killed and 1,874 were taken prisoner. Among the many studies of this battle and its aftermath are: Whitaker and Whitaker, *Dieppe: Tragedy to Triumph*; Loring Villa, *Unauthorized Action.*

49 QA: Botterell fonds, Box 5, Folder 34, Botterell, "Memories," 1–2.

50 Dates for John Counsell's admission to the Montreal Neurological Institute and his transferral to Toronto can be found in: NA, RG 38, volume 192, Rehabilitation Liaison with Services: W.S. Woods to The Honourable the Minister, Ottawa, 19 March 1943; NA, RG 38, vol. 243, Weekly Letters, D District, Toronto, vol. 4: A.C. Norwich, 29 March 1943, Weekly War Diary.

51 The time of his return to Hamilton can be found in VAC: File 31–15, volume 6, May 1942-June 1944, Prosthetic Services, Wheelchairs: R. Wilson, Toronto to C.A. Bell, Ottawa, 3 February 1944. Reference to Counsell's employment in 1944 Hamilton can be found in VAC: File 1–30, vol. 1

Lyndhurst Lodge: Civil Service of Canada [Job] Application Form, 4 pages, signed John Counsell, 16 November 1944.

52 NA, RG 38, volume 192, Rehabilitation Liaison with Services: W.S. Woods to The Honourable the Minister [J.L. Ralston], Ottawa, 19 March 1943. Counsell was awarded both the Order of the British Empire and the Military Cross: Tremblay, "Lieutenant John Counsell," 325.

53 NA, RG 38, volume 192, Rehabilitation Liaison with Services: W.S. Woods to The Honourable the Minister [J.L. Ralston], Ottawa, 19 March 1943. This was not an isolated incident. Related documents in this file refer to similar problems for other veterans, as well as John Counsell, and mention efforts to rectify this situation. It was obviously considered a serious problem by officials.

54 QA, Botterell fonds, Box 5, Folder 34, Botterell, "Memories," 1.

55 NA, RG 38, vol. 243, Weekly Letters, D District, Toronto, vol. 4: C. McMane, Weekly War Diary, Toronto, 29 March 1943, 1.

56 Ibid., 2.

57 ATJ: Jane Glassco, Toronto, Interview with author, 1 February 2002.

58 Ibid. Jane Glassco recalled this incident as taking place with World War 1 veteran Eddie Baker. Ken Langford said it involved Edward Dunlop and contacted his widow, Doreen Dunlop, to confirm details. Ken Langford, Communication with the author, 11 July 2003. For reference to the friendship that developed between Counsell and Dunlop while they were in commando training in Scotland in 1941 see Tremblay, "The Canadian Revolution in the Management of Spinal Cord Injury," n101, 155.

59 Ken Langford, who would work closely with Counsell in the post-war period, noted that "he rehabilitated himself" during this early period. Quoted in Tremblay, "Lieutenant John Counsell," 326.

60 QA: Botterell fonds, Box 5, Folder 34, E.H. Botterell, "Memories," 11.

61 VAC: File 31–15, volume 6, May 1942-June 1944, Prosthetic Services, Wheelchairs: William Z. Cone, Montreal, to Dr W. Lalonde, Montreal, 13 April 1943. This letter was written after John Counsell had left Montreal, though Cone refers to him in the letter. For a discussion of the history of this wheelchair, see the excellent article by Tremblay, "Going Back to Civvy Street."

62 ATJ: Ken and Mary Langford, Interview with author, Toronto, 29 May 2003.

63 VAC: File 31–15, vol. 6, Prosthetic Services, Wheelchairs, May 1942–June 1944: L.M. Wood makes reference to Cone's influence on Counsell in this regard in his letter to Major Austin Bell, Ottawa, 16 December 1943. See also: NA, RG 38, vol. 187, Demobilization and Rehabilitation Committee on Special Casualties: "W.S.W." [Walter S. Woods], Ottawa, to Dr A.W. Park, Calgary, 19 May 1944, in which Woods refers to Counsell, though not by name, when noting "Another man whose spinal cord was severed at Dieppe

was deliberately put into contact with a man engaged in business in Montreal who has a similar disability." Reference to Jimmy Darou's friendship with John Counsell can be found in Tremblay, "Lieutenant John Counsell," 325–6; Holleman, *From Darkness Into Light*, 13–14.

64 NA, RG 38, vol. 243, Weekly Letters, D District, Toronto, vol. 4: C. McMane, M.D., Toronto, Weekly Report, 13 December 1943. This report says he bought the wheelchair during a trip to the U.S. VAC: File 31–15, vol. 6, Prosthetic Services, Wheelchairs, May 1942–June 1944: L.M. Wood, Toronto, to Major Austin Bell, Ottawa, 16 December 1943, refers to help Counsell received from the son of the Canadian ambassador to the U.S.

65 ATJ: Glassco interview, 2002.

66 For biographical information on L.M. Wood, see: "Tribute to A Great Man," [no author], *The Caliper* 15:1 (Spring 1960): 5–6; Holleman, *From Darkness Into Light*, 15–16, 19–22; Tremblay, "Lieutenant John Counsell," 326–7.

67 QA: Botterell fonds, Box 5, Folder 34, Botterell, "Memories," 3.

68 ATJ: Ken Langford interview, 29 May 2003.

69 VAC: File 31–15, vol. 6, Prosthetic Services, Wheelchairs, May 1942–June 1944: C.A. Bell, Ottawa, to R. Wilson, Toronto, 9 December 1943; R. Wilson, Toronto, to C.A. Bell, Ottawa, 11 December 1943.

70 In addition to Counsell and Wood, participants at this meeting were: Dr C. McMane, Toronto District Administrator for Department of Pensions and National Health, Dr A.C. Norwich, Chief Medical Officer, Toronto, Drs McCormick, Orde, and Ryan, and Toronto District Orthopaedic Superintendent R. Wilson. VAC: File 31–15, vol. 6, Prosthetic Services, Wheelchairs, May 1942–June 1944: L.M. Wood, Toronto, to Major Austin Bell, Ottawa, 16 December 1943; R. Wilson, Toronto to Major C.A. Bell, Ottawa, 16 December 1943.

71 VAC: File 31–15, vol. 6, Prosthetic Services, Wheelchairs, May 1942–June 1944: quote is from G.H. Ryan to Dr A.C. Norwich, 13 December 1943; C.P. McCormick, Toronto, to R. Wilson, Toronto, 14 December 1943.

72 VAC: File 31–15, vol. 6, Prosthetic Services, Wheelchairs, May 1942–June 1944: C. McMane, Toronto, to T.D. Bain, Ottawa, 20 December 1943.

73 VAC: File 31–15, vol. 6, Prosthetic Services, Wheelchairs, May 1942–June 1944: L.M. Wood, Toronto, to Major Austin Bell, Ottawa, 16 December 1943.

74 VAC: File 31–15, vol. 6, Prosthetic Services, Wheelchairs, May 1942–June 1944: J.A. Catto, Toronto, to Director of Rehabilitation [A.M. Wright], Toronto, 20 December 1943.

75 VAC: File 31–15, vol. 6, Prosthetic Services, Wheelchairs, May 1942–June 1944: Quite a few letters in this file from December 1943–June 1944 deal

with this topic. In one letter, it was noted that since Everest and Jennings did not have patent rights in Canada it was all right to copy their design, though John Counsell said they should obtain permission to do this. See C.A. McMane, Toronto, to Major C.A. Bell, Ottawa, 2 June 1944.

76 VAC: File 31–15, volume 7, Prosthetic Services, Wheelchairs, June 1944–April 1945: C.A. Bell to R. Wilson, 22 August 1944.

77 VAC: File 31–15, volume 7, Prosthetic Services, Wheelchairs, June 1944–April 1945: H.A. Everest, Los Angeles, California, to Major C.A. Bell, Ottawa, 15 January 1945; T.D. Bain, Ottawa, to Major A.U. Meilke, 25 January 1945.

78 NA, RG 38, vol. 220, Treatment Services, volume 1: G.B. Chisolm, Director General of Medical Services, Ottawa, to District Medical Officers, All Military Districts, 4 May 1944. Federal approval for Special Treatment Centres came several months earlier: NA, RG 38, vol. 220, Treatment Services, vol. 2, G.B. Chisolm, Ottawa, to the Adjutant General, Ottawa, 4 January 1944.

79 VAC: File 1–30, volume 1, Lyndhurst Lodge, May 1944–April 1945: Dr R.E. Wodehouse, Ottawa, to Col. C. McMane, 30 May 1944.

80 VAC: File 1–30, volume 1, Lyndhurst Lodge, May 1944–April 1945: H.W. De Guerre, Toronto, to Col. C. McMane, Toronto, 9 June 1944, with report attached by A.C. Norwich, 8 June 1944.

81 VAC: File 1–30, volume 1, Lyndhurst Lodge, May 1944–April 1945: Memorandum to The Honourable the Minister from Deputy Minister R. Wodehouse, 26 June 1944.

82 Ibid.

83 VAC: File 1–30, volume 1, Lyndhurst Lodge, May 1944–April 1945: R.E. Wodehouse, Ottawa, to Colonel G. S. Currie, Ottawa, 4 July 1944; Extract from Minutes of a Meeting of the Wartime Committee on Hospitalization, 5 July 1944.

84 VAC: File 1–30, volume 1, Lyndhurst Lodge, May 1944–April 1945: Precis, Nathanson Property, 153 Lyndhurst Ave, Toronto, 6 June 1944–9 November 1944; Assistant Deputy Minister, Dept. of Justice, Ottawa, to W. Gunn, Dept. of Veterans Affairs, Ottawa, 14 December 1944; S. Cuddy, Department of Veterans Affairs, Ottawa, 22 December 1944; Austin G. Ross, Toronto, to Deputy Minister of Justice, Ottawa (with attachment), 20 January 1945. Numerous documents in this file detail these negotiations. The Treasury Board approved a total price of $48,000, with $3,000 from this amount to cover insurance and tax costs. The $45,000 offer for the property included some household furniture and equipment, as well as a "musical organ" and bowling-alley equipment, neither of which were to be used by the new occupants. Documents from the late 1940s indicate that a good deal of time and effort was spent trying to get rid of the "musical organ" because it

took up so much space. Still, the final price for 153 Lyndhurst was a bargain by 1944 standards and federal officials knew it, noting early on in the assessment of the property that an earlier attempt to sell it had shown there was "no buyer in sight," so they had plenty of room to manoeuvre. Lt Col. S.E. Lyons, Department of National Defence, Ottawa, to Dr R.E. Wodehouse, Deputy Minister, Dept. of Pensions and National Health, Ottawa, 15 August 1944, 2.

85 VAC: File 1–30, volume 1, Lyndhurst Lodge, May 1944–April 1945: A.G. Ross, Toronto, to Deputy Minister of Justice, Ottawa, 26 October 1944; W. Gunn, Ottawa, to Mr Barrow, Ottawa, 16 November 1944; H.W. De Guerre to W.H. George, 28 November 1944; C. McMane, Toronto, to W.S. Woods, Ottawa, 30 November 1944; C. McMane [Deputation to Property Committee], Toronto, 30 November 1944; Austin G. Ross, Toronto, to Deputy Minister of Justice, 23 and 25 November 1944; Robertson, Fleury and Lane, Barristers and Solicitors, to Col. Chas. McMane, Toronto, 1 December 1944; C. McMane to Robertson, Fleury and Lane, 2 December 1944; J.P. Kent, Deputy City Solicitor, Toronto, to Austin G. Ross, Toronto, 19 December 1944.

86 The exact date of the construction of 153 Lyndhurst is not cited in the sources examined, though one document notes that the land on which the property sits was subject to building restrictions that expired at the end of 1914, thus suggesting the approximate date. See: VAC: File 1–30, vol. 1, Lyndhurst Lodge, May 1944–April 1945: A.G. Ross, Toronto, to Deputy Minister of Justice, Ottawa, 26 October 1944. For the cost of original construction and later sales price see: VAC: File 1–30, vol. 1, Lyndhurst Lodge, May 1944–April 1945: Lt Col. S.E. Lyons, Department of National Defence, Ottawa, to Dr R.E. Wodehouse, Deputy Minister, Dept. of Pensions and National Health, Ottawa, 15 August 1944. For reference to home ownership and the brief tenancy of Hemingway see Saso, "Hemingway Slept Here."

87 VAC: File 1–30, volume 1, Lyndhurst Lodge, May 1944–April 1945: H.W. De Guerre, Toronto, to Col. C. McMane, Toronto, 9 June 1944, with report attached by A.C. Norwich, 8 June 1944; Lt Col. S.E. Lyons, Department of National Defence, Ottawa, to Dr R.E. Wodehouse, Deputy Minister, Dept. of Pensions and National Health, Ottawa, 15 August 1944.

88 VAC: File 1–30, volume 1, Lyndhurst Lodge, May 1944–April 1945: A.C. Norwich, Toronto, to Dr T.D. Bain, Ottawa, 17 November 1944.

89 VAC: File 1–30, volume 1, Lyndhurst Lodge, May 1944–April 1945: A.C. Norwich, Toronto, to Dr T.D. Bain, Ottawa, 1 December 1944. This document says this was done "on the thirty-day emergency clause."

90 VAC: File 1–30, volume 1, Lyndhurst Lodge, May 1944–April 1945: W. Herbert George to H. W. De Guerre, 11 November 1944; A.C. Norwich,

Toronto, to H.W. De Guerre, Toronto, 11 December 1944; S. Cuddy, Department of Veterans Affairs memo, 22 December 1944.

91 VAC: File 1–30, volume 1, Lyndhurst Lodge, May 1944–April 1945: C. McMane, Toronto, to Col. G.S. McFarlane, Ottawa, 16 December 1944. Within a few weeks requests were made to allow Mr Ford and an unnamed husband and wife who worked in the kitchen to live in the building. A.C. Norwich, Toronto, to A.J. Dixon, Ottawa, 9 and 19 January 1945.

92 VAC: File 1–30, volume 1, Lyndhurst Lodge, May 1944–April 1945: S.J. Dixon, Ottawa, to District Administrator, Toronto, "December 22, 1944" crossed out in original with "Jan. 15, 1945" written over it.

93 VAC: File 1–30, volume 1, Lyndhurst Lodge, May 1944–April 1945: "Setting Pace For World To Help War Paralytics," *Toronto Daily Star*, 13 January 1945.

94 Ibid. The quote is from Dr A.C. Norwich.

95 VAC: File 1–30, volume 1, Lyndhurst Lodge, May 1944–April 1945: Unsigned letter, though clearly written by an official in the Department of Pensions and National Health, Ottawa, to Francis Farwell, President, Wartime Convalescent Homes War Charities, Hamilton, Ontario, 4 July 1944.

96 VAC: File 1–30, volume 1, Lyndhurst Lodge, May 1944–April 1945: Extract from Minutes of a Meeting of the Wartime Committee on Hospitalization, 5 July 1944.

CHAPTER TWO

1 L/CP. T.A. Bullock, "C Squadron, 11 Troop, 8 Recce, 1942–1945" (Privately printed manuscript, undated, circa 2001), 47. This source was provided courtesy of Ken Langford.

2 NA, RG 38, vol. 209, Special Treatment Centres Correspondence, vol. IV: A.C. Norwich, Toronto, to DVA Deputy Minister, 9 February 1945. See also: VAC: File 1–30, vol. 1, Lyndhurst Lodge, May 1944–April 1945: *Toronto Daily Star*, "Setting Pace for World to Help War Paralytics," 13 January 1945, which mentions the six and four figure regarding patients from Christie Street and Red Chevron.

3 Andrew C. Clarke, 17 February 1977, In-service Education Talk, taped by Loma Stone, who kindly provided a copy of this tape.

4 VAC: File 1–30, vol. 1, Lyndhurst Lodge, May 1944–April 1945: C. McMane, Toronto, Memorandum Re – Fire Inspection, Lyndhurst Home, 26 January 1945. This memo is attached to a letter from A.E. MacGregor, Toronto, to Deputy Minister, Ottawa, 2 February 1945. The Deputy Chief's last name is spelled with and without an "a" in these documents.

5 In addition to the sources cited in note 4, see VAC: File 1–30, vol. 1, Lyndhurst Lodge, May 1944–April 1945: C. McMane, Toronto, to DVA Deputy Minister, Ottawa, 10 February 1945.

6 VAC: File 1–30, vol. 1, Lyndhurst Lodge, May 1944–April 1945: A.E. MacGregor, Toronto, to Colonel C. McMane, Toronto, 9 February 1945.

7 VAC: File 1–30, vol. 1, Lyndhurst Lodge, May 1944–April 1945: H.W. De Guerre, Ottawa, to A.J. Dixon, Ottawa, 8 February 1945; A.J. Dixon to H.W. De Guerre, 14 February 1945; W.S. Woods, Ottawa, to The Honourable The Minister, Ottawa, 16 February 1945; A.J. Dixon to Deputy Minister [Woods], 20 February 1945; F.L. Barrow, Ottawa, to DVA Chiefs of Divisions, et al., 24 February 1945.

8 All quotes are from the section of his memoirs in which this episode is discussed: QA, Botterell fonds, Box 5, Folder 34, "Memories," 18–24.

9 L/CP. T.A. Bullock, "C Squadron, 11 Troop, 8 Recce, 1942–1945," 43–4. Mr Bullock dates this episode from November 1944, though Botterell and other sources date his arrival as the following February.

10 Ibid., 25–8. For a discussion of the role and influence of W.P. Warner, see Tremblay, "The Right to the Best Medical Care."

11 QA: Botterell fonds, Box 5, Folder 34, "Memories," 29–31. Isabel (Wilson) Potter later worked with patients with spinal cord injuries at Sunnybrook Hospital in Toronto. She died in January 2002 at the age of 95.

12 All information about Dr Jousse's background, including quotes, is from NA, RG 32, Series C–2, vol. 1137, 1910.07.21, Jousse, A.T. [Federal Civil Service Employment File, 1945–50]: Civil Service of Canada Application Form, 20 February 1947.

13 Ibid. Another source in this same file says his disability was due to "post-anterior poliomyelitis": A.C. Norwich, Toronto, to Deputy Minister, DVA, Ottawa, 19 February 1945. Since Jousse would have been the person most familiar with his medical history, his interpretation is accepted as the most reliable.

14 NA, RG 32, Series C–2, vol. 1137, 1910.07.21, Jousse, A.T. [Federal Civil Service Employment File, 1945–50]: Civil Service of Canada Application Form, 20 February 1947.

15 ATJ: Eileen Jousse Woloshyn, Kingston, interview with author, 3 October 2001.

16 QA: Botterell fonds, Box 5, Folder 34, "Memories," 37.

17 Ibid., 36–8. Botterell wrote that there was a slight delay in the appointment because of Duncan Graham, head of medicine at the TGH, was opposed to Jousse getting a voluntary appointment in the TGH Neurology Clinic, which Botterell was trying to arrange. Jousse said he would take the Lyndhurst job

without the neurology appointment which "solved the impasse." Botterell
and Jousse had met briefly before his appointment. Botterell had been a lec-
turer in physiology at the University of Toronto during Jousse's third year in
medicine in the late 1930s and had once tested him. They had also met during ward rounds at the TGH in January or February 1945. See Interview with
Dr Al Jousse by Valerie Schatzker, 1979, 44.

18 NA, RG 32, Series C–2, vol. 1137, 1910.07.21, Jousse, A.T. [Federal Civil
Service Employment File, 1945–50]: A.C. Norwich, Toronto, to Deputy
Minister, DVA, Ottawa, 19 February 1945.

19 NA, RG 32, Series C–2, vol. 1137, 1910.07.21, Jousse, A.T. [Federal Civil
Service Employment File, 1945–50]: Department of Veterans Affairs,
Appointment to Staff, signed A.C. Norwich and H.W. De Guerre, 27–2–45.
This post was initially half-time, then increased to full-time medical director
on 1 April 1945. QA, Botterell fonds, Box 5, Folder 34, "Memories," 31.

20 Jousse interview, 1979, 46.

21 Ibid., 47.

22 NA, RG 38, vol. 209, Special Treatment Centres Correspondence, vol. VI:
Lyndhurst Lodge Report, August 1945, A.T. Jousse.

23 Years later Jousse recalled that officers were originally housed on the second
floor and lower ranks were on the first floor, but this soon ended at
Botterell's insistence, as he felt that mixing the ranks would improve rehabilitation efforts among otherwise "pampered" officers. Botterell was himself a
Lieutenant Colonel in the RCAMC and would have had more military clout to
do this than Jousse would have. Jousse interview, 1979, 47.

24 Ibid.

25 NA, RG 38, vol. 209, Special Treatment Centres Correspondence, vol. V:
Lyndhurst Lodge, Report for the Month of May 1945, A.T. Jousse; NA, RG
38, vol. 209, Special Treatment Centres Correspondence, vol. VI: Lyndhurst
Lodge Report, August 1945, A.T. Jousse.

26 L/CP. T.A. Bullock, "C Squadron, 11 Troop, 8 Recce, 1942–1945," 47–53.

27 NA, RG 38, vol. 208, Hospital Accommodation Survey – Beds – Wartime
Committee on Hospitalization: 1 June 1945 report; VAC: File 1–30, vol. 2,
Lyndhurst Lodge, April 1945–December 1946: Murray Dillon, Executive
Assistant to Deputy Minister, DVA, Ottawa, to Superintendent, Engineering
Division, W.H. George, Ottawa, 9 June 1945.

28 NA, RG 38, vol. 243, Weekly Letters, "To" District, vol. 6: Weekly War
Diary, 11 June 1945, H.W. De Guerre; VAC: File T–5260–01, vol. 1, Paraple-
gia General, November 1944–August 1945: Memorandum to Dr Warner by
Edward Dunlop, Ottawa, 13 June 1945 (containing quote from L.M. Wood);
W.P. Warner to Major Edward Dunlop, Ottawa, 15 June 1945.

29 In addition to the sources cited in this article about the early years of rehabilitation at Lyndhurst, a document written in the mid-1950s by James Burke, who was himself a paraplegic and was an out-patient of Lyndhurst during the late 1940s, provides a good deal of information about the program in Toronto and elsewhere in Canada. CPA, National Office, Ottawa: James Burke, "Return to Action: A Report on the Rehabilitation of Canadian Paraplegics," (Unpublished manuscript, circa 1954–55).

30 For reference to the two trips to New York, see: NA, RG 38, vol. 209, Treatment Services, vol. V: E.H. Botterell, Toronto, to A.C. Norwich, Toronto, 2 May 1945; NA, RG 38, vol. 210, Draft Copies Minutes, Dr Convery's File, vol. 3: Report on the Trip to New York, A.T. Jousse, 29 June 1945. Reference to the Toronto viewing in July 1945 of the film from the Institute for the Crippled and Disabled can be found in: NA, RG 38, vol. 209, Special Treatment Centres Correspondence, vol. VI: Report for July, A.T. Jousse, 27 July 1945. This same report also mentions that coloured film was taken of the Lyndhurst program at that time. No trace of this 1945 Lyndhurst Lodge film could be found.

31 NA, RG 38, vol. 209, Special Treatment Centres Correspondence, vol. V: Report on Lyndhurst Lodge for April 1945, A.T. Jousse; Lyndhurst Lodge, Report for the Month of May 1945, A.T. Jousse; Lyndhurst Report for July, A.T. Jousse, 27 July 1945; Lyndhurst Lodge Report, August 1945, A.T. Jousse.

32 Jousse and Nettlefield, "Physiotherapy and the Paraplegic Patient"; Botterell et al., "Paraplegia Following War"; Jousse and Botterell, "Paraplegia."

33 Ibid.

34 NA, RG 38, vol. 209, Special Treatment Centres Correspondence, vol. V: Lyndhurst Lodge report – Special Treatment Centre, Department of Neurosurgery at Christie Street Hospital, Month of June 1945, E.H. Botterell. Dr Jousse had been away in New York for much of this month, so Botterell wrote the report within his own monthly statement on Christie Street.

35 Botterell et al., "Paraplegia Following War," 257.

36 QA: Botterell fonds, Box 5, Folder 34, "Memories," 40.

37 Jousse and Nettlefield, "Physiotherapy and the Paraplegic Patient," 9.

38 NA, RG 38, vol. 209, Special Treatment Centres Correspondence, vol. V: Report on Lyndhurst Lodge for April 1945, A.T. Jousse; Lyndhurst Lodge, Report for the Month of May 1945, A.T. Jousse; Lyndhurst Report for July, A.T. Jousse, 27 July 1945; Lyndhurst Lodge Report, August 1945, A.T. Jousse. Reference to the employment of Jim Bartlett in June 1949 by the CPA can be found in: CPAN: CPA Fifth Annual Report, 1950, 4.

39 NA, RG 38, vol. 209, Special Treatment Centres Correspondence, vol. V:
    Report on Lyndhurst Lodge for April 1945, A.T. Jousse; Lyndhurst Lodge,
    Report for the Month of May 1945, A.T. Jousse; Lyndhurst Report for July,
    A.T. Jousse, 27 July 1945; Lyndhurst Lodge Report, August 1945,
    A.T. Jousse.

40 NA, RG 38, vol. 209, Special Treatment Centres Correspondence, vol. VI:
    Lyndhurst Report for July, A.T. Jousse, 27 July 1945; Lyndhurst Lodge
    Report, August 1945, A.T. Jousse.

41 VAC: File 31–15, vols. 9 and 10, Prosthetic Services, Wheelchairs, vol. 9,
    August 1945–May 1946, vol. 10, June 1946–December 1947: R. Wilson,
    Toronto, to Deputy Minister, Ottawa, 1 October 1945; Allocation of Wheel
    Chairs "D" District ["December 14, 1945" handwritten on page]; A.T.
    Jousse to Medical Assistant to D.A., DVA, Dr A.C. Norwich, 5 January 1946
    [re reference to shortage of wheelchairs the previous summer]; A.T. Jousse to
    Director of Prosthetic Services, Ottawa, 12 August 1946 [re use of wheel-
    chairs in rural areas]; A.T. Jousse to Director of Prosthetic Services, Ottawa,
    13 January 1947 [re quote]. This file and other related files in this series have
    information about different types of prosthetic products that patients tried
    out at Lyndhurst to see whether they were useful. For information about the
    patient population of Lyndhurst in December 1945 see the "Weekly Hospital
    Statement" produced for that month regarding all DVA hospitals in Canada:
    NA, RG 38, vol. 207, Treatment Services, vol. 8.

42 ATJ: Ken Langford, Interview with author, Toronto, 29 May 2003.

43 Whalley, "Driving the Ford with Hand Controls."

44 NA, RG 38, vol. 209, Special Treatment Centres Correspondence, vol. VI:
    Lyndhurst Report for July, A.T. Jousse, 27 July 1945; Lyndhurst Lodge
    Report, August 1945, A.T. Jousse.

45 ATJ: Jack Higman, Mississauga, Interview with author, 15 September 2001.
    Mr Higman mentioned that the trip was to the Muskoka region outside
    Toronto, though a source from the time indicates that it was further north to
    Algonquin Park: CPAN: CPA Third Annual Report, 1948, 16–17.

46 VAC: File T5260–01, vol. 2, Treatment Services, Paraplegic Cases, July
    1945–June 1947: [List of] Paraplegics, 9 January 1946; Nominal Role [sic] of
    Paraplegics at Lyndhurst Lodge, 14 January 1946, A.T. Jousse.

47 ATJ: Ken Langford, Toronto, Interview with author, 21 November
    2001.

48 NA, RG 38, vol. 209, Special Treatment Centres Correspondence, vol. V:
    Report on Lyndhurst Lodge for April 1945, A.T. Jousse; Lyndhurst Lodge,
    Report for the Month of May 1945, A.T. Jousse; A.C. Norwich, Toronto, to
    Dr Convery, Ottawa, 13 June 1945.

49 NA, RG 38, vol. 209, Special Treatment Centres Correspondence, vol. VI: Lyndhurst Lodge Report, August 1945, A.T. Jousse; Lyndhurst Lodge Report, September and October 1945.

50 VAC: File 3–26–2–1, vol. 1, Treatment Services, Paraplegic Cases, CPA Payments, March 1945–October 1947: John Counsell, Toronto, to Edward Dunlop, Ottawa, 14 November 1945.

51 VAC: File 3–26–2–1, vol. 1, Treatment Services, Paraplegic Cases, CPA Payments, March 1945–October 1947: John Counsell, Toronto, to Edward Dunlop, Ottawa, 28 November 1945.

52 VAC: File 3–26–2–1, vol. 1, Treatment Services, Paraplegic Cases, CPA Payments, March 1945–October 1947: Edward Dunlop, Ottawa, to John Counsell, Ottawa, 1 December 1945.

53 VAC: T5260–01, vol. 2, Treatment Services – Paraplegic Cases, July 1945–June 1947: Frayne, "Walking and Working, Paraplegics Zestful."

54 NA, RG 38, vol. 243, Weekly Letters, vol. 6: Minutes of the First Meeting of the Paraplegic Committee held at Christie Street Hospital at 3 p.m. on Tuesday, 16 January 1945.

55 NA, RG 38, vol. 209, Special Treatment Centres Correspondence, vol. IV: Report on Lyndhurst Lodge, 30 March 1945, A.T. Jousse.

56 Canadian Paraplegic Association, National Office, Ottawa (hereafter CPAN): CPA, undated two-page document, circa May–June 1945, which outlines the establishment of the CPA and issuance of 10 May 1945 Letters Patent; Meeting of Provisional Directors, CPA, 23 May 1945; First Meeting of Directors, 23 May 1945. For a national history of the CPA during its early years see Holleman, *From Darkness into Light*.

57 ATJ: Jack Higman, Mississauga, Interview with author, 15 September 2001.

58 CPAN: CPA Board Minutes, 6 June 1945. See also correspondence on this matter in: VAC, File 3–26–2–1, vol. 1, Treatment Services, Paraplegic Cases, CPA Payments, March 1945–October 1947.

59 VAC: File 3–26–2–1, vol. 1, Treatment Services, Paraplegic Cases, CPA Payments, March 1945-October 1947: Unsigned copy of a letter from Dr Jousse, addressed to Major Dunlop, 14 May 1945, appended to Dunlop's memo to Brig. General Warner, Ottawa, 18 May 1945.

60 CPAN: Dominion Charter, Canada [for the CPA], by Paul Martin, Secretary of State, Ottawa, signed W.P. J. O'Meara, 10 May 1945. Reprinted in CPA First Annual Report, 1946, 8–10.

61 CPAN: CPA Board Minutes, First Meeting of Directors, 23 May 1945; Minutes, 26 July 1945; Minutes, 17 September 1945.

62 CPAN: Board Minutes, 26 July 1945; 7 December 1945; *The Caliper* 2:1 (March 1947): 16–17.

63 VAC: File 3–26–2–1, vol. 1, Treatment Services, Paraplegic Cases, CPA
   Payments, March 1945–October 1947; DVA, Minutes of Conference on
   Paraplegics, 15 August 1945. These minutes list Toronto as having 67
   paraplegic veterans, but another report a few days later gives the figure as 64,
   with the breakdown as indicated in the text of this chapter. VAC: T5260–01,
   vol. 2, Treatment Services – Paraplegic Cases, July 1945–June 1947:
   E.H. Botterell, Toronto, to Dr A.C. Norwich, Toronto, 27 August 1945.

64 *The Caliper* "was originally conceived as a method of occupational therapy"
   for paraplegic veterans in Quebec's Ste Anne's Hospital, where it was first
   published as an internal newsletter in 1945. The word "Caliper" refers to leg
   braces. The CPA national magazine kept this name from 1946 to 1999, when
   it was changed to *Total Access*. For its origins, see: VAC: File 3–26–2–1, vol.
   1, Treatment Services – Paraplegic Cases – CPA Payments, March 1945–
   October 1947: D. George Petrie, Circulation Manager, Caliper Office, Ste
   Anne de Bellevue, Quebec, to Walter S. Woods, Ottawa, 24 December 1945,
   with attached issue of newsletter from 17 December 1945, vol. 1, no. 2.

65 VAC: T5260–01, vol. 2, Treatment Services – Paraplegic Cases, July
   1945–June 1947: E.H. Botterell to Superintendent Dr van Nostrand, 6
   December 1945; E.H. Botterell, Memorandum to J.W. Cluff, A.T. Jousse, 3
   May 1945; G.R.D. Farmer, Ottawa, Memorandum to Deputy Minister, DVA,
   14 August 1946; E.H. Botterell, et al., "Paraplegia Following War."

66 VAC: T5260–01, vol. 2, Treatment Services – Paraplegic Cases, July
   1945–June 1947: E.H. Botterell to Superintendent Dr van Nostrand, 6
   December 1945; CPAN: CPA Board Minutes, 7 December 1945.

67 VAC: File 3–26–1, vol. 1, Treatment Services, Paraplegic Cases, Individual
   Civilians, December 1945–August 1947: T.D. Bain, Ottawa, to Deputy
   Minister, DVA, 8 January 1945. The number of patients at Lyndhurst at this
   time can be found in VAC, T5260–01, vol. 2, Treatment Services – Paraplegic
   Cases, July 1945–June 1947: Dr A.T. Jousse, Toronto, to Dr T.D. Bain,
   Ottawa, Nominal Role [sic] Call of Paraplegics at Lyndhurst Lodge, 14
   January 1946.

68 VAC: File 3–26–1, vol. 1, Treatment Services, Paraplegic Cases, Individual
   Civilians, December 1945–August 1947: D.J. Galbraith, Vice-Chairman,
   Workmen's Compensation Board, to T.D. Bain, DVA, Ottawa, 21 January
   1946; T.D. Bain, Ottawa, to DVA District Administrator, Toronto, 23
   January 1946; J.W. Merritt, DVA, Toronto, to Deputy Minister, Ottawa,
   22 February 1946.

69 VAC: File 3–26–1, vol. 1, Treatment Services, Paraplegic Cases, Individual
   Civilians, December 1945–August 1947: G. Woodrow Bradford, Dundas,
   Ontario, to Hon. Ian McKenzie, Ottawa, 26 March 1946.

70 VAC: T5260–01, vol. 2, Treatment Services – Paraplegic Cases, July 1945–
    June 1947: E.H. Botterell, Memorandum to J.W. Cluff, A.T. Jousse, 3 May
    1945.

71 VAC: File 3–26–1, vol. 1, Treatment Services, Paraplegic Cases, Individual
    Civilians, December 1945–August 1947: Dr R.V. Chapple, Sudbury, to Dr H.
    Botterell, Toronto, 30 May 1946. The letter Chapple referred to was from
    J.T. Phair, Deputy Minister of Health, Toronto, to Dr J. D. McInnes,
    Sudbury, 21 May 1946. There are numerous letters in the file from Dr
    Chapple and his correspondents about trying to help Frank C.

72 VAC: File 3–26–1, vol. 1, Treatment Services, Paraplegic Cases, Individual
    Civilians, December 1945–August 1947: E.H. Botterell, Toronto, to R.V.
    Chapple, Sudbury, 3 June 1946.

73 VAC: File 3–26–1, vol. 1, Treatment Services, Paraplegic Cases, Individual
    Civilians, December 1945–August 1947: Dr R.V. Chapple, Sudbury, to J.L.
    Gauthier, M.P., 19 June 1946.

74 VAC: File 3–26–1, vol. 1, Treatment Services, Paraplegic Cases, Individual
    Civilians, December 1945–August 1947: A.C. Norwich, Toronto, to Deputy
    Minister, DVA, Ottawa, 14 June 1946.

75 VAC: File 3–26–1, vol. 1, Treatment Services, Paraplegic Cases, Individual
    Civilians, December 1945–August 1947: A.T. Jousse to E.H. Botterell, 17
    June 1946.

76 VAC: File 3–26–1, vol. 1, Treatment Services, Paraplegic Cases, Individual
    Civilians, December 1945–August 1947: Harry Botterell to Dr F. H. Van
    Nostrand, Superintendent, Christie Street Hospital, Toronto, 24 June 1946;
    W.P. Warner, Ottawa, to Deputy Minister, Ottawa, 26 June 1946; F. H. van
    Nostrand, Toronto, to Dr T.D. Bain, et al., Ottawa, 29 June 1946; F.L. Barrow,
    Acting Secretary, DVA, to Heads of Branches, et al., re Paraplegic Centres, 24
    August 1946. There is a good deal of additional correspondence from late June
    to late August 1946 about this matter, including some from the WCB.

77 VAC: File 3–26–1, vol. 1, Treatment Services, Paraplegic Cases, Individual
    Civilians, December 1945–August 1947: W.S. Woods, Deputy Minister, DVA,
    to Dr Warner, 4 October 1946; Frank C.'s admission and discharge dates are
    listed on a sheet for all Canadian paraplegic centres attached to a letter from
    W.P. Warner to Deputy Minister, DVA, 28 April 1947.

78 VAC: File 3–26–1, vol. 1, Treatment Services, Paraplegic Cases, Individual
    Civilians December 1945–August 1947: Sheet with list of civilian patients for
    all Canadian paraplegic centres attached to a letter from W.P. Warner to
    Deputy Minister, DVA, 28 April 1947.

79 Canadian Paraplegic Association, Ontario, Toronto (hereafter "CPAO")
    Newspaper Collection, "New Lease on Life Given to Paraplegic," *Chatham*

Daily News, 12 September 1947; "Paraplegic Opens Office to Handle Boom Business," *Chatham Daily News*, nd, June 1948; Clark, "Magazines Are My Business." The first Chatham newspaper story states that Clark was the first of two female patients treated at Lyndhurst, though the source cited in the preceding note indicates that this is incorrect.

80 CPAN: CPA Fourth Annual Meeting, 27 May 1949.

81 ATJ: Marjorie Bleasdell, Interview with author, Toronto, 1 April 2002.

82 ATJ: Dorothy Naylor, Interview with author, Toronto, 14 February 2002.

83 Katie Barton, Interview with author, Toronto, 2 July 2001.

84 CPAO Newspaper Collection: "No Handicap to Wedding: Bride to be Uses Canes, Groom in Wheelchair," *Toronto Telegram*, 15 March 1951.

85 CPAO Newspaper Collection: "Wedding Sets Town Agog, Bride and Groom Paraplegics," [newspaper source not cited, nor is year though it appear to be from the late 1940s, dateline February 9].

86 Ken Langford, Toronto, Interview with author, 21 November 2001.

87 Bullock, "C Squadron," 48–9. See also the following articles: "Unlimited Horizons," *The Caliper* 4:2 (Summer 1949): 12–13; CPAO Newspaper Collection, "Paraplegics Win Through: Four Are U of T Graduates," *The Toronto Telegram*, 28 May 1949; "Six Wounded Win Degrees," *The Globe and Mail*, 7 June 1949 [includes reference to two blind students].

88 ATJ: Evelyn Paul, Interview with author, Toronto, 15 February 2002.

89 CPAO Newspaper Collection, "Paraplegics Express Gratitude To Doctor by Gift of a Car" [newspaper source not cited], 1 November 1947; "War Paraplegics Surprise Doctor With Gift of Auto" [newspaper source not cited], 1 November 1947.

90 A.T. Jousse interview, 1979, 50.

91 Margaret Jousse, Interview with author, Ottawa, 17 October 2001.

92 CPAN: CPA Board Minutes, 20 May 1947.

93 CPAN: CPA Board Minutes, 25 May 1948; CPA Third Annual Meeting Minutes, 25 May 1948.

94 CPAN: CPA Fourth Annual Report, 1949, 13.

95 CPAN: CPA Board Minutes, 17 October 1947; CPA Third Annual Report, 1948, 20.

96 CPAN: CPA Fourth Annual Report, 1949, 16.

97 CPAN: CPA Fourth Annual Meeting, 27 May 1949.

98 CPAN: CPA Board Minutes, 15 March 1949; CPA Fifth Annual Report, 1950, 4.

99 VAC: File 1–30, vol. 3, part B, Lyndhurst Lodge, September 1949–December 1950: Agreement Between His Majesty the King in Right of Canada

[Department of Veterans Affairs] and Canadian Paraplegic Association, 31 March 1950, signed Milton F. Gregg, John G. Counsell, G.K. Langford.

100 VAC: File 1–30, vol. 3, part B, Lyndhurst Lodge, September 1949–December 1950: G.D. Lennox, Ottawa, to John Counsell, Toronto, 8 April 1950.

101 CPAN: CPA Fifth Annual Meeting, 12 May 1950.

102 Ibid.

103 CPAO Newspaper Collection: "Noted Officer: Lt.-Col. Hay, Dies in Toronto" [news clipping, source uncited], June 1949; "Lt.-Col. A.J. Hay" [news clipping, source uncited], June 1949; CPAN: "Lieut.-Col. A.J. Hay," *The Caliper* 4:2 (Summer 1949): 11.

CHAPTER THREE

1 ATJ: Myrll Jackson, Vancouver, Telephone Interview with author, 7 November 2001.

2 CPAN: CPA Board Minutes, 24 February 1950.

3 CPAN: CPA Board Minutes, 29 September 1950; 31 January 1951; CPAN: CPA 6th Annual Report, 1951, 4.

4 The new wing technically added eleven new beds to the overall capacity bringing the total to fifty-two. However, two bedrooms were subsequently eliminated in the older part of the building for use as physiotherapy and examining rooms. Thus there was an actual gain of nine beds when all the renovations and space allocation had been settled by the beginning of January 1956. It rose by two more beds by 1960. CPAN: CPA Executive Committee Minutes, 8 April 1953; Board Minutes, 11 February 1955; CPA Annual Meeting, 11 May 1956; CPA 10th Annual Report, 1955, 1–2; CPA 11th Annual Report, 1955–56, 9; Archives of Ontario (hereafter AO), RG 10–154, Hospitals and Institutions Central Files Reel Listing, Reel 165: M.E.J. Stalker to C.J. Telfer, Ontario Department of Health, 24 August 1955 [re quote about washrooms]; J.K. Jamieson to C.J. Telfer, Ontario Department of Health, 17 January 1956; L. Jamieson, two-page report on 2 November 1960 visit to Lyndhurst Lodge, 24 November 1960.

5 CPA 11th Annual Report, 1955–56, 7. The $1,185 elevator installation was paid for by the Atkinson Foundation: AO, RG 10–154, Hospitals and Institutions Central Files Reel Listing, Reel 165: G.K. Langford, CPA, to C.J. Telford, Ontario Department of Health, 15 February 1957.

6 ATJ: Ken Langford, Toronto, Interview with author, 21 November 2001.

7 AO, RG 10–154, Hospitals and Institutions Central Files Reel Listing, Reel 165: Memo from M. Phillips, Ontario Department of Health, to Leslie Frost, Ontario Prime Minister and Provincial Treasurer, 30 June 1954. The exact

date is provided by: C.J. Telfer, Director, Public and Private Hospitals Division, to L.B. Morrison, Lyndhurst Lodge, 15 July 1955. (See this reel for other related letters about this matter).

 8 AO, RG 10–154, Hospitals and Institutions Central Files Reel Listing, Reel 165: J. K. Jamieson to C.J. Telfer, Ontario Hospital Services Commission, 11 August 1956.

 9 ATJ: Ken Langford, Toronto, Interview with author, 21 November 2001, 29 May 2003.

10 CPAN: CPA 14th Annual Report, 1958, 9; ATJ: William O. Geisler, Toronto, Interview with author, 18 February 2002; CV, William O. Geisler.

11 Naylor, *Private Practice, Public Payment*; Duffin, *History of Medicine*, 128.

12 ATJ: William O. Geisler, Toronto, Interview with author, 4 March 2002.

13 CPAN: CPA Annual Meeting, 10 February 1959; CPA 14th Annual Report, 1958, 9.

14 ATJ: Ken Langford, Toronto, Interview with author, 21 November 2001.

15 CPAN: CPA 15th Annual Report, 1960, 11.

16 AO, RG 10–154, Hospitals and Institutions Central Files Reel Listing, Reel 165: R.W.I. Urquhart, Chairman, Ontario Hospital Services Commission, to I.S. Johnston, Chairman of the Board, Lyndhurst Lodge, 14 April 1960; John Horsal, Chairman of the Rate Board, to Dr A.T. Jousse, 11 July 1960. The rates for both of these years had earlier been slightly higher but were revised downwards, which cost the hospital $9,088.27, because the province had reimbursed them at a slightly higher rate in 1959 and during the first quarter of 1960. E.P. McGavin, OHSC Comptroller, to L.B. Morrison, Lyndhurst Lodge, 9 September 1960.

17 AO, RG 10–154, Hospitals and Institutions Central Files Reel Listing, Reel 165: R.M. Saunders, Regional Representative, OHSC, to Mr W.L. Clark, Consultant, Hospital Finance (Budgets), Toronto, 18 September 1962; AO, RG 10–154, Hospitals and Institutions Central Files Reel Listing, Reel 280, MS 6098: John B. Neilson, OHSC, to Brigadier I.S. Johnston, Chairman, Lyndhurst Lodge Hospital Board, 10 February 1964.

18 AO, RG 10–154, Hospitals and Institutions Central Files Reel Listing, Reel 165: R.M. Saunders, Regional Representative, OHSC, to Mr W.L. Clark, Consultant, Hospital Finance (Budgets), Toronto, 19 September 1961.

19 AO, RG 10–154, Hospitals and Institutions Central Files Reel Listing, Reel 280, MS 6098: Dr Gordon Caudwell to R.D. Beaman, OHSC, re Visit, Lyndhurst Lodge, Toronto, 18 March 1964.

20 CPAN: CPA 7th Annual Report, 1952, 7; CPAN: CPA 8th Annual Report, 1953, 6.

21 CPAN: CPA 11th Annual Report, 1955–56, 9; CPA 12th Annual Report, 1956, 7.

22 CPAN: CPA 13th Annual Report, 1957, 7; CPA 14th Annual Report, 1958, 9. This average length of stay remained consistent into the early 1960s; Jousse, "The Evolution of the Treatment Programme for Paraplegics," 136.

23 ATJ: Myrll Jackson, Vancouver, Telephone Interview with author, 7 November 2001.

24 ATJ: Bev Hallam, Toronto, Interview with author, 20 August 2001.

25 Rutty, "'Do Something! ... Do Anything!'"; Porter, *The Greatest Benefit to Mankind*, 695–6.

26 CPAN: CPA 9th Annual Report, 1954, 4.

27 Jousse, "Rehabilitation Following Poliomyelitis."

28 ATJ: Mabel C. Brown, Ottawa, Interview with author, 10 March 2002.

29 ATJ: Gordon Paterson, Scarborough, Interview with author, 2 November 2001.

30 ATJ: Anonymous interview with author, southwestern Ontario, 23 November 2001.

31 ATJ: Margaret Staton, Santa Barbara, California, Telephone Interview with author, 19 December 2001.

32 CPAN: CPA 12th Annual Report, 1956, 7.

33 Breithaupt, Jousse, and Wynne-Jones, "Late Causes of Death and Life Expectancy in Paraplegia."

34 AO, RG 10–154, Hospitals and Institutions Central Files Reel Listing, Reel 165: A.T. Jousse to Dr R.S. Peat, OHSC, 3 December 1959; R.S. Peat to Dr A.T. Jousse, 7 December 1959. This young man's type of disability is not mentioned in the correspondence.

35 AO, RG 10–154, Hospitals and Institutions Central Files Reel Listing, Reel 280, MS 6098: A.T. Jousse to Dr B.L. Brosseau, Commissioner of Hospitals, OHSC, Toronto, 29 September 1964; Dr B.L. Brosseau to Dr A.T. Jousse, 20 October 1964.

36 ATJ: Bev Hallam, Toronto, Interview with author, 20 August 2001.

37 ATJ: Ken Langford, Toronto, Interview with author, 29 May 2003.

38 Ibid.

39 CPAN: CPA 9th Annual Report, 1954, 6–7. Statistical analysis by gender is not possible in this survey, for while it lists eighty-seven female civilian casualties, and the numbers for each disability, there is no further data; Workmen's Compensation Casualties and War Casualties may have included some women by this time. The survey also noted that, of the 385 respondents, sixty-seven, or 17 per cent, were workmen's compensation casualties.

40 ATJ: Ken Langford, Toronto, Interview with author, 29 May 2003.

41 ATJ: Dr Megan Wynne-Jones, Toronto, Interview with author, 13 May 2002.

42 Jousse, "The Evolution of the Treatment Programme for Paraplegics in Canada," 135–6.

43 ATJ: Bev Hallam, Toronto, Interview with author, 20 August 2001.

44 CPAN: CPA 13th Annual Report, 1957, 7.

45 CPAN: CPA Board Minutes, 1958, Lyndhurst Lodge Payroll, 1956–58, CPA Head Office Payroll, 1958, signed John Counsell, 28 May 1960.

46 ATJ: Margaret MacDonald, Toronto, Interview with author, 20 March 2002.

47 ATJ: Evelyn O. Paul, Toronto, Interview with author, 15 February 2002.

48 AO, RG 10–154, Hospitals and Institutions Central Files Reel Listing, Reel 165: 3 April 1962 report of visit to Lyndhurst Lodge by Louise Jamieson, Consultant, Hospital Nursing Services, 3 April 1962.

49 AO, RG 10–154, Hospitals and Institutions Central Files Reel Listing, Reel 165: A.T. Jousse to Miss Louise Jamieson, Consultant, Hospital Nursing Services, OHSC, Toronto, 11 October 1962. There were two other recommendations: that the director of nursing enroll in a course on nursing unit administration, which was not done as of the fall of 1962 (it was noted that she "will do so in all probability"); and that an assistant director of nursing be hired, which was implemented.

50 AO, RG 10–154, Hospitals and Institutions Central Files Reel Listing, Reel 280, MS 6098: A.T. Jousse to Avon Kierstead, OHSC, 25 May 1964.

51 CPAN: CPA 13th Annual Report, 1957, 7.

52 CPAN: CPA 9th Annual Report, 1954, 5.

53 CPAN: CPA 18th Annual Report, 1962, 11.

54 CPAN: CPA 20th Annual Report, 1964, 4.

55 AO, RG 10–154, Hospitals and Institutions Central Files Reel Listing, Reel 165: L. Jamieson, two-page report about 2 November 1960 visit to Lyndhurst Lodge, 24 November 1960.

56 ATJ: Ken Langford, Toronto, Interview with author, 12 June 2001.

57 The hospital committee or board was set up after Lyndhurst was approved as a convalescent hospital under the Public Hospitals Act in 1954.

58 CPAN: CPA Board Minutes, 26 October 1960. See CPA Annual Report for 1965, which notes that Counsell resigned as CPA president after holding this position since its inception in 1945. He then became chairman and J.D. Woods became CPA president. CPAN: CPA 21st Annual Report, 1965, 4.

59 ATJ: Ken Langford, Toronto, Interview with author, 29 May 2003.

60 ATJ: Margaret MacDonald, Toronto, Interview with author, 20 March 2002.

61 ATJ: Evelyn O. Paul, Toronto, Interview with author, 15 February 2002.

62 ATJ: Betty Brooks, Toronto, Interview with author, 29 November 2001.

63 ATJ: Elizabeth Holman, Toronto, Interview with author, 1 February 2002. During this interview she recalled beginning work at Lyndhurst in the early

1960s, but the CPA payroll from 1957 states "Miss B. Holman" was employed at $245 per month. CPAN: CPA Board Minutes 1957, CPA Payroll, signed John Counsell, 30 May 1957.

64 CPA Board Minutes, 1958, Lyndhurst Lodge Payroll, 1956–58, CPA Head Office Payroll, 1958, signed John Counsell, 28 May 1958.

65 ATJ: Elizabeth Holman, Toronto, Interview with author, 1 February 2002.

66 ATJ: Dr William O. Geisler, Toronto, Interview with author, 4 March 2002.

67 ATJ: Anonymous interview with author, southwestern Ontario, 23 November 2001.

68 AO, RG 10–154, Hospitals and Institutions Central Files Reel Listing, Reel 165: Name of correspondent is omitted from source due to privacy legislation. The letter is addressed simply to "Dear sir," 6 October 1959. Based on the response, this refers to the Minister of Health; M. B. Dymond, Ontario Minister of Health, to correspondent, 7 October 1959.

69 ATJ: Anonymous interview with author, southwestern Ontario, 23 November 2001.

70 ATJ: Margaret Staton, Santa Barbara, California, Telephone Interview with author, 19 December 2001.

71 ATJ: Dr Henry Barnett, Toronto, Interview with author, 5 April 2002.

72 ATJ: Gordon Paterson, Toronto, Interview with author, 2 November 2001.

73 ATJ: Margaret Staton, Santa Barbara, California, Telephone Interview with author, 19 December 2001.

74 Noell, *Another Path to My Garden*, 71. She mentions that the ramp was built on top of the original twenty steps going down to the basement level.

75 ATJ: Evelyn O. Paul, Toronto, Interview with author, 15 February 2002.

76 ATJ: Betty Brooks, Toronto, Interview with author, 29 November 2001.

77 ATJ: Margaret Staton, Santa Barbara, California, Telephone Interview with author, 19 December 2001.

78 ATJ: Betty Brooks, Toronto, Interview with author, 29 November 2001.

79 ATJ: Gordon Paterson, Toronto, Interview with author, 2 November 2001.

80 ATJ: Bev Hallam, Toronto, Interview with author, 20 August 2001.

81 ATJ: Margaret MacDonald, Toronto, Interview with author, 20 March 2002.

82 ATJ: Evelyn O. Paul, Toronto, Interview with author, 15 February 2002.

83 ATJ: Donna Walters, Toronto, Interview with author, 8 March 2002. Donna Walters, the long-time secretary of Dr Geisler (since 1971), was told this story by the late Peggy Hicks.

84 ATJ: Mabel Brown, Ottawa, Interview with author, 10 March 2002.

85 ATJ: Ken and Mary Langford, Toronto, Interview with author, 29 May 2003; Katie Barton, Toronto, Interview with author, 2 July 2001. Katie Barton also recalled going with Lyndhurst patients to Christie Street Hospital in the late

1940s to hear Paul Robeson sing. For reports about the CPA annual dinner see Burke, "Among Those Present;" and James, "Annual Dinner."

86 ATJ: Ken Langford, Toronto, Interview with author, 21 November 2001.

87 ATJ: John Yaremko, Toronto, Interview with author, 5 July 2001.

88 ATJ: Gordon Paterson, Toronto, Interview with author, 2 November 2001.

89 CPAN: Burke, "Readin', Ritin' and ... Calculus."

90 ATJ: Margaret MacDonald, Toronto, Interview with author, 20 March 2002; Elizabeth Holman, Toronto, Interview with author, 1 February 2002.

91 CPAN: CPA Board Meeting, 23 June 1964, 5.

92 ATJ: Ken Langford, Toronto, Interview with author, 23 November 2001.

93 Burke, "This is Your Announcer – Cam Langford"; "Lyndhurst on the Air," *The Caliper* 8:3 (Fall 1953): 5–6; ATJ: William O. Geisler, Toronto, Interview with author, 27 May 2003. Cam Langford was a cousin of Ken Langford.

94 "Lyndhurst Lodge Graduate Wins President Eisenhower Award," *The Caliper* 12:3 (Summer 1957): 12.

95 *The Caliper* 10:3 (Fall 1955): 14 [photo caption]. ATJ: William O. Geisler, Toronto, Interview with author, 27 May 2003.

96 Jamieson, "Life at Lyndhurst."

97 ATJ: Bev Hallam, Toronto, Interview with author, 20 August 2001.

CHAPTER FOUR

1 ATJ: Kathy Drummond, Toronto, Interview with author, 25 September 2001.

2 CPAN: CPA Board Minutes, 31 May 1961; 7 June 1962; 25 November 1962; 19 November 1963.

3 CPAN: CPA 21st Annual Report, 1965, 7.

4 CPAN: CPA 23rd Annual Report, 1967, 3.

5 CPAN: CPA 23rd Annual Report, 1967, 5.

6 AO, RG 10–154, Reel 369, MS 6112: K.E. Bennett, Auditor to Mr Good, OHSC (names of correspondents are obscured on the copies), 4 April 1966. The name of this accountant is not mentioned in the documents.

7 AO, RG 10–154, Reel 369, MS 6112: [Names of correspondents are obscured] O. Clusian (?) Hospital Operating Standards, OHSC, to Mr J. Normal(?), OHSC, 11 May 1966.

8 ATJ: Ed Ratelle, Ottawa, Interview with author, 9 December 2001.

9 ATJ: Gavin Shanks, Kingston, Interview with author, 2 October 2001.

10 ATJ: Lucille Fortier Owen, Toronto, Telephone Interview with author, 27 June 2002 [revised June 2003].

11 ATJ: Kathy Drummond, Toronto, Interview with author, 25 September 2001.

12 AO, RG 10–154, Reel 369, MS 6112: K.A. Torrance, OHSC, to Mr K. Box, OHSC, 2 June 1966. This report also noted that the person responsible for linen was caught stealing sheets, which could help to explain why these costs were higher than they should have been.

13 L.B. Morrison was Lyndhurst administrator from 1952 to 1966, when he was replaced by J.S.T. Rajan. These dates are from: CPAN: CPA 7th Annual Report, 1952, 1; "Senior Appointment," *Caliper* 21:3 (Autumn 1966): 7.

14 AO, RG 10–154, Reel 369, MS 6112: K. Torrance to A.C. Longmoore, OHSC, 20 July 1966; W.L. Clark to A.T. Jousse, 22 July 1966.

15 AO, RG 10–154, Reel 369, MS 6112: S.G. Blair, OHSC, to Mr A.C. Laugharne, OHSC, 13 February 1967.

16 AO, RG 10–154, Reel 369, MS 6112: A.T. Jousse to S. Blair, OHSC, 28 June 1967, with four-page attachment. The Archives of Ontario have cut the gardener's name from the document for reasons of confidentiality.

17 AO, RG 10–154, Reel 369, MS 6112: S.G. Blair, OHSC, to A.T. Jousse, 29 September 1967.

18 AO, RG 10–154, Reel 369, MS 6112: J.C. Cross, Auditor, OHSC, to D.W.M. Jenkins, Lyndhurst Lodge Hospital, 17 July 1967 and 2 August 1967. Lyndhurst tried to change this assessment but it stood, with S.G. Blair stating that "if depreciation on elevators was allowable because of their use by patients then, for example, depreciation on the parts of the hospital used by patients should also be allowable." AO, RG 10–154, Reel 369, MS 6112: S.G. Blair to A.C. Laugharne, OHSC, 13 September 1967.

19 AO, RG 10–154, Reel 369, MS 6112: [Nursing staff inspection report] Lyndhurst Lodge Hospital, L. Jamieson, undated letter reporting on 12 and 20 October 1967 visits. See also: Louise Jamieson to Dr Jousse, 9 November 1967. Jamieson noted that written personnel policies still had to be provided for staff members, something she had raised several years earlier; that an organizational chart was required to set out the duties of nurses in the hospital; and that policy manuals should be provided. She recommended changes in all of these areas. Dr Jousse wrote back that he was "in agreement with all" of the changes recommended: A.T. Jousse to Louise Jamieson, OHSC, 21 November 1967.

20 CPAN: CPA Board of Directors Meeting, 28 March 1968.

21 CPAN: CPA 24th Annual Report, 1968, 5.

22 CPAN: CPA 25th Annual Report, 1969, 6.

23 CPAN: CPA 21st Annual Report, 1965, 8; CPA 23rd Annual Report, 1967, 5. The remaining 7 per cent of the in-patient population discharged in 1967 included five hemiplegics, one person each with a head injury, multiple sclerosis, peripheral neuritis, muscular atrophy, and polio. The average in-stay of

people who were re-admitted was forty-three days. Males made up 80 per cent of all discharges, and females 20 per cent.

24 CPAN: CPA 25th Annual Report, 1969, 6. Quadriplegics made up just under 32 per cent of all discharged patients, while paraplegics made up just over 65 per cent. Polio vaccines, mentioned in chapter 3, explain the dwindling numbers of polio patients.

25 CPAN: CPA 26th Annual Report, 1970, 7.

26 CPAN: CPA 27th Annual Report, 1971, 6–7. Males made up 78 per cent and females 22 per cent of the in-patient population, while people above the age of thirty comprised 58 per cent of the total; the remaining 42 per cent of in-patients were under thirty.

27 CPAN: CPA 29th Annual Report, 1973, 7–8. There were 154 in-patients in 1973; 80.5 per cent had spinal cord injuries; the remaining 19.5 per cent were simply listed as "Other." No average stay data was published for 1973. During 1974, with the move taking place in July, 102 people were discharged, with their average stay being 7.5 months. CPAN: CPA 30th Annual Report, 1974, 6–7. The statistics for this year are slightly off in the published report, which states that 99 people were discharged, though the column adds up to 102.

28 E.H. Botterell, et al. "Acute Spinal Cord Injuries." Falls not related to industry comprised 14 per cent, gunshot wounds made up 3 per cent, stab wounds and airplane mishaps caused 1 per cent each; the last 3 per cent were miscellaneous. Of the sports accidents, over 65 per cent were caused by a person diving into shallow water; most of these were young men, and almost half were under twenty. This study looked at 224 people injured in 1969–70. A few years before, a study on mortality showed that the death rate among partial paraplegics was not much different from that of the rest of the population. However, partial quadriplegics died at twice the rate expected for everyone else; the death rate for complete paraplegics was four times greater than that of the general population; and, for complete quadriplegics, mortality rates were twelve times higher than normal death rates. See Jousse, Wynne-Jones, and Breithaupt, "A Follow-up Study of Life Expectancy and Mortality in Traumatic Transverse Myelitis." Kidney failure was the primary cause of death among 36 per cent of the total, which indicated that the 1960s had not seen a notable decline in this cause of death among people with this disability. The authors suggested that more effective means of preventing bladder infection were essential to improve these numbers. This 1968 publication focused on 965 paraplegics and quadriplegics who were treated in Toronto between 1945 and 1966; 203, or 21 per cent, had died.

29 Botterell, et al., "Acute Spinal Cord Injuries," 379–80.

30 ATJ: Dr Gavin Shanks, Kingston, Interview with author, 2 October 2001. Soon after his internship at Lyndhurst ended, Gavin Shanks remembered that the use of in-dwelling catheters stopped and short-term catheters were used instead. Urine was drained after a few hours rather than weeks. This practice reduced infections significantly and helped to reduce hospital stays.

31 CPAN: CPA Board of Directors Meeting, 28 March 1968.

32 ATJ: David Symington, Kingston, Interview with author, 18 March 2002. Symington arrived from the University of Washington in Seattle, where he held a similar position from 1962 to 1966; prior to that he had worked at the G.F. Strong Centre in Vancouver from 1957 to 1962, after arriving from Scotland.

33 CPAN: CPA 22nd Annual Report, 1966, 9.

34 CPAN: CPA Board of Directors Meeting, 7 October 1968.

35 CPAN: CPA Board of Directors Meeting, 23 January 1969.

36 CPAN: CPA 24th Annual Meeting, 27 March 1969.

37 LH: Lyndhurst Hospital Board Minutes, 29 September 1970.

38 LH: Lyndhurst Hospital Board Minutes, 12 January 1972.

39 AO, RG 10–154, Reel 280, MS 6098: A.T. Jousse to Dr John Neilson, Chairman, OHSC, Toronto, 3 March 1965. Dr Jousse had requested coverage by the province for dental care of long-term patients at Lyndhurst, but this was not agreed to.

40 QA: Botterell fonds, Box 5, Folder 2 – Toronto General Hospital, Neurosurgery, 1948–79: "Memorandum re Neurosurgical Division, Department of Surgery, Toronto General Hospital at University of Toronto," undated document, 3.

41 The exact date of the opening of this TGH department is not clear from the sources consulted for this book. For the dates cited here, see University Health Network, Toronto General Hospital, Archives, TGH fonds inventory, 128.

42 ATJ: Dr William O. Geisler, Toronto, Interview with author, 4 March 2002.

43 ATJ: Dr William O. Geisler, Toronto, Interview with author, 27 May 2003.

44 ATJ: Bev Hallam, Toronto, Interview with author, 20 August 2001.

45 Barnett et al. "Post-Traumatic Syringomyelia."

46 ATJ: Henry Barnett, Interview with author, Toronto, 5 April 2002. Dr Barnett travelled to London, England, in 1967 at CPA expense, to retrieve the spine of this ex-Lyndhurst patient, Mrs B., for medical research. CPAN: CPA Board of Directors Meeting, 26 October 1967.

47 ATJ: Therese Proietti, Etobicoke, Ontario, Interview with author, 11 February 2002.

48 ATJ: Lucille Fortier Owen, Toronto, Telephone Interview with author, 27 June 2002 [revised June 2003]. Less than two years after Lucille Fortier

(Owen) left Lyndhurst, an enormous controversy erupted in Toronto when surgeon Gordon Murray claimed in late 1967 that he had a "cure" for paraplegia. Dr Jousse initially supported him, but, along with other physicians, this support evaporated when Murray's claim that he could make "paraplegics walk again" was proven false. See McKellar, *Surgical Limits*, 132–60.

49 ATJ: Lucille Fortier Owen, Toronto, Telephone Interview with author, 27 June 2002 [revised June 2003].

50 ATJ: Bill Owen, Toronto, Interview with author, 24 June 2002. Lucille Fortier Owen mentioned tensions between younger patients at Lyndhurst and the CPA executive who worked there. For example, some of the younger male patients felt the CPA should help them to start small businesses, but this was not agreed to. "Everyone felt that the veterans were entitled to the benefits a grateful nation granted them." However, younger patients felt that there was an "economic disparity between the veterans and civilians," which these opposing views reflected. ATJ: Lucille Fortier Owen, Toronto, Telephone Interview with author, 27 June 2002 [revised June 2003].

51 ATJ: Kathy Drummond, Toronto, Interview with author, 25 September 2001.

52 Geisler et al., "Vocational Re-Establishment of Patients with Spinal Cord Injury." People from urban locales had a somewhat better chance of getting a job or going back to school within the overall sample group of 1,204 ex-Lyndhurst patients surveyed. This was especially so in comparison to people who lived in the countryside or a village, where the figure was 43 per cent; towns, small cities, and larger cities were virtually the same at 54 per cent, when both employment and school are added together.

53 ATJ: Kathy Drummond, Toronto, Interview with author, 25 September 2001.

54 ATJ: Tom Bailey, Burin, Newfoundland, Telephone Interview with author, 25 November 2001.

55 ATJ: William O. Geisler, Toronto, Interview with author, 27 May 2003.

56 ATJ: Betty Brooks, Toronto, Interview with author, 29 November 2001. Newspaper photo with caption about Ronald McInnes showing his new book to Betty Brooks in *The Toronto Star*, 11 January 1973, 42. Thanks to Betty Brooks for providing a copy of this item.

57 ATJ: Bill Owen, Toronto, Interview with author, 24 June 2002.

58 ATJ: ALPHANEWS Newsletter, March 1972, Fall 1972. Thanks to Bill Owen for providing copies of these newsletters.

59 ATJ: Bill Owen, Toronto, Interview with author, 24 June 2002.

60 CPAN: CPA 23rd Annual Report, 1967, 1; CPA Board of Directors Meeting, 7 October 1968; Ken Langford, Communication with author, 11 July 2003.

61 ATJ: Myrll Jackson, Vancouver, Telephone Interview with author, 7 November 2001.

62 ATJ: Bev Hallam, Toronto, Interview with author, 20 August 2001.

63 ATJ: Bev Hallam, Toronto, Interview with author, 20 August 2001.

64 ATJ: William O. Geisler, Toronto, Interview with author, 27 May 2003.

65 ATJ: Gavin Shanks, Kingston, Ontario, Interview with author, 2 October 2001.

66 ATJ: Gavin Shanks, Kingston, Ontario, Interview with author, 2 October 2001.

67 AO, RG 10–154, Reel 369, MS 6112: K.E. Bennett, Auditor to Mr Good, OHSC (names of correspondents are obscured on the copies), 4 April 1966.

68 AO, RG 10–154, Reel 280, MS 6098: A.T. Jousse to Dr John Neilson, Chairman, OHSC, Toronto, 29 April 1965. A visit to Lyndhurst on 23 April 1965 by an OHSC representative seemed to prompt Jousse's letter, as the report filed from this visit noted that the OHSC was "extremely reluctant" to agree to their request for orderly salaries to be increased: AO, RG 10–154, Reel 280, MS 6098: K. A. Torrance to A.C. Laugharne, OHSC, 26 April 1965.

69 AO, RG 10–154, Reel 280, MS 6098: Financial Advisor Varty to Mr Box, OHSC, 12 May 1965 (the names of the correspondents are obscured on this document). For Riverdale orderly salaries at this time see K. A. Torrance to A.C. Laugharne, OHSC, 26 April 1965.

70 AO, RG 10–154, Reel 280, MS 6098: K. A. Torrance to A.C. Laugharne, OHSC, 14 September 1965.

71 CPAN: CPA Board of Directors Meeting, 26 October 1967.

72 AO, RG 10–154, Reel 369, MS 6112: J.S.T. Rajan, Administrator, Lyndhurst Lodge Hospital, to Mr R. Gardner, OHSC, 16 June 1967.

73 AO, RG 10–154, Reel 369, MS 6112: [Nursing staff inspection report] Lyndhurst Lodge Hospital, L. Jamieson, undated letter reporting on 12 and 20 October 1967 visits. See also Louise Jamieson to Dr Jousse, 9 November 1967.

74 CPAN: CPA Board of Directors Meeting, 21 October 1966. In 1973 the director of rehabilitation counselling services was given four weeks paid vacation after one year's employment. CPAN: CPA Board of Directors Meeting, 4 October 1973.

75 CPAN: CPA Board of Directors Meeting, 12 January 1968.

76 CPAN: CPA Board of Directors Meeting, 7 April 1970.

77 LH: Lyndhurst Hospital Board Meeting, 14 October 1971.

78 LH: Lyndhurst Hospital Board Meeting, 12 January 1972. Evelyn O. Paul recalled the death of George White in 1972 during her interview: E.O. Paul, Toronto, Interview with author, 15 February 2002.

79 LH: Lyndhurst Hospital Board Meeting, 12 January 1972. This former employee later filed a complaint with the provincial Human Rights Commission over his lost job; the outcome of this complaint is not known.

80 ATJ: Lucille Fortier Owen, Toronto, Telephone Interview with author, 27 June 2002 [revised June 2003].

81 LH: Lyndhurst Hospital Board Minutes, 14 October 1971, 12 January 1972; CPAN: CPA Board of Directors Meeting, 8 January 1974; 9 April 1974.

82 LH: Lyndhurst Hospital Board Minutes, 5 June 1974.

83 ATJ: Evelyn O. Paul, Toronto, Interview with author, 15 February 2002.

84 CPAN: CPA 25th Annual Report, 1969, 7.

85 CPAN: CPA 28th Annual Report, 1972, 2; CPA Executive Committee Meeting, 12 January 1972.

86 CPAN: CPA 26th Annual Report, 1970, 3.

87 ATJ: Charlie Saso, Ottawa, Interview with author, 22 October 2001.

88 Wilson, "Life Doesn't End In A Wheelchair," 6. Thanks to both Sheila Avery, Toronto, and Loma Stone, Toronto, for providing a copy of this article.

89 ATJ: Charlie Saso, Ottawa, Interview with author, 22 October 2001.

90 ATJ: Ed Ratelle, Ottawa, Interview with author, 9 December 2001.

91 ATJ: Loma Stone, Toronto, Interview with author, 22 November 2001.

92 ATJ: Dr Gavin Shanks, Kingston, Interview with author, 2 October 2001.

93 CPAN: CPA 22nd Annual Meeting, 11 April 1967.

94 CPAN: CPA 25th Annual Meeting, 7 April 1970. Dr Tran had come to Lyndhurst after a year's training at the Montreal Rehabilitation Institute.

95 ATJ: Dr Nimmi Bharatwal, Toronto, Interview with author, 10 April 2002.

96 CPAN: CPA 25th Annual Meeting, 7 April 1970.

97 CPAN: CPA 26th Annual Report, 1970, 3.

98 CPAN: CPA 27th Annual Report, 1971, 5.

99 CPAN: CPA Board of Directors Meeting, 26 May 1970.

100 CPAN: CPA Board of Directors Meeting, 29 September 1970.

101 CPAN: CPA Board of Directors Meeting, 2 December 1970.

102 CPAN: CPA Board of Directors Meeting, 8 February 1971.

103 CPAN: CPA Board of Directors Meeting, 5 April 1971.

104 LH: Lyndhurst Hospital Board of Directors Meeting, 20 July 1971.

105 CPAN: CPA Board of Directors Meeting, 18 November 1971.

106 CPAN: CPA 28th Annual Report, 1972, 7.

107 CPAN: CPA 28th Annual Meeting, 10 April 1973.

108 CPAN: CPA 28th Annual Meeting, 10 April 1973.

109 CPAN: CPA Board of Directors Meeting, 12 December 1972.

110 CPAN: CPA Board of Directors Meeting, 27 August 1974.

111 CPAN: CPA Board of Directors Meeting, 10 April 1973.

112 CPAN: CPA 29th Annual Report, 1973, 7.

113 CPAN: CPA Board of Directors Meeting, 25 June 1973. As it turned out, this laboratory was not used for the purposes originally intended.

114 ATJ: Ken Langford, Toronto, Interview with author, 21 November 2001.

115 ATJ: Betty Brooks, Toronto, Interview with author, 29 November 2001.

116 ATJ: Ken Langford, Toronto, Interview with author, 21 November 2001.

117 CPAN: CPA Board of Directors Meeting, 27 August 1974.

118 ATJ: Kathy Drummond, Toronto, Interview with author, 25 September 2001. Lucille Fortier Owen mentioned that she thought the new building should have been built in a more urban environment closer to amenities, such as main roads and "city life" for people in wheelchairs, rather than in the more isolated area where it is located. She also said that her former roommates would have liked the more open, airy feeling of the new hospital in contrast to the old cramped building. ATJ: Lucille Fortier Owen, Toronto, Telephone Interview with author, 27 June 2002 [revised June 2003].

119 ATJ: Charlie Saso, Ottawa, Interview with author, 22 October 2001.

120 CPAN: CPA 30th Annual Report, 1974, 5–6.

CHAPTER FIVE

1 ATJ: Barbara Turnbull, Toronto, Interview with author, 1 March 2002. The art that Barbara Turnbull referred to was bought with $25,000 donations from each of the Gordon and Gardiner Foundations, which were in turn matched by the provincial Wintario corporation, thus raising $100,000 for a permanent art collection at Lyndhurst. Board member Helen Phelan, sister of the founder of the Gardiner Foundation, and Elizabeth Gordon, from the wealthy Gordon family, were a "committee of two" who made the art selections, which have risen in value since their original purchase in the mid-1970s. ATJ: Ken and Mary Langford, Toronto, Interview with author, 29 May 2003.

2 AO: RG 10–1, File 81.24, Box 81, Letter to Frank Miller, Minister of Health, Toronto, from a correspondent whose name is withheld for privacy reasons, 29 April 1975. Other similar letters in this file, making the same point and written in the spring of 1975, all have a near identical response from the same MOH official.

3 CPAN: CPA 32nd Annual Report, 1976, 5; LH: Board Minutes, 23 January 1979, 2; CPA 38th Annual Report, 1982–83 (1 April to 31 March), published in *Caliper* 38 (September 1983); LH: "Building Hope," Newsletter, Spring 1997, 3.

4 CPAN: CPA Board Minutes, 29 January 1975; "New Medical Director," *Caliper*, 30:1 (Spring 1975): 2. For reference to his resignation from the Lyndhurst Board see: LH: Lyndhurst Board Minutes, 22 July 1980.

5 CPAN: A.C. Clarke, memo to D. Jenkins, CPA, Toronto, 6 July 1977; CPA Executive Committee Meeting, 22 July 1977. Ken Langford was on the hospital board into the 1990s.

6 LH: Lyndhurst Board Minutes, 5 July 1978.

7 CPAN: CPA 34th Annual Report, 31 March 1979, v.

8 LH: Lyndhurst Board Minutes, 21 November 1978; 23 January 1979. In early 1983 this issue came up again when it was noted that 85 per cent of all beds were occupied, though if those being held in reserve for people receiving acute care at other local hospitals were factored in, it would have been a 100 per cent occupancy rate. Twenty patients who had completed their rehabilitation program remained in the hospital as they has nowhere to go; accessible housing was in short supply and so too were spaces at chronic-care facilities. This impeded the smooth transfer of people in and out of the hospital. These were difficult times, as the hospital operated without a medical director, staff shortages continued, no funding was offered by the province for eleven more staff positions, and, most importantly, no money was forthcoming to open up beds on the empty fourth unit of the hospital. However, with the opening of the patient-initiated Nucleus Housing project in northwestern Toronto, eleven long-stay patients had a home to go to (as is discussed elsewhere in this chapter). While this helped to get people back into the community and opened up more bed space, the waiting list continued to remain stable at twenty-five to thirty patients. LH: Lyndhurst Board Minutes, 23 March, 27 April, 25 May, 22 June, 31 August, 26 October 1983.

9 ATJ: Betty Brooks, Interview with author, Toronto, 29 November 2001.

10 The primary concerns that gave rise to this union drive were job security and patient-to-nurse ratio. By August 1977 the ONA had been certified by the province to represent registered and graduate nurses at Lyndhurst, except for three head nurses, people above the rank of head nurse, the hospital staff health nurse, and nurses employed for less than twenty-four hours per week. During the late 1970s the ONA and SEIU represented approximately sixty employees. LH: Lyndhurst Board Minutes, 17 May and 23 August 1977; 21 March 1978. In 1984 twenty-four part-time employees became part of the SEIU bargaining unit: LH: Lyndhurst Board Minutes, 28 March 1984.

11 Several of their representatives presented a list of fourteen "demands and complaints" to the hospital. Though they were not unionized, an SEIU representative was present during their initial two-and-a-half hour meeting with board chairman Jack Blain on 14 April 1977. Their concerns related to having a say in staffing matters, job security, safety issues particularly in regard to heavy lifting, extended maternity care, salaries, and internal staffing relationships. The physiotherapists decided to withdraw their practice of lifting

patients between wheelchair and mat in the gym until these issues were dealt with. A few weeks later, it was reported that some staffing issues were changed, such as vacation periods and earlier maternity leaves but the crucial issue of lifting was left the same as before, so this continued to be a point of contention. Eventually, the job action ended when physiotherapists began to lift patients again five months after they had stopped; no resolution to their concerns on this issue was recorded. LH: Lyndhurst Board Minutes, 17 May, 5 July, 23 August, and 20 September 1977.

12 LH: Lyndhurst Board Minutes, 9 October 1979. Frustration with "conservative" hospital practices at Lyndhurst may have been partly responsible for turnover among staff such as physiotherapists during the early 1980s. Another factor in the departure of some employees, as was explained at the beginning of this chapter, was that some well-respected colleagues lost their jobs during this period, notably long-time PT head, Barbara Duffin. As well, some staff in the allied health professions were at that time considering whether or not to "move on," because of tensions over getting a response to their proposals to update and change things. LH: Lyndhurst Board Minutes, 25 March 1981. By early 1981, when the significant turnover rates in this department were noted, sixteen physiotherapists were employed at Lyndhurst, eleven of them full-time. LH: Lyndhurst Board Minutes, 25 February 1981. One vacancy in the PT Department was also noted. The turnover rate was supposed to "settle down" by early March of that year.

13 ATJ: Betty Brooks, Interview with author, Toronto, 29 November 2001.

14 LH: Lyndhurst Board Minutes, 23 September 1980. Staff changes led to fewer admissions by the spring of 1980, when the average bed occupancy for April was recorded as being 65.5. However, these numbers were somewhat distorted because beds had to remain unoccupied to await the return of in-patients away for acute care at one of the local hospitals – five to seven beds at a time were kept open like this. Nevertheless, occupancy continued to decline – by September 1980 the average was sixty-seven beds, fifteen fewer than two years earlier.

15 A number of long-time employees departed under considerably more amicable terms than some of their colleagues during the early years on Sutherland Drive. After granting extensions for five years past his retirement date, in early 1976 the board declined to renew a half-time employment contract for Jim Bartlett, who retired after 29 years. Dorothy Waddell was another staff departure that spring when she resigned after seven years of being in charge of volunteers. LH: Lyndhurst Board Minutes, 23 February 1976. In June 1982 Arthur James retired as the director of maintenance after thirty-seven years on the job. LH: Lyndhurst Board Minutes, 24 March 1982. Two years later,

Basil Thomas also retired after thirty-nine years as an orderly, a position he had held since Lyndhurst opened in 1945. LH: Lyndhurst Board Minutes, 25 April 1984.

16 CPAN: CPA 30th Annual Report, 1974, 6–7. CPA 38th Annual Report, 1982–83 (April to March), published in *Caliper*, 38 (September 1983). Thirty-nine re-admitted patients had an average in-hospital stay of sixty-five days.

17 LH: Lyndhurst Board Minutes, 4 February 1975.

18 LH: Lyndhurst Board Minutes, 18 October 1976; 15 November 1977; 17 January 1978. After Dr Geisler resigned as medical director in 1979, Dr Nirmala Bharatwal became acting medical director and was appointed to this position, which she held until 1982, the following year. Both Dr Geisler and Dr Bharatwal (who was hired full-time in 1975) remained on active medical treatment staff for the rest of the period covered by this chapter. Geisler retired in 1998; Bharatwal remained after amalgamation. A general practitioner, Dr Terence Brown, was hired on a part time basis to work under Dr Claude Vipond, who had been hired as associate medical staff in 1976.

19 LH: Lyndhurst Board Minutes, 25 March 1981.

20 The agreement between the University of Toronto and Lyndhurst was renewed in 1988 and 1990. LH: Lyndhurst Board Minutes, 30 January, 27 February 1985; 22 October and 26 November 1986; 26 October 1988; 26 September 1990. A formal teaching agreement with the University of Toronto was reached in 1990. It was renewed every two years thereafter. The agreement allowed medical students to train in rehabilitation medicine. LH: Lyndhurst Board Minutes, 26 April 1990; 28 October 1992.

21 LH: Lyndhurst Board Minutes, 23 February and 18 October 1976.

22 ATJ: Dr Charles Tator, Interview with author, Toronto, 20 December 2001.

23 ATJ: Dr Ron Tasker, Interview with author, Toronto, 27 July 2002. He mentioned that, when it came to relief of pain, "We are in a position that we could really help a small percentage, thirty to forty percent" of people with spinal cord injuries.

24 Geisler et al., "Survival in Traumatic Spinal Cord Injury"; see also the earlier studies: Geisler et al., "Survival in Traumatic Transverse Myelitis"; Jousse et al., "Life Expectancy and Mortality in Traumatic Transverse Myelitis"; Breithaupt et al., "Late Cause of Death and Life Expectancy in Paraplegia." The statistics included here are from the first publication.

25 ATJ: Dr Nirmala A. Bharatwal, Toronto, Interview with author, 10 April 2002; William O. Geisler, Conversation with author, 8 October 2003.

26 LH: Annual Report, 1987–88, 13; 1991, 2.

27 ATJ: Dr Nirmala A. Bharatwal, Toronto, Interview with author, 10 April 2002.

28 In 1976 the total number of staff had increased by 18 per cent (twenty-nine), for a total of 158; bed spaces had increased by over 33 per cent with increased provincial funding. CPAN: CPA 32nd Annual Report, 1976, 5–6. By 1977 the total number of staff had climbed to 185. CPAN: CPA 33rd Annual Report, 1977, 9.

29 LH: Lyndhurst Board Minutes, 16 August 1976; 22 April 1981; Dr William O. Geisler, Conversation with author, 8 October 2003.

30 LH: Lyndhurst Board Minutes, 27 November 1985.

31 LH: Lyndhurst Board Minutes, 22 January 1986.

32 LH: Lyndhurst Board Minutes, 23 November 1988.

33 LH: Lyndhurst Board Minutes, 25 June 1986; Dr William O. Geisler, Conversation with the author, 8 October 2003.

34 ATJ: Bill Brown Interview with author, Toronto, 22 March 2002. Eventually, Bill Brown decided to leave Lyndhurst to work as a psychiatric nurse at Toronto's Queen Street Mental Health Centre.

35 LH: Lyndhurst Board Minutes, 28 January 1987.

36 LH: Lyndhurst Board Minutes, 29 April 1987.

37 LH: Lyndhurst Board Minutes, 24 June 1987.

38 Allowing same-sex staff to change a patient's catheters had been a major issue only five years before, as is discussed elsewhere in this chapter. However, with this change in policy this was no longer possible for most male patients since most nurses were females. Unlike in 1982, this development was not successfully challenged.

39 ATJ: Lloyd Charles, Toronto, Interview with author, 15 February 2002.

40 ATJ: Michael O'Brien, Toronto, Interview with author, 8 July 2002.

41 LH: Lyndhurst Board Minutes, 1 December 1993, 31 March and 6 October 1994; 28 February and 26 September 1996; 16 January 16 and 25 September 1997. LH: "Building Hope," Newsletter, Spring 1997, 3.

42 For example, during 1975, the first full year of Lyndhurst's operation on Sutherland Drive, ninety-seven patients were discharged, of whom 82.5 per cent were first-time admissions. Quadriplegics made up 41 per cent of the overall group (thirty-one males, nine females); 48.5 per cent were paraplegics (thirty-six males, eleven females); and the remainder consisted of four people with multiple sclerosis, three with hemiplegia, two with Friedereich's ataxia, and one with Parkinson's disease. The average stay of first-admission patients was seven-and-a-half months, while for re-admissions it was two-and-a-half months. CPAN: CPA 31st Annual Report, 1975, 6–7. The following year saw 129 patients discharged of whom 68 per cent, or 88 people, were first-time admissions. Of the overall total in 1976, 43 per cent were quadriplegics (46 males, 9 females); 40 per cent were paraplegics (38 males, 14 females); and

the remaining 17 per cent included 10 people with hemiplegia, 6 with multiple sclerosis, 3 with head injuries, 2 with polio, and one with dystonia musculotum deformans. CPAN: CPA 32nd Annual Report, 1976, 6–7. In 1977, 153 people were discharged from Lyndhurst, of whom almost 78 per cent, or 119, were first-time admissions. Quadriplegics made up 37 per cent of this group (45 males, 12 females); 43 per cent were paraplegics (51 males, 15 females); the remaining 20 per cent included 10 people each with hemiplegia and multiple sclerosis, 5 with head injuries, 2 with polio, 2 with forms of peripheral neuritis, and one with Kugelberg Welander syndrome. The average stay of the 119 first-time admissions was the shortest in seven years: 5.6 months. CPAN: CPA 33rd Annual Report, 1977, 10–12. In 1978 Lyndhurst had provincial approval for 95 beds with an average of 82 being occupied. A total of 163 patients were discharged, of whom 119, or 73 per cent, had been admitted for the first time; 98 or 82 per cent of the first-time admissions were people with spinal cord injuries, while the remaining 21 had other unlisted disabilities. The average length of stay was 6.6 months for the 119 first-time admissions, of whom 12 people, or 10 per cent, were discharged to chronic-care facilities. CPAN: CPA 34th Annual Report, 31 March 1979, v. Statistics are for the calendar year, though the fiscal year had changed.

43 LH: Lyndhurst Hospital Annual Report, 1987–88, 8. Quadriplegics made up 45 per cent of first-time admissions, while paraplegics made up 30 per cent. The remaining 25 per cent comprised "spinal cord related conditions." Seventy-one per cent of first-time admissions came from hospitals within Toronto, 15 per cent were from other hospitals outside Toronto in Ontario, 13 per cent arrived from home, and 1 per cent came from other health-care facilities. Males made up 81 per cent of these first admissions, females 19 per cent. Their average age was twenty-eight.

44 LH: "Building Hope," Newsletter, Fall 1996, 3. During the mid-1990s, new admissions ranged from 133 in 1995 to 114 in 1996. The occupancy rate was fairly stable as well, with sixty-six, or 84 per cent, of seventy-nine beds being used in 1995. A year later, when the bed complement was reduced to seventy by provincial cuts, the occupancy rate was sixty-one beds, or 87 per cent. LH: Annual Report, 1995, 2; 1996, 2 (1996 Annual Report is printed in "Building Hope," Newsletter, Fall 1996).

45 LH: "Building Hope," Newsletter, Fall 1996, 13. Mark Tonack, a researcher at Lyndhurst, also reported on some revealing statistics for all of North America in the mid-1990s. He noted that the divorce rate among married people with spinal cord injuries was between 70 and 80 per cent. This population group had an unemployment rate of 50 to 90 per cent and as many as 20 per cent committed suicide. However, he also noted that many people

with this disability were able to live on their own in the community. In North America by the late twentieth century, 11,000 people a year suffered a spinal cord injury; approximately 225,000 people across the continent had this disability. LH: "Building Hope," Newsletter, Summer 1996, 4.

46 Dr William O. Geisler, Conversation with author, 16 October 2003.

47 ATJ: Kirby Rowe, Interview with author, Kingston, Ontario, 3 October 2001. Dr Geisler mentioned that partying happened on all wards. The Laird Tavern was promoted by staff to get some of the partying out of Lyndhurst. Dr William O. Geisler, Conversation with author, 16 October 2003.

48 In 1977, of 119 first-time admissions, 45 per cent (fifty-four people) were discharged to their own homes; 30 per cent (thirty-six people) went to live with relatives or friends; 13.5 per cent (sixteen people) were sent to general hospitals; and 6.5 per cent (eight people) were transferred to chronic-care facilities. The remaining 5 per cent included two people who were lost track of, one who went to a group home, one who was transferred to another rehabilitation facility, and one who died at Lyndhurst. As well, twenty-seven (22.5 per cent) of 119 first-time discharged patients had found full-time employment, four (3 per cent) had part-time jobs, and seven (6 per cent) went back to school. CPAN: CPA 33rd Annual Report, 1977, 10–12.

49 LH: Lyndhurst Board Minutes, 17 March 1975.

50 LH: Lyndhurst Board Minutes, 13 May 1975.

51 LH: Lyndhurst Board Minutes, 9 September 1975.

52 Ryan, "Organizations of, and For, the Disabled."

53 "The Disabled Citizen," *The Caliper* 36 (Autumn 1981): 12–14; Ryan, "I.Y.D.P.: Fourth Quarter Report"; McLeod, "CPA: Achieving Dignity." For a good summary of activism during this period, see Driedger, *The Last Civil Rights Movement*.

54 AO: RG 10–57, TB 7, File 898–3: Letter to Minister of Health, Larry Grossman, Toronto, from correspondent whose name has been withheld for privacy reasons, 21 October 1982 (attachment to letter re charter of Patients Transportation Corporation).

55 LH: Lyndhurst Board Minutes, 25 March and 22 July 1980.

56 LH: Lyndhurst Board Minutes, 30 September, 27 October, 24 November 1982; 26 October 1983.

57 AO: RG 10–57, File 898–2: R.F. Swan, Administrator, Lyndhurst Hospital, to Ms M. Risk, Executive Director, College of Nurses of Ontario, Toronto, 7 February 1983. Randy Swan was administrator of Lyndhurst from 1980 to 1998. He succeeded Douglas Perkins, who held this post from 1975 to 1980.

58 AO: RG 10–57, TB 7 898–3, fourteen-page letter, including survey, to Paul Stirling, director, psychological services, Lyndhurst Hospital, from a corre-

spondent whose name has been withheld for privacy reasons, 21 September 1982. A copy of this report was sent on the same date to Larry Grossman, Minister of Health, Toronto. Dr Geisler recalled hearing people say they were "inmates rather than patients" from the 1950s to the 1980s. Dr William O. Geisler, Conversation with author, 16 October 2003.

59 AO: RG 10–57, TB 7, File 898–3: Letter to Minister of Health, Larry Grossman, Toronto, from a correspondent whose name has been withheld for privacy reasons, 21 October 1982 (attachment to letter re survey findings and Report to Board of Directors, Lyndhurst Transportation Corporation and Patients of Lyndhurst Hospital.

60 AO: RG 10–57, TB 7, File 898–3: Letter to Minister of Health, Larry Grossman, Toronto, from a correspondent whose name has been withheld for privacy reasons, 23 November 1982.

61 AO: RG 10–57, TB 7, File 898–3: Letter from Minister of Health, Larry Grossman, Toronto, to a correspondent whose name has been withheld for privacy reasons, 20 January 1983.

62 LH: Lyndhurst Board Minutes, 30 September, 27 October, 24 November 1982; 26 October 1983.

63 LH: Lyndhurst Board Minutes, 22 February 1984. Computers began to be used at Lyndhurst for administrative purposes beginning in the 1960s: Dr William O. Geisler, Conversation with author, 16 October 2003.

64 LH: Annual Report, 1987–88, 9. LH: "Building Hope," Newsletter, Fall 1996, 18 (quote). The acronym PARTY was changed slightly by 1996 to mean "Prevent Alcohol and Risk Related Trauma in Youth."

65 LH: Lyndhurst Board Minutes, 22 August and 28 November 1984.

66 LH: Lyndhurst Board Minutes, 30 January 1985.

67 LH: Lyndhurst Board Minutes, 28 October 1987.

68 LH: Lyndhurst Board Minutes, 3 February 1994.

69 LH: Lyndhurst Board Minutes, 4 May 1995. This legislation was part of wide-ranging changes enacted under the Ontario Advocacy Commission, which came into existence at this time. It was abolished by the Harris Conservatives shortly after their election in June 1995.

70 LH: Lyndhurst Board Minutes, 25 April 1996.

71 LH: Lyndhurst Board Minutes, 26 September 1996.

72 LH: Lyndhurst Board Minutes, 30 July 1998.

73 LH: Lyndhurst Board Minutes, 24 September 1998.

74 ATJ: Michael O'Brien, Toronto, Interview with author, 8 July 2002.

75 Turnbull, *Looking in the Mirror*. For more information on her work, see the web site: www:barbaraturnbull.org.

76 ATJ: Barbara Turnbull, Interview with author, Toronto, 1 March 2002.

77 ATJ: Carmen Mobbs, Interview with author, Toronto, 21 April 2002.

78 LH: Annual Report, 1986–87, 58–9.

79 LH: Annual Report, 1987–88, 9.

80 LH: Annual Report,, 1988–89, 15.

81 LH: Lyndhurst Board Minutes, 18 October 1976.

82 LH: Lyndhurst Board Minutes, 17 January 1977.

83 LH: Lyndhurst Board Minutes, 28 April 1982; 26 January 1983. The Workmen's Compensation Board also helped to find houses for WCB patients, as did the Department of Indian Affairs for a Native Canadian Lyndhurst patient: Dr William O. Geisler, Conversation with author, 30 October 2003.

84 ATJ: Lise Desrochers, Interview with author, Toronto, 26 March 2002.

85 ATJ: Kirby Rowe, Interview with author, Kingston, Ontario, 3 October 2001.

86 A 1950s Cottage Program similar to the one developed at Lyndhurst in the 1990s was mentioned by Dr William O. Geisler in conversation with the author, 30 October 2003.

87 LH: "Building Hope," Newsletter, Winter 1994, 10–11.

88 LH: Annual Report, 1993, 6.

89 LH: Lyndhurst Board Minutes, 27 February, 25 June, 18 December 1997.

90 LH: Lyndhurst Board Minutes, 19 September 1978. Prior to this period, dating back to at least the 1950s, issues pertaining to sexuality were talked about with individual patients by medical staff in the course of regular consultations at Lyndhurst: Dr William O. Geisler, Conversation with author, 30 October 2003.

91 LH: Annual Report, 1989, 2; 1990, 2; 1991, 2; 1993, 2; LH: Lyndhurst Board Minutes, 31 January 1990; 12 May and 2 June 1993.

92 LH: "Building Hope," Newsletter, Spring 1997, 2.

93 LH: Lyndhurst Board Minutes, 29 October 1985.

94 LH: Lyndhurst Board Minutes, 2 February 1993.

95 LH: Annual Report, 1993, 6. Quote is from: LH: "Building Hope," Newsletter, 12.

96 LH: Annual Report, 1990, 2, 6. The Lyndhurst Research Department was funded by the A. T. Jousse Foundation, CPA, Man in Motion Legacy Fund, Ontario Ministry of Community and Social Services, Ontario Ministry of Health, National Health Research and Development Program, and Natural Sciences and Engineering Research Council. John Labatt Ltd "funded a clinical research program aimed at evaluating the utility of the Lyndhurst Adaptive Robotic Aid (LARA) for use by disabled individuals." LH: Annual Report, 1991, 6.

97 LH: Lyndhurst Board Minutes, 30 May, 26 September 1990; 29 May 1991.

98 LH: Lyndhurst Board Minutes, 7 December 1995.

99 LH: Lyndhurst Board Minutes, 28 November 1996. Accreditation was a major issue that was debated on and off at the board level from 1976 to the second half of the 1980s. Early in 1987, after a visit by a surveyor the previous fall, Lyndhurst was approved for the maximum allowed three-year accreditation by the Canadian Council on Hospital Accreditation. LH: Lyndhurst Board Minutes, 29 April 1987. Accreditation was approved every three years thereafter for the remainder of the period covered in this chapter.

100 ATJ: Michael O'Brien, Interview with author, Toronto, 8 July 2002.

101 LH: Lyndhurst Board Minutes, 25 September 1997.

102 Not getting anywhere with the province did not stop Lyndhurst from looking somewhere else for income. To help raise money for both spinal cord injury research and the operation of the hospital, the Lyndhurst Foundation was established on 31 December 1987. The foundation solicited private-sector funding for this purpose. It began with $1.2 million taken from the hospital's unused equity funds. During its first year, the foundation raised $138,000 from 167 donors. Much of this was used for research and for equipment for the new Robson Urology Clinic. LH: Annual Report, 1987–88, 15; LH: Annual Report, 1989, 3. Within five years, almost $1 million had been raised by the foundation for "research and patient care equipment needs." LH: Annual Report, 1992, 5. One former board member, Helen Phelan, decided to help out with funding problems by donating $50,000 to buy new beds for patients. LH: Lyndhurst Board Minutes, 24 June 1992. A number of successful fundraising events were also organized to raise money for the hospital during this period; a gala organized by the Lyndhurst Foundation brought in $125,000. LH: Lyndhurst Board Minutes, 4 May 1995. By 1996 other funding sources outside the provincial government included the CPA, the University of Toronto, the Toronto Board of Education, the Lyndhurst Foundation, and Home Care services. LH: Lyndhurst Board Minutes, 28 February 1996.

103 LH: Lyndhurst Board Minutes, 23 March 1988.

104 CPA 37th Annual Report, 1981–82 (April-March) published in *Caliper* 37 (Summer 1982): v; LH: Lyndhurst Board Minutes, 18 December 1997. The changing nature of the relationship between the CPA and Lyndhurst from the late 1970s to 1990s happened, according to Dr Bharatwal, because the CPA was looked upon as "an outside agency." Issues around access to patient records and confidentiality came up. The CPA "could not have access to the chart of the patient, which is the private property of the patient and the hospital. But I think the importance of CPA staff being involved earlier in patients' rehabilitation was slowly realized. [CPA Ontario Executive Director] Bill Adair again made an effort to bring CPA closer to Lyndhurst and therefore the referral system got started again almost as soon as the patients were

admitted and definitely before they were discharged. So now CPA does get to know everyone as they are admitted." Dr Nirmala Bharatwal, Toronto, Interview with author, 10 April 2002.

105 During the late 1970s, the ONA and SEIU represented approximately sixty employees. LH: Lyndhurst Board Minutes, 17 May and 23 August 1977; 21 March 1978. In 1984 twenty-four part-time employees became part of the SEIU bargaining unit: LH: Lyndhurst Board Minutes, 28 March 1984. Improvements made in unionized employees' benefits package were reflected among non-unionized workers during the 1980s. In early 1981 an arbitrator awarded SEIU members an 18 to 24 per cent wage increase over fourteen months. To respond to the gains made by unionized employees, non-unionized staff in the "clerical-management-professional group" had improvements made in their dental plan, bereavement leave, and vacation period (four weeks after ten years; five weeks after twenty years), and a 3 per cent wage increase. LH: Lyndhurst Board Minutes, 24 June and 28 October 1981. Nurses who were part of the ONA bargaining unit at Lyndhurst saw their salaries rise by 8.25 per cent over two years in 1986–87. LH: Lyndhurst Board Minutes, 28 January 1987. Beginning in late 1986 non-unionized employees had their vacations pegged at four weeks after eight years and five weeks after seventeen years. A pay equity program was instituted in 1987 to coincide with the SEIU program. If an employee was seriously sick during a vacation this would be recorded as sick days, not as part of an employee's vacation time. LH: Lyndhurst Board Minutes, 26 November 1986.

106 In 1992, when there was only a 1 per cent raise in provincial funding, the Ministry of Health policy ordered the "downsizing of institutional care." In response to this, Lyndhurst cut $300,000 from their budget; $200,000 was for salaries and benefits and $100,000 was for hospital supplies. This led to the loss of five full-time jobs, though no jobs in spinal cord rehabilitation were eliminated. LH: Annual Report, 1992, 2; Annual Report, 1995, 2. LH: Lyndhurst Board Minutes, 15 September 1993. Unpaid days were an annual part of work-life for public employees up until 1996, as had been negotiated under the 1993 "Social Contract." LH: Annual Report, 1996, 2. As occurred across Ontario from 1993 to 1996, the Social Contract Act stipulated that provincially funded employees who earned more than $30,000 per year had their wages held at the same level; they were also required to work twelve unpaid days annually in a legislated attempt to reduce the provincial deficit. Two more full-time positions were cut in 1995 as $240,000 was cut. LH: Annual Report, 1995, 2.

107 LH: "Building Hope," Newsletter, Spring 1997, 3.

108 LH: Lyndhurst Board Minutes, 25 June 1997.

109 LH: Lyndhurst Board Minutes, 14 August 1997.

110 LH: Lyndhurst Board Minutes, 30 October 1997.

111 LH: Lyndhurst Board Minutes, 30 October 1997; 26 February and 15 April 1998.

112 LH: Lyndhurst Board Minutes, 28 May 1998.

113 LH: Lyndhurst Board Minutes, 18 December 1997.

114 LH: Lyndhurst Board Minutes, 24 September 1998.

115 LH: Lyndhurst Board Minutes, 25 September 1997.

116 LH: Lyndhurst Board Minutes, 26 February 1998.

117 LH: Lyndhurst Board Minutes, 24 September and 20 October 1998.

CHAPTER SIX

1 Dr Botterell died at the age of 91 on 23 June 1997. Schatz et al., "E. Harry Botterell."

2 Dr Botterell received the Order of Canada for his overall medical work: Rasbach, "Lives Lived: Edmund Henry (Harry) Botterell." John Counsell was named to the Order of Canada in 1968. "His Legacy to the Handicapped: John Gibbons Counsell, O.C., O.B.E., M.C." [no author], *Caliper* 31:4 (Winter 1976): 4–5.

3 Dr Jousse was named to the Order of Canada in 1969. "In Memoriam: Albin T. Jousse, Order of Canada (1969), B.A., M.D., LL.D., F.R.C.P. [C]" [no author], *Caliper* 48:4 (Winter 1993): 4; Geisler, "Obituary: Albin Theophile Jousse." Dr Geisler was named to the Order of Canada in 2001: "Coutts appointed to Order of Canada [appointment list]," *The Globe and Mail,* 24 August 2001.

4 As one example, see citation in DeVivo and Stover, "Long-Term Survival and Causes of Death."

5 LH: "Research at Lyndhurst: Recommendations from Stakeholders," June 1997, 1.

6 "Driving their own care: Toronto Rehab patients can choose complementary and alternative therapies," no author, *Toronto Rehab* (Winter 2002): 6–7 (quote is on 7).

7 Dr William O. Geisler, Conversation with the author, 8 October 2003. The issue of spinal cord regeneration is widely reported and debated in the press, as the following citations indicate: Foss, "Paraplegic regains movement after cell procedure"; Immen, "Spinal implants give hope to disabled"; Abraham, "Man of steel." For various perspectives on this topic by people with spinal cord injuries see Vargo, "Superman's Folly"; Letters in response, *Caliper* 53:2

(Fall 1998): 4, Vargo, "Biting the Magic Bullet"; Letters in response, *Total Access* 1:3 (Spring 2000): 3 and *Total Access* 2:1 (Fall 2000): 5.

8 ATJ: Michael O'Brien, Interview with author, Toronto, 8 July 2002; revised, September 2003.

.

Bibliography

The following are used as abbreviations for Archives and Collections in the notes:

ATJ   A.T. Jousse Foundation, Toronto
AO   Archives of Ontario, Toronto
CPAN   Canadian Paraplegic Association National Office, Ottawa
CPAO   Canadian Paraplegic Association Ontario Office, Toronto
LH   Lyndhurst Hospital, Toronto Rehabilitation Institute, Toronto
QA   Queen's University Archives, Kingston, Ontario
NA   National Archives of Canada, Ottawa
VAC   Archives for Veterans Affairs Canada, Charlottetown, Prince Edward Island

NOTE ON SOURCES

Since the primary sources consulted for this book are too numerous to list here, only the basic record type is noted below. Readers are directed to the notes for specific archival file and record group references as well as collections that are held in various locations noted herein. The University Health Network, Toronto General Hospital Archives, TGH fonds, were consulted, but access restrictions prevented any useful research in their records for the history covered in this book.

ARCHIVES AND COLLECTIONS

A.T. Jousse Foundation (ATJ), Toronto
   All interviews indicated in acknowledgments and notes.

Donated material from personal collections indicated in acknowledgments
and notes.
Archives of Ontario (AO), Toronto
  Ministry of Health records
  Ministry of Community and Social Service records
Canadian Paraplegic Association National Office (CPAN), Ottawa
  The Caliper: The Journal of the Canadian Paraplegic Association
    (1946–99)
  Total Access: Canadian Paraplegic Association (1999–2001)
  Canadian Paraplegic Association National Board Minutes, 1945–98
  Canadian Paraplegic Association Annual Reports, 1946–98
  Published CPA reports
  Various historical documents, published and unpublished, on CPA and
    Lyndhurst
Canadian Paraplegic Association Ontario Office (CPAO), Toronto
  Canadian Paraplegic Association Ontario Board Minutes, 1979–1998
  Historical newspaper collection
  Published CPA reports
  Various historical documents, published and unpublished, on CPA and
    Lyndhurst
Lyndhurst Hospital, Toronto Rehabilitation Institute (LH), Toronto
  Lyndhurst Board Minutes, 1958–98
  Annual Reports, 1986–98
Queen's University Archives (QA), Kingston, Ontario
  Edmund Henry ("Harry") Botterell fonds, 1927–97
National Archives of Canada (NA), Ottawa
  Department of Health records
  Department of Veterans Affairs records
  Public Service Commission records
Archives for Veterans Affairs Canada (VAC), Charlottetown, Prince Edward
  Island
  Lyndhurst Lodge records
  Prosthetic Services records
  Treatment Services, Paraplegic Cases records

PUBLISHED SOURCES

Abraham, Carolyn. "Man of steel uses his will and electricity to beat odds: In
the world of spinal-cord injuries, Reeve's recovery equals leaping a tall
building in a single bound," *Globe and Mail*, 13 September 2002.

ALPHANEWS Newsletter, March 1972, Fall 1972.

Barnett, H.J.M., A.T. Jousse, T.P. Morley, and W.M. Lougheed. "Post-Traumatic Syringomyelia," *Paraplegia* 9:1 (May 1971): 33–7.

Barton, Len, ed. *Disability and Society: Emerging Issues and Insights.* Harlow, England: Addison Wesley, Longman, 1996.

Bors, Ernest. "Veterans Administration Technical Bulletin TB10–503 Spinal Cord Injuries." Washington, 15 December 1948.

Botterell, E.H., A.T. Jousse, Carl Aberhart, and J.W. Cluff. "Paraplegia Following War," *Canadian Medical Association Journal* 55 (1946): 249–59.

– A.T. Jousse, A.S. Kraus. M.G. Thompson, M. Wynne-Jones, and W.O. Geisler. "A Model for the Future Care of Acute Spinal Cord Injuries," *The Canadian Journal of Neurological Sciences* (November 1975): 361–80.

Breithaupt, D.J., A.T. Jousse, and Megan Wynne-Jones. "Late Causes of Death and Life Expectancy in Paraplegia," *Canadian Medical Association Journal* 85 (8 July1961): 73–7.

"Building Hope." Lyndhurst newsletter, 1994–1998.

Bullock, T.A. L/CP. "C Squadron, 11 Troop, 8 Recce, 1942–1945." Privately printed manuscript, undated, circa 2001.

Burch, Susan. *Signs of Resistance: American Deaf Cultural History, 1900–1942.* New York: New York University Press, 2002.

Burke, James. "Readin', Ritin' and ... Calculus," *The Caliper* 11:1 (Spring 1956): 5–6, 16.

– "Return to Action: A Report on the Rehabilitation of Canadian Paraplegics." Unpublished manuscript, circa 1954–55.

– "Among Those Present," *The Caliper* 8:2 (Summer 1953): 10–11, 18.

– "This is Your Announcer – Cam Langford," *The Caliper* 8:1 (Spring 1953): 9–10.

Caliper: The Journal of the Canadian Paraplegic Association. 1946–99.

Clark, Ruth K. "Magazines Are My Business," *The Caliper* 4:1 (March 1949): 16–17, 26.

DeVivo, Michael J. and Samuel L. Stover. "Long-Term Survival and Causes of Death," in S.L. Stover et al., eds, *Spinal Cord Injury: Clinical Outcomes from the Model Systems.* Gaithersburg, Maryland: Aspen Publishers, 1995, 289–316.

Driedger, Diane. *The Last Civil Rights Movement: Disabled People's International.* New York: St. Martin's Press, 1989.

Duffin, Jacalyn. *History of Medicine.* Toronto: University of Toronto Press, 1999.

"Facilities of Lyndhurst Lodge Used by WCB [Workmen's Compensation Board] Patients: Lyndhurst Lodge in Toronto Provides Outstanding Treatment for Paraplegics," WCB *News Bulletin* (March 1964): 2–3.

Foss, Krista. "Paraplegic regains movement after cell procedure," *Globe and Mail*, 15 June 2001.

Frayne, Trent. "Walking and Working, Paraplegics Zestful," *Globe and Mail*, 15 November 1945.

Geisler, Wm. O. "Obituary: Albin Theophile Jousse, MD, FRCP (C)," *Paraplegia* 32 (1994): 634.

– A.T. Jousse, Megan Wynne-Jones, and D. Breithaupt. "Survival in Traumatic Spinal Cord Injury," *Paraplegia* 21:6 (1983): 364–73.

– A.T. Jousse, and Megan Wynne-Jones. "Survival in Traumatic Transverse Myelitis," *Paraplegia* 14:4 (February 1977): 262–75.

– A.T. Jousse, and Megan Wynne-Jones. "Vocational Re-Establishment of Patients with Spinal Cord Injury," *Medical Service Journal* 22:7 (July–August 1966): 698–709.

Gerber, D.A., ed. *Disabled Veterans in History*. Ann Arbor: University of Michigan Press, 2000.

Globe and Mail, Toronto. 19 January 2002. Obituary for Jack Higman, 1923–2002.

Guttmann, Ludwig. *Spinal Cord Injuries: Comprehensive Management and Research*. Oxford: Blackwell, 1973.

Heaman, Elsbeth. *St Mary's: The History of a London Teaching Hospital*. Montreal: McGill-Queen's University Press, 2003.

Hockenberry, John. *Moving Violations: War Zones, Wheelchairs, and Declarations of Independence*. New York: Hyperion, 1995.

Holleman, Marian Patterson. *From Darkness Into Light: The Founding of the Canadian Paraplegic Association*. Toronto: Canadian Paraplegic Association, 1991.

Husson, Therese-Adele. *Reflections: The Life and Writings of A Young Blind Woman in Post-Revolutionary France*. Translated with commentary by Catherine Kudlick and Zina Weygand. New York: New York University Press, 2001.

Immen, Wallace. "Spinal implants give hope to disabled," *Globe and Mail*, 1 February 2002.

James, Don. "Annual Dinner," *The Caliper* 9:2 (Summer 1954): 9–10.

Jamieson, George. "Life at Lyndhurst," *The Caliper* 12:3 (Summer 1957): 12.

Jousse, A.T. "The Evolution of the Treatment Programme for Paraplegics in Canada," *The Journal of the Association for Physical and Mental Rehabilitation* 16:5 (September–October 1962): 131–6.

- "Rehabilitation Following Poliomyelitis," *University of Toronto Medical Journal* 31:4 (January 1954): 159–61.
- Megan Wynne-Jones, and D.J. Breithaupt. "A Follow-up Study of Life Expectancy and Mortality in Traumatic Transverse Myelitis," *Canadian Medical Association Journal* 98 (20 April 1968): 770–2.
- and E.H. Botterell. "Paraplegia," *Treatment Services Bulletin, Department of Veterans Affairs* 11:6 (June-July 1947): 60–4.
- and Ruth Nettlefield. "Physiotherapy and the Paraplegic Patient," *The Journal of the Canadian Physiotherapy Association* 1:14 (August 1946): 4–9.

Kidd, Frank. "The Treatment of the Bladder in Gunshot Injuries of the Spinal Cord," *British Medical Journal* (5 April 1919): 397.

Kudlick, Catherine J. "Disability History: Why We Need Another 'Other'," *The American Historical Review* 108:3 (June 2003): 763–93.

Linton, Simi. *Claiming Disability: Knowledge and Identity*. New York: New York University Press, 1998.

Longmore, Paul K. *Why I Burned My Book and Other Essays on Disability*. Philadelphia: Temple University Press, 2003.

- and Lauri Umansky, eds, *The New Disability History: American Perspectives*. New York: New York University Press, 2001.

Loring Villa, Brian. *Unauthorized Action: Mountbatten and the Dieppe Raid*. rev. ed. Don Mills, Ontario: Oxford University Press, 1994.

McDonald, Irene. *For the Least of My Brethren: A Centenary History of St Michael's Hospital*. Toronto: Dundurn Press, 1992.

McKellar, Shelley. *Surgical Limits: The Life of Gordon Murray*. Toronto: University of Toronto Press, 2003.

McKenzie, Kenneth G. "Fracture, Dislocation, and Fracture Dislocation of Spine," *Canadian Medical Association Journal* 32:3 (March 1935): 263–9.

McLeod, Joanne E. "CPA: Achieving Dignity for Disabled Persons," *The Caliper* 37 (September 1982): 4.

McPherson, Kathryn. *Bedside Matters: The Transformation of Canadian Nursing, 1900–1990*. Toronto: Oxford University Press Canada, 1996.

Michalko, Rod. *The Difference That Disability Makes*. Philadelphia: Temple University Press, 2002.

Morton, Desmond and Glenn Wright. *Winning the Second Battle: Canadian Veterans and the Return to Civilian Life, 1915–1930*. Toronto: University of Toronto Press, 1987.

Munro, Donald. "Care of the Back Following Spinal-Cord Injuries: A Consideration of Bed Sores," *New England Journal of Medicine* 223 (1940): 392–8.

- "The Treatment of the Urinary Bladder in Cases with Injury of the Spinal Cord," *American Journal of Surgery* 38 (1937): 120–36.

Naylor, David C. *Private Practice, Public Payment: Canadian Medicine and the Politics of Health Insurance*. Kingston and Montreal: McGill-Queen's University Press, 1986.

Neilsen, Robert. *"Total Encounters," The Life and Times of the Mental Health Centre Penetanguishene*. Hamilton, Ont.: McMaster University Press, 2000.

Noell, Marilyn. *Another Path to My Garden: My Life as a Quadriplegic*. Toronto: Dundurn Press, 1992.

Oliver, Michael. *Understanding Disability: From Theory to Practice*. New York: St. Martin's Press, 1996.

Porter, Roy. *The Greatest Benefit to Mankind: A Medical History of Humanity*. New York and London: W.W. Norton & Co., 1997.

Rasbach, Noreen. "Lives Lived: Edmund Henry (Harry) Botterell," *Globe and Mail*, 21 July 1997.

Reaume, Geoffrey. *Remembrance of Patients Past: Patient Life at the Toronto Hospital for the Insane, 1870–1940*. Toronto: Oxford University Press Canada, 2000.

Rioux, Marcia and Michael Bach, eds. *Disability Is Not Measles: New Research Paradigms in Disability*. North York, Ontario: Roeher Institute, 1994.

Robertson, Terence. *The Shame and the Glory: Dieppe*. Toronto: McClelland and Stewart, 1962, 1967.

Russell, Marta. *Beyond Ramps: Disability at the End of the Social Contract*. Monroe: Common Courage Press, 1998.

Rutty, Christopher J. "'Do Something! ... Do Anything!' Poliomyelitis in Canada, 1927–1962." PhD thesis, University of Toronto, 1995.

Ryan, Michael E. "I.Y.D.P.: Fourth Quarter Report," *The Caliper* 36 (Winter 1981–82): 4.

- "Organizations of, and For, the Disabled," *The Caliper* 36 (Autumn 1981): 4.

Saso, Charles J. "Hemingway Slept Here," *The Caliper* 25:4 (Winter 1970): 7.

Schatz, S.W. et al. "E. Harry Botterell: A Series of Papers Commemorating His Life and Contributions," *Canadian Journal of Neurosurgical Sciences* 26:3 (August 1999): 230–46.

Silver, John Russell. *History of the Treatment of Spinal Injuries*. New York: Kluwer Academic/Plenum Publishers, 2003.

Titchkosky, Tanya. *Disability, Self, and Society*. Toronto: University of Toronto Press, 2003.

Total Access: Canadian Paraplegic Association (formerly *The Caliper*). 1999–2002.

Tremblay, Mary. "Lieutenant John Counsell and the Development of Medical Rehabilitation and Disability Policy in Canada," in David A Gerber, ed., *Disabled Veterans in History*. Ann Arbor: University of Michigan Press, 2000, 322–46.

– "Going Back to Main Street: The Development and Impact of Casualty Rehabilitation for Veterans with Disabilities, 1945–1948," in Peter Neary and J.L. Granatstien, eds, *The Veterans Charter and Post World War II Canada*. Montreal and Kingston: McGill-Queen's University Press, 1998, 160–78.

– "The Right to the Best Medical Care: Dr. W.P. Warner and the Canadian Department of Veterans Affairs, 1945–55," *Canadian Bulletin of Medical History* 15:1 (1998): 3–25.

– "Going Back to Civvy Street: a historical account of the impact of the Everest and Jennings wheelchair for Canadian World War II veterans with spinal cord injury," *Disability and Society* 11:2 (1996): 149–69.

– "The Canadian Revolution in the Management of Spinal Cord Injury," *Canadian Bulletin of Medical History* 12:1 (1995): 125–55.

– "Living with Disability: The Early Pioneers. A Life History Account of the Experience of Individuals with Spinal Cord Injury before 1967 who Lived in the Community in Ontario." PhD thesis, State University of New York at Buffalo, 1993.

– Audrey Campbell, and Geoffrey L. Hudson. "When elevators were for pianos: an oral history account of the civilian experience of using wheelchairs in Canadian society. The first twenty-five years: 1945–1970," *Disability & Society* 20:2 (March 2005): 103–16.

Turnbull, Barbara. *Looking in the Mirror*. Toronto: The Toronto Star, 1997.

Vargo, Jim. "Biting the Magic Bullet: Why we need to be realistic about 'cures' for spinal cord injury," *Total Access* 1:2 (Winter 1999): 40.

– "Superman's Folly: Why Christopher Reeve's well publicized beliefs about SCI are unrealistic – and potentially damaging," *The Caliper* 53:1 (Summer 1998): 36.

Walker, J. W. Thomson. "Ureters and Their Orifices in Gunshot Wounds of the Spine," *British Medical Journal* (15 March 1919): 325.

Whalley, George W. "Driving the Ford with Hand Controls," *The Caliper* 3:4 (December 1948): 9–11, 22.

Whitaker, Denis and Shelagh Whitaker. *Dieppe: Tragedy to Triumph*. Toronto: McGraw-Hill Ryerson, 1992.

Wilson, Renate. "Life Doesn't End in a Wheelchair," *Weekend Magazine* 17:23 (10 June 1967): 2–4, 6–7.

Index

A.T. Jousse Appreciation Foundation, 4, 237n96
Aberhart, Carl, 36, 45, 76
accreditation, of Lyndhurst, 238n99
Acquired Immune Deficiency Syndrome (AIDS), 176
Action League for Physically Handicapped Advancement (ALPHA), 140–1
acupuncture, 185, 196
Adair, Bill, 189, 238n104
Addiction Research Foundation, 185
Agnew, Don, 24
alcoholism and social drinking, 98, 113–14, 162, 170–1, 172–3, 185, 235n47
Allen, Jocelyn Botterell, 202n27
Anonymous, 97–8, 111–12
Arnold, Vi, 74
Ash, Clifford, 36
Associate Medical Services (AMS), 87
attendant care, 137, 167, 183–4, 187
Au, P., 168
Avery, Sheila, 228n88

Bach, Michael, 6
Bagnato, Tony, 67
Bailey, Tom, 137–9, 162
Bain, T.D., 31, 59
Baker, Eddie, 204n58
Bank of Canada, 20
Barnett, Henry, 112, 130, 225n46
Bartlett, Jim, 48, 66, 107, 117, 118, 142, 145, 187, 211n38, 231n15
Barton, Katherine (nee Cassels), 65–6, 115, 221n85

Barton, Len, 6
Basingstoke, No. 1 Neurological Hospital, Royal Canadian Army Medical Corps, 19, 21, 24, 34
Beggs, Ross, 117, 118, 133–4, 140, 146, 187
Bellevue Hospital, New York City, 44
Bent, Phyllis, 117–18
Bharatwal, Nirmala, 150, 163, 179, 232n18, 238n104
Bickle, E.W., 56
Bigelow, Wilfrid, 15, 201n27
Bill V., 117
Blain, Jack, 171, 230n11
Bleasdell, Marjorie, 62–4, 65
Boston, Glenna, 178
Botterell, E.H. (Harry), 46–7, 64, 65, 76, 80, 90–1, 127, 129, 152, 192–3, 240n2; early career, 15; 1936–39 treatment of spinal cord injury, 16–19, 201n26, 202n28, 202n31, 202n33, 203n41, 211n34; World War II service, 19–20; and John Counsell, 20–1, 22; and Christie Street Hospital, 34–7, 58, 209n9; and A.T. Jousse, 38–9, 42, 60, 68, 210n23; and Lyndhurst, 36–7, 39, 57, 58–61, 68; death of, 191, 240n1
Bradford, G. Woodrow, 59, 70
Breithaupt, D.J., 161, 195
Broadfoot, Dave, 115
Brooks, Betty, 74, 109, 112–13, 139, 153, 158, 159, 226n56
Brosseau, B.L., 100
Brown, Bill, 164–5
Brown, Mabel C., 92–5, 115

Brown, Terence, 232n18
Bullock, Theo, 32, 35–6, 41–2, 66–7, 209n9
Burch, Suzanne, 6
Burin, Newfoundland, 137
Burke, James: early 1940s experiences as a person with paraplegia, 13–14; 211n29
Byrnes, Nora, 66

Caliper, The, 14, 58, 214n64
Cameron, Peter, 127
Cameron, Walter, 78
Canadian Arthritis and Rheumatism Society, 25
Canadian Breweries, Ltd, 84
Canadian Charter of Rights and Freedoms, 172
Canadian Council on Hospital Accreditation, 238n99
Canadian Medical Association, 15, 201n26
Canadian National Institute for the Blind, 25
Canadian Paraplegic Association (CPA), 7, 9, 14, 20, 33, 99, 109, 115, 117, 120, 124, 134, 146, 148, 157, 171, 175, 179, 193, 214n64, 220n58, 221n85; formation of, 53–6, 213n56; DVA and, 57, 68–71; Lyndhurst and, 55, 59, 68–71, 85, 86, 107, 116–17, 120, 123, 128, 129, 141, 183–4, 186, 188, 189, 190, 237n96, 238n102, 238n104; surveys and, 102, 219n39, 226n52; University of Toronto and, 106, 151, 158, 160, 188; support of former Lyndhurst residents by, 137; access issues and, 141; wheelchair sports and, 141; sexuality counselling and, 142, 184–5; new building and, 151–3, 228n113; spinal cord research and, 161, 225n46; human rights and, 172; tensions between younger Lyndhurst residents and executive, 226n50
cars: disability access of for people with spinal cord injuries, 26–7, 41, 50, 101–2, 183
Casa Loma, 28
Cassels, Katherine (Katie Barton), 65–6
Cassels, Nanette, 115
Catto, J.A., 26–7
Caudwell, Gordon, 88–9
Chapple, R.V., 60, 215n71

Charles, Lloyd, 165–7
Children's Aid Society of Toronto, 115
Christie Street Hospital (Dominion Orthopaedic Hospital), 11, 26, 27, 28, 30, 32, 42, 43, 44, 45, 48, 50, 58–9, 60–1, 68, 70, 208n2, 211n34, 221n85; 1945 crisis, 34–7, 209n9; closing of, 69
chronic care, 99–101, 171, 234n42, 235n48
Clark, Ruth, 62, 215–16n79
Clarke, Andrew, 9, 32–3, 54, 55, 66, 83, 107, 152, 153, 159, 192
Clarkson Gordon (accounting firm), 20
Clemenceau, Georges, 25
Cluff, Joe, 34, 45
Cole, Ted, 77
College of Nurses of Ontario, 173
Community Advisory Committee (CAC), Lyndhurst, 176, 184
computers: first used at Lyndhurst, 236n63
Cone, William, 24, 204n63
Connable, Ralph, 29
Cottage Program, 184, 237n86
Counsell, John, 12, 53, 72, 73, 76, 83, 101, 192, 193, 203n50, 204nn58, 61, 204n63, 240n2; personal and military background, 21–2, 204n52; purchases and promotes Everest and Jennings wheelchair, 24–7, 49, 206n75; L.M. Wood and, 25–6, 42, 204n63, 205nn64, 70; and purchase of Lyndhurst property, 29–30; hired as rehabilitation officer and Lyndhurst administrative director, 30, 31; influence on operation of Lyndhurst Lodge, 33–4, 42–3, 59, 84; influence on patients, 41; leg-braces and, 47; formation of CPA and, 53–6, 57; steps down from CPA, 107, 220n58; death of, 191

Darou, Jimmy, 24, 205n63
Darryl M., 183
Deer Lodge, Winnipeg, 57
De Guerre, H.W., 28
Department of Indian Affairs, 237n83
Department of Veterans Affairs (DVA), 23, 26, 33, 38, 50, 52, 57, 59–61, 68–71, 85, 128, 151, 193
depression, 131, 138, 162
Desrochers, Lise, 183–4

Diemer, Alphonsus, 66
Dieppe raid, 1942, 21, 203n48
Dillon, Murray, 42
Disability policy re spinal cord injury: federal, 12, 57–8, 58–61; provincial, 68; municipal, 68, 140
discrimination, racial, 168
Divadale Convalescent Hospital, 49, 83, 120, 151, 152
divorce rate, of people with spinal cord injuries, 234n45
Don Jail, Toronto, 147
Douglas, Tommy, 86
Drew, George, 76
drug use, 142–3, 172–3, 179, 185
Drummond, Kathy, 119, 122, 134–7, 153–4, 195
Duffin, Barbara, 74, 75, 81, 109, 135, 153, 158, 231n12
Dunlop, Doreen, 204n58
Dunlop, Edward, head of DVA Rehabilitation Division, 23, 34, 53, 204n58

education: and Lyndhurst residents, 66–7, 84, 101, 116–17, 136–7, 182–3, 226n52, 235n48
Eisenhower, Dwight D., 117
employment: Lyndhurst former patients and, 102–3, 104 (Table 3), 117–18, 136, 140, 185, 186, 187, 193–4, 226n52, 234n45
Euclid Hall, Toronto, 11
Everest and Jennings wheelchair. See wheelchair

Famous Players Theatres, 29
Ferguson, T.G., 84, 151
Ford, Douglas, first employee hired at Lyndhurst, 31, 208n91
Frank C., man, treated by Botterell, 1937, 15,16; leaves TGH, 202n30
Frank C., boy, first civilian admitted to Lyndhurst, 1946, 60–1, 215nn71, 77
Frost, Leslie, 115

G.F. Strong Centre, Vancouver, 225n32
Gallie, W.E., 15, 76
gardener, labour of at Lyndhurst, 123, 223n16
Gardiner Foundation, 229n1
Gardiner, W.J., 129

Gartshore, John, 21
Gauthier, J.L., 60
Geisler, William, 79, 82, 90, 92, 110, 114, 139, 147, 160, 161, 163, 164, 167, 191, 192, 195, 197, 240n3; hired at Lyndhurst, 86; as medical director, 157, 180, 181, 232n18, 235n47, 236n58, 237n86; works on TGH paraplegic unit, 129, 142;
Gilleland, Barbara, 78
Glassco, Jane, 23, 24–5, 204n58
Globe and Mail, The, 53, 72, 86, 135
Gordon, Elizabeth, 20, 22, 23, 229n1
Gordon, Walter, 20, 22, 56, 153
Graham, Duncan, 209n17
Grossman, Larry, 175
Guttman, Ludwig, 10, 20

Hallam, Bev, 91, 101, 103–4, 114, 118, 135, 141–2, 195
Hanson, Bert, 65
Harris, Mike, 188, 236n69
Harris, R.I., 15
Hartley I., 17
Harvard Medical School, 157
Hay, Arthur John, 54, 55, 70–1
Health Department: federal, 22, 23, 24, 26, 27, 28, 31; provincial, 84, 111, 120, 124, 151, 152, 154, 156, 164, 175, 183, 187–8, 237n96, 239n106; municipal, 111
Health Services Restructuring Commission Report, 188
Heaman, Elsbeth, 3
Hemingway, Ernest, 29, 207n86
Herbie (orderly), 96
Herd, Peter, 33
Hicks, Peggy, 114–15
Higginbottom, Ted, 42, 53, 54
Higman, Jack: 1944 experiences at Basingstoke Hospital, 19–20; memories of Lyndhurst, 50–1; memories of founding of CPA, 54–5, 195, 203n43, 212n45
Hockenberry, John, 6
Hodgson, John, 151
Hoffman, Dave, 169
Holman, Elizabeth, 110, 220–1n63
Home Care services, 238n102
Hospital for Sick Children, Toronto, 139
housing, disability access to, 101–2, 183–4, 230n8, 237n83

Human Rights Commission (Ontario),
  227n79
hydrotherapy, 83

Institute for the Crippled and Disabled
  (New York City): influence on
  Lyndhurst program, 43–5, 211n29
insurance: health care coverage, 85. *See
  also* AMS, OHIP, PSI
International Year of Disabled Persons
  (1981), 172

Jackson, Myrll, 83, 89–91, 141
James, Art, 110–11, 134, 231n15
Jamieson, J.K., 85
Jamieson, Louise, 105, 124, 223n19
Janet H., 94–5
Jefferson, Geoffrey, 20
Jewett, Glenn, 116–17, 136
Joe S., 16
Johnston, Ian, 83
Jousse, Albin Theophile, 57, 76, 79, 80,
  88, 90, 99, 105, 107, 110, 164, 192,
  193, 195, 225n48, 240n3; background
  and pre-Lyndhurst career, 37–8,
  209n11; disability of, 38, 209n13;
  appointment as Lyndhurst's first
  medical director, 38, 209n17, 210n19;
  E.H. Botterell and, 38–9, 42, 43, 60,
  68, 209n17, 210n23; early impressions
  of Lyndhurst, 39–40; early articles
  published, 45; rehabilitation program
  at Lyndhurst and, 43–53, 92–5, 101,
  211n34; John Counsell and, 55;
  admission policies and, 88–9; patients'
  memories of, 63, 64–5, 92, 95, 103–4,
  114, 134, 138, 141; staff memories of,
  67, 107, 108–9, 142–3, 146, 147,
  149–50; chronic care and, 99–101;
  building plans and, 120; as
  administrator, 122–3, 144–5, 223n19,
  225n39, 227n68; concern about cost
  cutting, 128; medical research and,
  130, 161; new building and, 151–3;
  retires, 157; death of, 191
Jousse, Margaret, 68

Kerr, Mary Lou, 97
King, William Lyon Mackenzie, 20
Kingston General Hospital, 127
Kiwanis Club, 172, 174
Kudlick, Catherine, 5

Laird Tavern, 170–1, 235n47
Langford, Cam, 117, 222n93
Langford, Ken, 25, 49–50, 56, 65, 73, 79,
  82, 84, 87, 101–02, 171, 192, 208n1,
  222n93; wounded in Holland,
  admitted to Lyndhurst, 51; meets with
  Tommy Douglas, 86; managing
  director, CPA, 107; adoption barriers,
  115–16; new building and, 152–3;
  retires, 157
Langford, Mary, 51, 101–2, 115–16
Lawrence, Mabel, 39
Linton, Simi, 6
Longmore, Paul, 5
Lyndhurst, 3, 4, 5, 6, 7, 9, 20, 23,18, 75,
  81, 82, 207n86, 223n19; rehabilitation
  centre, original ideas about, 23, 26–7,
  33–4; acquisition of 153 Lyndhurst
  Avenue, 27–9, 206n84; physical
  environment of, 29–30, 111–13,
  121–2, 153–4, 221n74; name of, 30,
  34, 152, 189; composition of staff, 31,
  40, 104–5, 233n28; opening of facility
  and first patients, 32–3; renovations of,
  and additions to, original building, 33,
  51–2, 83–5, 217nn4, 5; appointment of
  A.T. Jousse as medical director, 38–9;
  patients' routine and daily life at, 40–1,
  46, 48–9, 92, 130–9, 168–82, 210n23,
  221n85, 233n38, 236n58; future plans
  for, 42–3; rehabilitation program,
  43–53, 87–9, 90–1, 92–5, 98, 101–3,
  112–13, 126–8, 148–9, 157–8, 160,
  182–7, 188–9, 193–4; discharge of first
  patient, 48; patients' councils at, 54,
  133, 171–7, 178; CPA and 55, 59,
  68–71, 85, 86, 107, 116–17, 120, 123,
  128, 129, 141, 183–4, 186, 188, 189,
  190, 237n96, 238nn102, 104; veterans
  to civilians, 58–61, 215nn71, 76, 77;
  first women patients, 62, 215n79;
  women patients on second floor, 113,
  120–1; patient population, 68–9, 88–9,
  91–2, 95, 96 (Table 1), 99, 101–2, 103
  (Table 2), 124, 125–6, 219nn22, 39,
  223n23, 233n42, 234n43, 235n48;
  education and, 84, 101, 116–17,
  126–7, 226n52, 232n20; classified as
  convalescent hospital, 1954, 85; health
  insurance and, 85–7; staff salaries and
  benefits, 86–7, 104–5, 110, 123,
  143–6, 159, 160, 227nn68, 74,

239nn105, 106; per diem rate, 87, 218n16; chronic care and, 99–101, 234n42, 235n48; employment prospects of former patients, 102–3, 104 (Table 3), 136, 171, 185, 226n52, 234n45, 235n48; medical training and, 106, 232n20; complaints about conditions at, 111; alcohol drinking at, 113–14, 170–1, 172–3, 235n47; building plans, 119–20, 124; categorized as rehabilitation centre, 124; dental care and, 128–9, 225n39; depression and suicide, 131, 138, 162, 234n45; wheelchair sports and, 141; smoking "dope" and drug use at, 142–3, 172–3, 179; "telephone mechanics," 143; staff team, 147, 150; new building, 151–4, 163, 228n113, 229n118; pressure for bed space at, 155–6, 230n8, 231n14, 232n16, 233nn28, 42, 234n44; consultants and, 160–1; sexual harassment, racial discrimination and, 168; Lyndhurst Foundation, 177, 238n102; amalgamation, 187–90; missing 1945 film of, 211n30; prosthetic products tried out by early patients at, 212n41; establishment of hospital board at, 220n57; Research Department, 237n96; accreditation of, 238n99

MacDonald, Margaret, 104, 105, 106, 107–8, 114, 135
MacFarlane, Joseph A., 76
MacGregor, A.E., 208n4
MacMillan, R., 185
maintenance staff, 145–6. See also James, Art
Man in Motion Legacy Fund, 237n96
Manufacturers Life Insurance Company, 102, 161
Maple Leaf Gardens, 40, 49, 56, 84
Marley, Bob, 166
Martindale, Richard (Dick, orderly), 110, 143, 149
Mathers and Haldenby (architects), 151
McCarthy, John, 24
McDonald, Irene, 3
McDougall, E. Peter, 161
McEwan, A.D., 66
McHaffie, Gerald, 74
McInnes, Ronald, 139, 226n56

McKenzie, Kenneth G., 14, 15, 17, 18, 38, 201n19, 202n31
McMane, Charles, 23, 25, 29, 205n70
medical training, 106, 232n20
Meek, Charles, 151
Memorial University, 139
Metro Integrated Health Delivery Network, 188
Michalko, Rod, 6
Millar, Ross, 12
Miller, Frank, 154
Ministry of Community and Social Services, 184
Mobbs, Carmen, 179–82, 195
Moffat, Murray, 184
Montreal Neurological Institute, 22, 24, 203n50
Montreal Rehabilitation Institute, 228n94
Morrison, L.B., 122, 223n13
Mount Sinai Hospital, 158
Mrs B., 130, 225n46
Munro, Donald, 14, 201n19
Munro Tidal Irrigator, 14, 15, 45
Murray, Gordon, 225n48

Nathanson, Irene, 28, 30, 31
National Health Research and Development Program, 237n96
National Hospital, London, England, 15
National Society for the Deaf and Hard of Hearing, 25
Natural Sciences and Engineering Research Council, 237n96
Naylor, Dorothy, 64–5
Neilsen, Robert, 3
Nettlefield, Ruth, 43, 47
Nightingale School of Nursing, 106
Noell, Marilyn, 112, 221n74
Noptanya, Dr, 150
Norvaisza, Joe, 144
Norwich, A.C., 28, 32, 38, 52, 60, 205n70
Nucleus Housing, 183–4
nursing staff, 76, 105–6, 107–8, 132, 135–6, 144, 145, 148–9, 164–5, 166–7, 178, 220n49, 239n105

O'Brien, Michael, 167, 177, 186, 197
occupational therapy and therapists, 45, 145, 163–4, 178
O'Connor, Bill (William), 66, 118
Oliver, Michael, 6

Ontario Advocacy Commission, 236n69
Ontario Hospital Insurance Plan (OHIP), 86, 87, 105, 218n16
Ontario Hospital Services Commission (OHSC), 85, 100, 119, 120, 122, 123, 124, 128, 143, 144, 145, 151, 153, 227n68
Ontario Institute for Studies in Education (OISE), 137
Ontario Labour Relations Board, 168
Ontario Ministry of Community and Social Services, 237n96
Ontario Nurses Association (ONA), 159, 230n10, 239n105
orderlies, 96, 105, 108, 143–4, 145, 148–9, 165–7, 227n68
Oshidari, Alborz, 186
Owen, Bill, 134, 140–1
Owen, Lucille (Fortier), 121–2, 132–4, 145, 184, 189, 225n48, 226nn50, 58, 229n118

paraplegia: history of treatment up to World War I, 9–12; in inter-war period, 12, 14–19; causes and treatment of, 126–7, 130, 168–9; Lyndhurst population of, 58, 88–9, 95, 96 (Table 1), 98, 99, 101–2, 103 (Table 2), 104 (Table 3), 109, 116, 117, 125, 137, 138, 163–4, 168, 173–4, 179, 224nn24, 26, 27, 233n42, 234n43; life expectancy study, 161–3, 224n28; veteran population of in Toronto, 1945, 214n63
Paterson, Gordon, 95–7, 112, 113–14, 116, 195
patients' councils, 54, 133, 171–7, 178
Paul, Evelyn, 67, 104–5, 108–9, 112, 114, 146, 227n78
Pearse, Robin, 15
Peat, R.S., 100
Penetanguishene Mental Health Centre, Ontario, 3
per diem rate, 87
Perkins, Douglas, 172, 235n57
Phelan, Helen, 157, 229n1, 238n102
Physicians Services Incorporated (PSI), 86–7
physiotherapy and physiotherapists, 41, 45, 46, 73, 74, 75, 81, 97, 104–5, 106, 108–9, 131, 132, 135, 138, 139, 144,

145, 151, 158–9, 164, 165, 177, 178–9, 217n4, 230n11, 231n12
Pilon, Marie, 76
polio, 62, 65, 91–5, 96 (Table 1), 101, 103 (Table 2), 110, 117, 121, 125
Port Arthur General Hospital, Thunder Bay, Ontario, 169
post-traumatic syringomyelia, 130
pregnancy, 179–81
Prevention of Alcohol- Related Trauma in Youth (PARTY): Lyndhurst program, 176, 236n64
Professional Association of Interns and Residents of Ontario, 150
Proietti, Therese, 131–2
psychologist, need for at Lyndhurst, 157
Purchase, Ken, 48, 53, 66

quadriplegia: causes and treatment of, 9–10, 126–7, 130; Lyndhurst population of, 88–91, 96 (Table 1), 99, 101–2, 103 (Table 2), 104 (Table 3), 109, 117, 125, 131, 132, 134–7, 138, 139, 147–8, 163–4, 169–70, 173–4, 177–8, 179, 183–4, 224nn24, 26, 27, 233n42, 234n43; waiting list for Lyndhurst, 155–6; life expectancy study and, 161–3, 224n28
Queen Elizabeth's Hospital, Toronto, 13, 158
Queen's University, Kingston, Ontario, 127
Quirt, Douglas, 32, 54, 66

Rajan, J.S.T., 122, 123, 223n13
Ratelle, Ed, 121, 146, 148, 187
Red Chevron (Christie Street Hospital Annex), 32, 208n2
Reeve, Charles (Chuck), 49, 63
Rehabilitation Institute of Toronto, 188
rehabilitation program: at Lyndhurst, 43–53, 87–9, 90–1, 92–5, 98, 101–3, 112–13, 126–8, 148–9, 157–8, 160, 182–7, 188–9; in Ontario regional centres, 126–8, 148–9, 162, 170. See also Lyndhurst and Jousse, Albin Theophile
Ridley College, St Catharines, Ontario, 20–1
Rioux, Marcia, 6
Riverdale Convalescent Hospital, 144, 227n69

Robeson, Paul, 221n85
Robson, Charles, 185
Robson Urology Clinic, 184–5, 195, 238n102
Roosevelt, Franklin, 65
Rossier, Alain, 157–8
Rotary Club, 60, 184
Rotenberg, Brenda, 170
Rowe, Kirby, 169–71, 175, 184
Royal Canadian Air Force, 9
Royal Canadian Army Medical Corps (RCAMC), 19, 21, 210n23
Royal College of Physicians and Surgeons of Ontario, 139
Russell, Marta, 6
Ryerson Polytechnic (University from 1993), 118, 134, 140

St John's General Hospital, St John's, Newfoundland, 137
St Joseph's Hospital, Toronto, 3, 131
St Mary's Hospital, London, England, 3
St Michael's Hospital, Toronto, 4, 13, 158
Ste Anne de Bellevue Hospital, Quebec, 57, 214n64
Saso, Charlie, 146–8, 154, 159, 187
Saunders, Sally, 185
Scarborough, Ontario, 136
Service Employees International Union (SEIU), Local 204, 145–6, 165, 166, 230nn10, 11, 239n105
sexual harassment, 168
sexuality, 97, 129–30, 142, 184–5, 237n86
Shanks, Gavin, 121, 126, 142–3, 149–50, 225n30
Sharpe, Jean, 41, 43
Shaughnessy Hospital, Vancouver, 57
sidewalk wheelchair access ramps, 140
Silver, John Russell, 4
Smythe, Conn, 49, 56
Social Contract Act (1993–96), 239n106
staff salaries and benefits, 86–7, 104–5, 110, 123, 143–6, 227nn68, 74, 239nn105, 106
Staton, Margaret, 98–9, 112, 113, 134
Stoke Mandeville Spinal Centre, Aylesbury, United Kingdom, 20
Stone, Loma, 148–9, 228n88
stryker frame, 169
suicide, 131, 138, 162, 234n45

Sunnybrook Hospital, 37, 69, 70, 90, 99, 115, 120, 128, 129, 158, 169, 170, 176
Swan, Randy, 173, 175, 235n57
Symington, David, 127–8, 225n32

Tasker, Ron, 161, 232n23
Tator, Charles, 161
technology: accessibility and, 133, 181–2, 185–6, 237n96
Tepperman, P., 160
Thomas, Basil (Tommy, orderly), 110, 143, 149, 231n15
Thomson, J.S.H., 83
Titchkosky, Tanya, 6
Tonack, Mark, 234n45
Toronto Board of Education, 238n102
Toronto Daily Star, 18, 29
Toronto General Hospital (TGH), 37, 59, 64, 69, 90, 95–6, 99, 129, 158, 173, 193, 209n17, 225n41
Toronto Rehabilitation Centre, 188
Toronto Rehabilitation Committee, 25
Toronto Rehabilitation Institute (TRI), 190, 196
Toronto Star, 179, 226n56
Toronto Western Hospital, 129, 161
Torrance, K.A., 122
Total Access, 214n64
"toughness," culture of at Lyndhurst, 133
Tran, Dr, 150, 228n94
Transitional Living Program, 184
transportation, public: disability access to, 141
Tremblay, Mary, 4–5, 16, 201n17
Tri-Hospital Rehabilitation Corporation, 190
Truscott, Elizabeth, 77
Turnbull, Barbara, 155, 161, 177–9, 184, 229n1

United Nations, 172
University of Manitoba, 15
University of Toronto, 15, 52, 66, 106, 128, 140, 150, 151, 158, 160, 188, 232n20, 238n102
University of Washington, 225n32
Upper Canada College, 135

Vaughan Theatre, 116
Victorian Order of Nurses, 143
Vipond, Claude, 232n18

Waddell, Dorothy, 146, 231n15
Walker, J.W. Thomson, 10
Warner, W.P., 36, 42, 209n10
Weaves, Marlene, 178
wheelchairs: Everest and Jennings, 24–7, 49–50, 71, 205n75; power, 133; access issues for, 140–1, 178, 181
wheelchair sports, 141
White, George, 52, 73, 91, 97–8, 112, 145, 227n78
Whittle, Douglas, 52
William, M., 16, 18
William P., World War I veteran with a spinal cord injury, 10–11
Wilson, Isabel, 36, 209n11
Wilson, R., 26, 205n70
Wodehouse, R.E., 28
Woloshyn, Eileen, 38
Wood, L.M. (Lewis), 12, 30, 53, 73, 84, 193; background, 25; John Counsell and, 25–6, 42, 204n63, 205nn64, 70; Lyndhurst and, 42–3, 61; CPA and, 54, 57; death of, 84, 205n66 (obituary in *The Caliper*)
Woods, J.D., 83, 120, 220n58
Woods, Walter S., 22, 204n63
Workmen's Compensation Board (WCB), 59, 60, 69, 74, 77, 78, 129, 237n83
Wrangham, Joseph, 54
Wynne-Jones, Megan, 79, 102, 161, 195

Yale University, 15
Yaremko, John, 115–16
York County Hospital, Newmarket, Ontario, 180
York University, 137

Zohra, 145